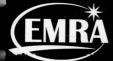

TOP
Pediatric
Clinical
PROBLEMS

Dale P. Woolridge, MD, PhD
Hans Bradshaw, MD
Editors-in-Chief

P9-AGU-572

Joshua Nchama

EMERGENCY MEDICINE RESIDENTS' ASSOCIATION

Introduction

This book was designed as a clinical primer on key topics in the emergent/urgent care of children. It is our hope that the emergency medicine resident or student will keep this book on their person and use it as a quick reference during a case or during downtime. Each chapter is by no means a complete review and, therefore, offers suggestions for additional readings. We've also provided review questions at the end of each chapter, which we hope will be helpful in preparing you to care for the patients you will encounter.

This book stemmed conceptually through combined emergency medicine/pediatrics dual training. These training programs exist within and are complementary to categorical emergency medicine and categorical pediatric training. Combined training has, since its conception, fostered education between the two departments. This book is an attempt to compile the educational material and networking inherent to this dual training.

Acknowledgments

This project is dedicated to my family, who inspires me to be the best that I can be. I would also like to thank all those in the specialties of emergency medicine, pediatrics – or both – who contributed directly and indirectly to this endeavor. It has been a true pleasure to work with all of these authors. The complementary nature of dual training in emergency medicine and pediatrics has allowed me to take part in the areas of medicine that I love most. I am doubly blessed to be able to enjoy colleagues and residents in two departments and participate in the training of combined emergency medicine/pediatric residents, who are also of two departments.

Dale P. Woolridge

Editors-in-Chief

Dale P. Woolridge, MD, PhD, FACEP, FAAEM, FAAP
Director, Emergency Medicine/Pediatrics Residency Program
Associate Professor of Emergency Medicine and Pediatrics
University of Arizona

Hans Bradshaw, MD
Assistant Professor of Emergency Medicine and Pediatrics
University of Arizona

Notice

Emergency medicine is an ever-changing field. Although every effort has been made to ensure dosages and treatment guidelines are accurate, ultimate responsibility remains with the treating physician. Neither the authors nor the publisher assumes any responsibility for injury to persons or property. Every effort has been made to follow diagnostic and therapeutic guidelines of ACEP, AHA, ACA, NIH, AHCPR, AAP, actual clinical practices, and the most recent and respected current clinical texts in pediatric medicine and emergency medicine.

Printed in the USA. ISBN: 978-1-929854-33-2

Additional copies of this publication are available from EMRA, 1125 Executive Circle, Irving, TX 75038-2522, 972-550-0920, **www.emra.org**.

Please send comments or suggestions to **emra@emra.org**.

EMRA Staff

Cathey B. Wise
Executive Director

Leah Stefanini
Meetings and Advertising Manager

Rachel Donihoo
Publications and Communications
Coordinator

Linda Baker
Marketing and Operations Manager

Chalyce Bland
Administrative Coordinator

Authors and Contributors

Sara Aberle, MD
Mayo Clinic
Department of Emergency Medicine

Barrett Adams, MD
Providence Health & Services

Hans Bradshaw, MD
University of Arizona
Department of Emergency Medicine

Lisa Chan, MD
University of Arizona
Department of Emergency Medicine

Stephen Charbonneau, MD, JD
University of Arizona
Department of Emergency Medicine

Brian Clothier, MD, MS
Salem Emergency Physician Service
Department of Emergency Medicine

James Colletti, MD
Mayo Clinic
Departments of Emergency Medicine
and Pediatrics

Larry Deluca, MD
University of Arizona
Department of Emergency Medicine

Becky Doran, MD
Baylor College of Medicine
Department of Pediatric Emergency
Medicine

Lisa Doyle, MD
Utah Emergency Physicians

Josh Ennis, MD
Stanford University
Division of Emergency Medicine

Albert Fiorello, MD
University of Arizona
Department of Emergency Medicine

Sean M. Fox, MD
Carolinas Medical Center
Department of Emergency Medicine

Charles Gillespie, MD
University of Arizona
Department of Emergency Medicine

Steve Groke, MD
University of Arizona
Department of Emergency Medicine

Emily Grover, MD
University of Arizona
Department of Emergency Medicine

Thomas Hellmich, MD
Mayo Clinic
Departments of Emergency Medicine
and Pediatrics

Melanie S. Heniff, MD
Indiana University
Department of Emergency Medicine

Katherine Hiller, MD
University of Arizona
Department of Emergency Medicine

Nathan Holman, MD
University of Arizona
Department of Emergency Medicine

Nicholas B. Hurst, MD
University of Arizona
Department of Emergency Medicine

Elisabeth Jannicky, MD
University of Maryland
Department of Emergency Medicine

Parisa P. Javedani, MD
University of Arizona
Department of Emergency Medicine

Nathaniel Johnson, MD
University of Arizona
Department of Emergency Medicine

Mi Jin Kim-Ley, PharmD
University of Arizona
College of Pharmacy

James Lehman, MD
Emergency Physicians Manhattan

Ben Leeson, MD
Texas A&M – Christus Spohn
Department of Emergency Medicine

Kimberly Leeson, MD
Texas A&M – Christus Spohn
Department of Emergency Medicine

Merlin C. Lowe, MD
University of Arizona
Department of Pediatrics

Alice Min, MD
University of Arizona
Department of Emergency Medicine

Abby Massey, MD
Professional Emergency Physicians

Garrett S. Pacheco, MD
University of Arizona
Department of Emergency Medicine

Kevin Reilly, MD
University of Arizona
Department of Emergency Medicine

Farshad "Mazda" Shirazi, MD, PhD
University of Arizona
Department of Emergency Medicine

Brittany Shutes, MD
University of Arizona
Department of Pediatrics

Mary Thiessen, MD
University of Arizona
Department of Emergency Medicine

Ryan Young, MD
Phoenix Children's Hospital
Pediatric Emergency Medicine

Chad Viscusi, MD
University of Arizona
Department of Emergency Medicine

Anna L. Waterbrook, MD
University of Arizona
Department of Emergency Medicine

Drew Watters, MD
Indiana University School of Medicine
Department of Emergency Medicine

Elizabeth Weinstein, MD
Indiana University
Department of Emergency Medicine

Dale P. Woolridge, MD, PhD
University of Arizona
Department of Emergency Medicine

Mark D. Wright, MD
University of Arizona
Department of Emergency Medicine

Giselle Zagari, MD
University of Arizona
Department of Emergency Medicine

Melissa Zukowski, MD
University of Arizona
Department of Emergency Medicine

EMRA Staff Editor

Rachel Donihoo, Publications and Communications Coordinator

Table of Contents

The Normal Newborn Examination

Merlin C. Lowe, MD

Critical Knowledge

- A newborn examination in the emergency department should be quick, yet thorough. A systematic approach to the exam will ensure nothing is missed.
- A thorough physical examination can help determine how best to proceed with evaluation of the infant.
- Recognizing age-appropriate variations in the examination, especially regarding vital signs, can be difficult. Using a quick-reference card can help provide easy recall.
- Recognizing common anatomical variations during the newborn examination can prevent an unnecessary workup.

Background

Newborns will present to the ED for many reasons. Evaluation of the newborn can be challenging due to the patient's inability to communicate and often nonspecific presenting signs. A quick, yet thorough, examination will allow the provider to proceed with the workup of the infant in an organized, effective fashion. Some infants will be brought to the ED when they are well; others will present with true illnesses. Being able to distinguish between a normal and abnormal neonatal exam can provide clues to guide further evaluation.

Epidemiology

Minor anomalies will be found in 15%-20% of newborns. These infants have a 3% chance of having a major anomaly. When the number of minor anomalies rises to 2 or 3, the risk of a major anomaly rises to 10% or 20%, respectively.

Infant Vital Signs

Age	Heart Rate	Respiratory Rate	Systolic Blood Pressure
Newborn	90-180	40-60	60-90
1 month	110-180	30-50	70-104
3 months	110-180	30-45	70-104
6 months	110-180	20-35	72-110
1 year	80-170	20-30	72-115

- Temperature is a crucial part of the vital-sign evaluation. One should be equally aware of high temperatures *and* low temperatures, as either can be an indicator of infection. Keep in mind that infection is not the only cause of temperature fluctuation. Hypothermia may be a sign of hypoglycemia, hypothyroidism, or hypoxia. Hyperthermia also may represent adrenal hemorrhage, intracranial hemorrhage, or drug withdrawal.
- Knowing appropriate vital signs for age is crucial to the ability of the clinician to recognize potential problems.
- A quick-reference chart for pediatric vital signs should be kept available.

General Evaluation

- One of the clinician's greatest tools to evaluate a newborn is the general impression one gets of an infant.
- Does the infant appear vigorous and alert, or ill and toxic?
- Look for signs of distress, including labored breathing, persistent crying, and irritability, with difficulty consoling the infant.
- A non-vigorous infant should be a red flag; seek an underlying issue.

Evaluation of the Head

- The anterior fontanel can remain open until approximately 18 months, although it often is quite small by age 12 months. An enlarged anterior fontanel can be an indication of hypothyroidism.
- Generally, the posterior fontanel is fully closed by 12 months, although it often becomes unpalpable months before this.
- The fontanel should be examined to ensure that it is soft and flat.
  - ▶ A bulging fontanel is an indicator of increased intracranial pressure.
  - ▶ A sunken fontanel may indicate dehydration.
- Significant molding can follow a vaginal birth. This generally resolves in 3 to 5 days.
- One should also examine for any evidence of a caput succedaneum or hemorrhages (such as a cephalhematoma) related to birth trauma (*Figure 1*). Extraction deliveries increase the risk of developing such a bleed.
  - ▶ Significant blood loss can occur from a subgaleal bleed.
  - ▶ The presence of *any* bleed increases the risk of future hyperbilirubinemia.

- Suture lines should be examined for evidence of excessive widening as an indicator of increased intracranial pressure, possibly from an underlying hydrocephalus.

Figure 1. Scalp Hematomas[6]

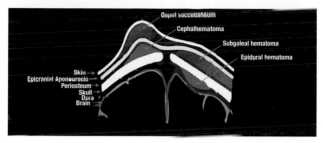

Eyes

- Red reflexes are assessed by viewing the pupil through the ophthalmoscope at least a few inches back from the eye. One should note color and symmetry of the red reflexes bilaterally.
  - ▶ A white reflex (leukocoria) may be indicative of several processes, including retinoblastoma, glaucoma, cataracts, or vitreous opacities.
  - ▶ A finding of leukocoria requires evaluation by an ophthalmologist.
- Extra-ocular movements should also be examined. Dysconjugate gaze at birth is not particularly concerning. This finding should resolve by 2 months of age. Persistent dysconjugate gaze should be evaluated.
- Subconjunctival hemorrhages are quite common following birth and are not dangerous. They typically will resolve within 1-2 weeks.

Ears

- Ear positioning should be evaluated. Low-set ears have been associated with several genetic syndromes.
- Preauricular skin tags or pits are quite common and often will run in families. New research has shown that they are generally inconsequential and do not require further workup.
- Ear anomalies (such as malformed auricles) can be associated with other anomalies—in particular, anomalies of the genitourinary tract. A renal ultrasound generally is recommended in these patients.

Mouth

- The mouth should be examined for any oral lesions. A finger can be inserted into the mouth to check for a cleft palate.
- About 1 in 3,000 infants will have a natal tooth. These need not be removed unless they pose a risk for aspiration or prevent proper feeding.
- Epstein pearls or Bohn's nodules may be seen in the mouth of an infant, as well. These are yellowish or white and slightly raised nodules located near the midpalatal raphe at the junction of the hard and soft palates. These resolve spontaneously.

Neck

- Congenital muscular torticollis has an incidence of 1 in 250 live births and is known to be more common in breech and forceps deliveries. It presents with the infant keeping the head flexed and turned, with the chin toward the unaffected side. Two-thirds of cases will have a palpable mass within the involved sternocleidomastoid muscle.
- Thyroglossal duct cysts may present as a midline neck mass.
- Branchial cleft anomalies can present as cysts, sinuses, or pits along the ear, preauricular space, and lateral neck.

Chest/Lungs

- When examining the chest, one must remember to examine all structures of the chest, including bones, lungs, and heart.
- Clavicle fractures following birth have an incidence of 0.2%-3.5%. Crepitus can be felt when palpating the fractured clavicle. X-ray can confirm its presence. No specific treatment is needed since they heal quite well.
- The lung exam should start by visualizing the infant breathe, while looking for nasal flaring, grunting, retractions, symmetrical chest rise, etc.
- Transient tachypnea of the newborn will often follow Cesarean section births but also can be seen with vaginal births. Infants may need some ventilatory support; however, full recovery is expected within 24 to 72 hours.
- The combination of fever and tachypnea is very concerning for pneumonia. In the absence of tachypnea, pneumonia is unlikely in pediatric patients.

Cardiovascular

- At birth, a complex series of events must occur for the neonatal circulatory system to function properly.
  - ▶ The foramen ovale must close.
  - ▶ The ductus arteriosus must close.
  - ▶ Pulmonary pressures must drop.

- The patent ductus arteriosus (PDA) functionally closes around 10 to 15 hours after birth. It permanently fuses closed by approximately 3 weeks. In infants with ductal dependent lesions, the PDA may remain open longer, causing the patient's presentation to be outside this 5-hour window. (It would not be uncommon for the duct to remain open for nearly a week.)

- Due to increased pulmonary pressures, S2 may not be split. As pressures *decrease* to baseline, S2 will become more physiologically split. An S3 may be heard near the apex and is considered normal. An S4 is *never* normal in a newborn.

- The cardiac exam in a newborn relies very much on information beyond the auscultation of the heart. Palpation of peripheral pulses can detect coarctation of the aorta, for example.

- Newborns can present with several murmurs. Distinguishing between innocent murmurs and pathological ones can be difficult. When uncertain, it is always best to request a cardiology evaluation and echocardiogram.

- Innocent murmurs are quite common at birth. They typically are heard best at the left lower sternal border and have a vibratory sound. They typically do not radiate and are graded as I-II/VI in nature. Innocent murmurs include venous hums, pulmonary ejection murmurs, peripheral pulmonic stenosis, and Still's murmurs.

- Harsh-sounding murmurs should not be attributed to innocent murmurs; neither should holosystolic or diastolic murmurs.

- Ventricular septal defects (VSD) are the most common cause of holosystolic murmurs. Other possibilities include mitral or tricuspid regurgitation or other variations of VSDs, such as atrioventricular septal defects (AVSD).

- Some syndromes are more commonly associated with heart defects. For example, approximately 30% of those with an AVSD have Down syndrome.

Abdomen

- Assessment should include examination for hepatomegaly, splenomegaly, and enlarged kidneys. The umbilical cord should also be inspected in newly born infants, noting for the presence of three vessels.

- The liver edge of a newborn will often be palpable approximately 1 cm below the costal margin. This is considered acceptable for neonates. Tables exist for appropriate liver spans in neonates and should be referenced when questions exist. In general, a liver span greater than 3.5 cm below the costal margin is considered enlarged.

- A spleen generally should not be palpable. A palpable spleen in the setting of jaundice could indicate a hemolyzing state such as cell-type incompatibility (e.g., ABO or Rh) or a defect in red cell morphology (spherocytosis, etc.).

- One should also remember that lung hyperinflation can move the liver and spleen downward, leading to an exam consistent with hepatosplenomegaly (but, liver and spleen spans will be normal).

- 0.2%-1% of infants will have a single umbilical artery (two-vessel cord). These infants have an increased incidence (threefold and sixfold, respectively) of severe renal anomalies and renal malformation.

- A scaphoid abdomen in a newly delivered infant should alert the physician to the possibility of a congenital diaphragmatic hernia (CDH). CDH is an indication for immediate intubation following delivery to minimize chances of air inflating the stomach and further compressing thoracic structures. Bag-valve mask ventilation is contraindicated with CDH.

Genitourinary Tract

- Boys should be examined for inguinal hernias, varicoceles, hydroceles, normal testes, and urethral anomalies (such as hypospadias).

- Inguinal hernias present as a bulge in the inguinal area or in the scrotum. If a hernia is detected, light, constant pressure should be applied to reduce it.

- Girls can present with inguinal hernias, as well, although the male-to-female ratio is 6:1. Presentation is as a bulge in inguinal area.

- Varicoceles develop from a dilation of the pampiniform plexus and internal spermatic vein. They are more common on the left and are more easily seen with the patient in an upright position.

- Hydroceles form from a failure of the processus vaginalis to fully close, allowing fluid, but not bowel, into the scrotum. Transillumination of the scrotum will allow differentiation. Hydroceles transilluminate; varicoceles do not.
- Ambiguous genitalia can be the result of girls who are virilized or boys who are undermasculinized. Phenotypes can be "nearly normal female" to "nearly normal male"— or anywhere in between.
  - ► Boys present with ambiguous genitalia due to defective androgen synthesis or end-organ resistance to androgens.
  - ► Girls most commonly present with ambiguous genitalia due to congenital adrenal hyperplasia (often due to 21-hydroxylase deficiency).
- Examination for ambiguous genitalia should include evaluation for clitoromegaly, micropenis, fused labia, or bifid scrotum.
- When ambiguous genitalia are found at birth, assignment of sex should be delayed pending confirmation by other means.

Extremities

- Examination should include evaluation for polydactyly, most commonly involving the "pinky" finger. Extra digits may range from a skin tag to fully formed phalanges. Toes also may be involved.
- A unilateral single, transverse palmar crease is found in approximately 4% of the general population. 1% will have a bilateral single crease. Single creases are associated with several syndromes; when present, other anomalies should be evaluated on physical exam.
- Unilateral club foot is found in 1 in 1,000 live births. Bilateral club feet are found in 30% to 50% of cases. Treatment is initially with serial casting. If this fails, surgery may be needed.

Neurological

- Time may not permit a full neurological exam, but a general assessment of neurological status should be done on all infants, with emphasis on tone, primitive reflexes, and a gross evaluation of cranial nerves, as well as muscular and sensory status.
- One should assess for symmetric facies and movement of all extremities.
- The infant should react to stimuli (light touch and pinprick).

- Hypotonia is an important finding to note, as it is the most common neurological sign seen in infants and is associated with various syndromes.
- Assess whether or not the infant is meeting developmental milestones.
- Focal deficits may be an indication of plexus palsy.

Primitive Reflexes (Limited Listing)

Reflex	Actions
Rooting reflex	Touch newborn's cheek; infant turns toward side touched
Walking reflex	When held upright, baby makes walking movements when foot touched.
Tonic neck reflex (Fencing reflex)	Turn baby's head to one side; the chin-side arm will extend, and the occiput-side arm will flex above the shoulder.
Moro reflex	Baby will extend then contract arms and grimaces when gently released to fall a few inches.
Palmar reflex	Stroking or lightly pressing the palm/sole causes the fingers/toes to curl.
Babinski reflex	Stroking the outer edge of the sole causes the toes to spread and the great toe to dorsiflex.

Timing of Primitive Reflexes

Reflex	Appears (time in gestational age)	Disappears (time post 40 weeks gestation in term infants)
Rooting reflex	30-34 weeks	3-4 months (fading by 1 month)
Walking reflex	32-36 weeks	1-2 months
Fencing reflex	Approximately 35 weeks (may be weak until 1 month after birth.)	3-4 months
Moro reflex	Approximately 32 weeks	3-6 months
Palmar reflex	20-26 weeks, well established by 32 weeks	2-3 months
Babinski reflex	At birth (due to need to stroke foot)	Resolution by the time of walking; normal up to 24 months in a non-ambulatory child

Skin

- Several common neonatal skin conditions should be recognized in order to prevent an extensive, unnecessary evaluation of the infant for pathology.

- Erythema toxicum will affect up to 50% of full-term infants. It typically presents within the first 2-3 days of life and resolves within a week. Lesions have a central papule surrounded by an erythematous base.

- Pustular melanosis affects approximately 5% of black infants and less than 1% of white infants. The pustules are present at birth or develop within 24 hours. The pustules subsequently rupture, leaving a classic collarette of skin with hyperpigmentation of the area. At birth, the pustules may have all ruptured, leaving only the collarettes.

- Milia classically are found on the nose, but may also be seen on other parts of the body. They are small cysts filled with keratinocytes and skin debris.

- Neonatal acne typically will develop between the second and fourth week of life. It peaks in intensity around 8-12 weeks and subsequently resolves. Typically, intervention is not needed; however, some cases may progress to severe nodulocystic acne. In those cases, medical management can help prevent scarring.

- "Angel kisses" and "stork bites" (seen on the eyelids and nape of the neck, respectively) represent nevi simplex. These typically will fade with increasing age, though some will remain.

- Nevus flamus, or port-wine stain, often will be more extensive than a nevus simplex and typically does not resolve. A nevus flamus that involves the ophthalmic and/or maxillary region should alert the examiner to the possibility of Sturge-Weber syndrome.

- Dermal melanosis – formerly referred to as "Mongolian spots" – are quite common. They represent increased areas of melanocytes and generally fade as the child ages. It is important not to mistake these for bruises.

Review Questions

1. **A single transverse palmar crease is:**
   A. Always associated with a genetic syndrome.
   B. Found in approximately 20% of the population.
   C. Should prompt further evaluation only when present bilaterally.
   D. Found in approximately 4% of the general population, but should still prompt a careful evaluation for other anomalies.

2. **On auscultation of the heart, you hear an S4 in a term newborn. Which of the following statements are correct?**
   A. An S4 can be normal in a newborn.
   B. S4s are pathologic by definition and require a full cardiac evaluation.
   C. An S4 is indicative of cardiac valvular problems.
   D. An S4 is indicative of a stiff pericardium.

3. **An 8-day-old infant arrives in the emergency department with obvious respiratory distress and central cyanosis. Saturations in the left arm are 65%. No murmur is heard on exam, but parents report the pediatrician noted a murmur at birth. Application of oxygen does not improve the hypoxia. Your next step should be:**
   A. Feel for a pulse and start chest compressions if the heart rate is less than 100.
   B. Start a prostaglandin E (PGE) infusion.
   D. Check four extremity blood pressures.
   D. Consult cardiology for a STAT echocardiogram.

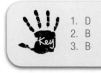

1. D
2. B
3. B

Apparent Life-Threatening Event

Sean M. Fox, MD

Critical Knowledge

- Apparent life-threatening event (ALTE) is not a diagnosis but rather a description of symptoms that generates considerable anxiety and concern for a child's caregiver.

- The National Institutes of Health Consensus Statement defines ALTE as: An episode that is frightening to the observer and that is characterized by some combination of apnea (central or obstructive); color change (usually cyanotic or pallid, but occasionally erythematous or plethoric); marked change in muscle tone (usually marked limpness); choking; or gagging. In some cases, the observer fears that the infant has died.[1]

- Apnea is a common clinical problem in infants and can be normal or pathologic.

  ▶ *Periodic breathing* is a normal pattern of breathing that involves three or more respiratory pauses, each being more than 3 seconds, with less than 20 seconds total duration. There is normal breathing between these episodes.

  ▶ *Apnea of prematurity* is pathologic apnea that occurs in preterm infants and often resolves by 37 weeks gestational age.

  ▶ *Pathologic apnea* is associated with **cyanosis**, **bradycardia**, **abrupt marked pallor, or hypotonia**, or being **>20 seconds in duration**.

- Since ALTE is a collection of symptoms, the etiologies are vast and diverse.

- The evaluation in the emergency department first must focus on detecting any immediate life-threatening causes.

- After determining medical stability, a thorough history and physical – looking for any signs that will help direct the further evaluation– is paramount.

- Often, the initial evaluation will be of a normal-appearing child in no apparent distress; yet, a low threshold for admission is still appropriate.

Background and Epidemiology

- The true incidence is difficult to determine, given the heterogeneity of the group that comprises it.

  ▶ Incidence of ALTE for all infants is between 0.2% and 6%.[2,3]

- ▶ 45% to 50% of the ALTE patients are classified as idiopathic.[4]
- Morbidity and mortality of ALTE:
  - ▶ Primarily associated with the underlying etiology
    - Morbidity and mortality of bacterial meningitis or that associated with pertussis
    - Child abuse is one etiology that leads to significant morbidity and mortality and needs to be conscientiously considered in each case.[5]
    - Even idiopathic ALTEs, however, have documented long-term neurological sequelae.[1,6]
      - — The mortality for idiopathic ALTE is classified as 0%-6%.[1]

Risk Factors
- Factors associated with an increased mortality are:
  - ▶ *Sleep-onset of apnea requiring resuscitation*
  - ▶ *Similar episode prior*
  - ▶ *A sibling who was the victim of sudden infant death syndrome (SIDS)*
  - ▶ *Development of a seizure disorder during monitoring*[7]
- Sudden infant death and apparent life-threatening events
  - ▶ While similarities exist, an association between ALTE and SIDS has *not* been demonstrated.[1]
  - ▶ Following the initiation of the national "Back to Sleep" program in 1992, there was *no* noted decrease in the incidence in ALTE, while the incidence of SIDS *did* decline.[8]

Differential Diagnosis and Critical Concepts
- ALTEs have a multitude of identifiable causes. Changes in color, muscle tone, and respirations may be symptoms of various specific diseases.[1,2]
  - ▶ **GI** (most common diagnosed pathology)
    - GERD
      - — Accounts for 20%-54% of cases
      - — Evidence that 1 in 10 admissions are due to repeat GERD events[9]
    - Intussusception
    - Volvulus

- **Neurologic** (second most common diagnosed pathology)
  - Seizure disorder
  - CNS bleed
  - Malformation/tumors
- **Respiratory** (third most common diagnosed pathology)
  - Obstructive sleep apnea
  - Airway abnormalities (i.e., laryngotracheomalacia, vocal cord masses)
  - Foreign-body aspiration
- **Infectious**
  - Serious bacterial infections (SBI)
    - Sepsis, meningoencephalitis, bacteremia, urinary tract infection, pneumonia
    - Prematurity (GA <37 wks) is a significant risk factor for SBI causing ALTE in patients ≤ 60 days of age.[10]
      - Lack of fever should not reduce concern for SBI.
      - Low body temperature (temp <35°C) is also concerning.
    - Pertussis should also be considered.
  - Viral illnesses
    - Respiratory syncytial virus (RSV) and upper respiratory infections
    - Croup
- **Cardiac**
  - Arrhythmia
  - Congenital heart disease
  - Tamponade
- **Metabolic**
  - Dehydration and electrolyte derangements
  - Inborn errors of metabolism
  - Endocrine abnormalities
- **Child Abuse**
  - Constitutes a small but very significant proportion of ALTE cases
  - Associated with high mortality (9%-32%)[5]

- ▶ **Accidental Poisoning**
  - One study found 8.4% of patients presenting with ALTE in the ED had positive comprehensive drug screens.
  - 4.7% were positive for OTC cold medications, despite the fact that no guardian reported giving these medications.[11]
- ▶ **50% of ALTE cases have no identifiable etiology.**[1]
- Dual diagnoses (i.e., a patient with respiratory infection and gastro-esophageal reflux) may exist.

Treatment/Evaluation

- Address the ABCDEs first!
  - ▶ Take care not to be cavalier with a patient that looks well.
  - ▶ Address the most life-threatening etiologies first.
- Currently there is no standard management strategy for ALTE.
  - ▶ There is no advocated minimal evaluation for patients presenting with apparent life-threatening events.[12]
  - ▶ First, determine whether the presentation fits the definition of an ALTE.
  - ▶ Next, assess for clues that may illuminate a *cause* of the ALTE.
- The most important initial diagnostic tool is a thorough **history and physical examination**.
  - ▶ History Points
    - Who was present, what was observed, and what actions were taken?
    - What kind of apnea was the patient having?
      - — **Central apnea** may be seen as a lack of respiratory effort.
      - — **Obstructive apnea** describes choking or gagging, or may even describe significant chest-wall excursion efforts or abdominal wall muscle contractions without successful ventilation.
      - — **Mixed apnea** – signs of both central and obstructive apnea. GERD can induce bronchospasm and also alter respiratory drive by affecting chemoreceptors.
    - Previous events and their similarities and differences
    - Timing
      - — Was the patient asleep?

- — Was the patient eating?
- — Was the patient playing?
- What type of bedding was the child in and was there any co-sleeping?
- Recent illnesses and feeding difficulties
- Recent medications given
  - — Ask specifically about OTC cold preparations.
  - — Often, use will not be reported.[11]
- Birth history (prematurity?), weight gain, and developmental milestones
- History of SIDS or infant deaths within the family
- Family history of cardiovascular, genetic, metabolic, or seizure disorders; also, any familial psychiatric illnesses should be inquired.
- Family's social circumstances

► **Physical Exam Points**
- Airway, breathing, and circulation
- A full set of vital signs, including finger-stick and height and weight
  - — *Hypoglycemia is easily treated and can often present with symptoms that could be classified as an ALTE.*
- Dysmorphisms
- Airway abnormalities
- Significant murmurs
- Presence of emesis
- Abdominal distention
- Hernias
- Thorough neurologic assessment, including a fundoscopic exam
- >50% of ALTE patients have normal initial physical examinations.[3,13,14]

► While there is no minimal workup, the evaluation can be rather extensive, given the vast differential for ALTE.[3,12,15]
- Numerous studies can be beneficial when based upon the history and physical.
- The initial assessment of ~70% of ALTE patients directed the further evaluation.[15]

- **Serious bacterial infection** should be highly considered in:
    - Patients less than 1 month old
    - Patients who are ≤ 60 days of age and have history of prematurity (<37 weeks GA)
    - Patients presenting with multiple ALTEs on the same day[10]
    - Investigating specifically for pertussis also may be warranted.
- There will be more utility in obtaining a nasopharyngeal swab for RSV in patients with URI signs than in those without symptoms.
- The child with URI symptoms may also benefit from comprehensive toxicology screen to look for unreported OTC cold preparation medications.[11]
- **Non-accidental trauma** should be highly considered in:
    - Patients with any physical exam findings or history concerning for abuse
    - Patients presenting with history of repeat ALTEs
    - This concern should lead to skeletal survey, head CT, and consultation of Child Protective Services
- Patients with significant murmurs may benefit from echocardiograms.
- An abnormal fingerstick may point to an underlying genetic or metabolic pathology and should generate an appropriate workup.
- ~30% of ALTE patients have inconclusive histories and physicals.[15]
    - ▶ In these patients, broad evaluations for systemic infections, metabolic diseases, or blood chemistry abnormalities are generally not productive.
    - ▶ Only 6% of tests contributed to the final diagnosis in one study.[15]
    - ▶ A period of observation can offer an opportunity to better characterize the patient's risk factors and determine a more tailored approach.
- **Disposition**
    - ▶ Most of these cases, without obvious benign etiologies, deserve a period of observation in the hospital in a monitored setting.[12,14]
        - ■ The presenting symptoms correlate poorly with the final diagnosis.[13]

- 7.8% of those who later had a negative ED evaluation required medical intervention while in the hospital.[14]
▶ Even patients with a diagnosis of GERD were shown to benefit from hospitalization; 6% had events during hospitalization; 9% had recurrent ALTEs; and 3% were given a significant new diagnosis.[9]
▶ The benefit of being able to observe the patient to better characterize the events, in addition to the possible extensive workup and the emotional stress that the event and the process of evaluation places upon the family, all favor admitting the patient to the hospital.

Review Questions

1. **When listening to a description of events that occurred to a child, which of the following would be LESS concerning and LESS likely to imply the event was an ALTE?**
   A. The child lost musculoskeletal tone during the event.
   B. The child strained and had a pause in breathing without changes in color or tone.
   C. There was a pause in breathing, and the child's face and lips looked blue during the event.
   D. The child's eyes rolled up and would not respond to stimulation during the event.

2. **In regard to the pathologic cause of ALTE, which is the most common?**
   A. GI
   B. Infectious
   C. Neurologic
   D. Respiratory

3. **Which of the following is correct?**
   A. Most patients evaluated for ALTE eventually have an identifiable cause for the event.
   B. Children who present to the ED with a reported ALTE can be discharged to home following a normal physical exam and workup.
   C. Most patients admitted to observation following an ALTE will require further medical intervention during admission.
   D. The presenting symptoms correlate poorly with the final diagnosis.

Key

1. B
2. A
3. D

The Febrile Child

Kimberly Leeson, MD
Ben Leeson, MD

Critical Knowledge

- Fever is defined as a temperature above 38.0°C (100.4°F).
- Fevers reported by guardians should be considered true fevers.
- Acute otitis media should never be considered a source for fever.
- ALL neonates (<28 days) with fever should be admitted and have a full sepsis workup.
- "Fever without localized source" algorithms should be used for low-risk infants and are not meant for use on high-risk infants.

Background

- A fever is defined as a temperature above 38.0°C (100.4°F) and may be an indication of a serious bacterial infection.
- As many as 20% of pediatric ED patients present with fever.
- Workup and treatment depend on many factors, including the child's age, appearance, risk factors for serious infections, and availability of follow up.
- Newborns and young children up to 3 years old are at increased risk for bacteremia and serious infections.
- The risk decreases with age, with the highest incidence during the first 3 months of life; children younger than 2 months have additional risks.
- Because of this, the pediatric patient with a fever is usually grouped by age:
  - ▶ The neonatal period (<28 days)
  - ▶ Young infants (28-60 days)
  - ▶ 2 months and older
- A life-threatening event occurs in up to 1% of children presenting with fever.
- While most illnesses in young children are viral in nature, as many as 5% of children without an obvious source will have bacteremia.
- Infants often present with nonspecific symptoms with no localizing sign; assessment of a child's behavior and appearance often provide the best clues about illness severity.
- The degree of fever, rapidity of rise, or response to antipyretics do not predict seriousness of illness.

- Performing a thorough history and physical are *vital*.
- Any child under 3 who appears ill requires a workup and admission, regardless of whether or not a fever exists.

Differential Diagnosis

- **Infectious** (Causative agent varies by age)
  - ► Meningitis
  - ► Pyelonephritis
  - ► Bacterial or viral pneumonia
  - ► Otitis media
  - ► Localized skin infections (i.e., cellulitis/abscess)
  - ► Osteomyelitis
  - ► Oral infections such as pharyngitis from *S. pyogenes* and viral herpetic gingivostomatitis
  - ► Generalized viral illness
- **Noninfectious**
  - ► High ambient temperature (especially in warmer months)
  - ► Overbundling children in cooler months (controversial)
  - ► Malignancy
  - ► Rheumatologic disease
  - ► Recent vaccination (especially with DTaP and MMR)
  - ► Ingestion, including aspirin and anticholinergics (especially in toddlers)

Diagnostics and ED Treatment

- Establish if patient is "low risk" or "high risk."
- Criteria for **low risk** include:
  - ► Previously healthy infants
  - ► Nontoxic appearance without an obvious focal bacterial infection
  - ► Reassuring UA (negative nitrites and less than 10 WBC/hpf)
  - ► Serum WBC count between 5,000 and 15,000
  - ► Negative CSF gram stain and less than 8 WBC/mm3, if obtained
  - ► Stool negative, and few WBCs in stool if diarrhea is present
  - ► No pulmonary infiltrate, if CXR is obtained

- Factors that indicate an **increased risk** of bacteremia or sepsis include:
  - ▶ Age less than 2 months
  - ▶ Immunocompromised state
  - ▶ Unvaccinated or undervaccinated state
  - ▶ Hypothermia (core temp <36.8°C or 98°F) or hyperthermia (core temp >40.5°C, 105°F)
  - ▶ History of sickle cell disease or HIV
  - ▶ Patients with inserted medical devices (pacemakers, VP shunts, long-term IVs)
- Important historical features:
  - ▶ Immunization history (including number of doses and dates of pneumococcal and *H. influenzae* vaccines)
  - ▶ Exposure to sick contacts, antibiotics
  - ▶ Recent travel
  - ▶ Previous hospitalizations
  - ▶ History of neglect or abuse
- Document presence of fever at home, duration, and treatment (subjective reports of fever at home are reliable indicators).
- Complete exam looking for signs of infection, including:
  - ▶ **Vitals:** abnormal vitals, including rectal fever or hypothermia, tachycardia or bradycardia, hypotension, tachypnea, hypoxia
  - ▶ **General:** irritability, inconsolability, lethargy, toxicity
  - ▶ **Skin:** including classic rashes; cellulitis; Osler nodes; pale, mottled or cool skin; and increased capillary refill >2 seconds
  - ▶ **HEENT:** pharyngitis, peritonsillar abscess, lymphadenitis, eye discharge, dry mucus membranes, and abnormal anterior fontanelle (sunken= dehydration, raised = can be associated with meningitis)
  - ▶ **Cardiovascular:** tachycardia or bradycardia, murmur or rub
  - ▶ **Respiratory:** tachypnea, wheezing, stridor, nasal flaring, grunting
  - ▶ **Abdomen:** umbilical infections, ridged abdomen (concerning for necrotizing enterocolitis in newborns, malrotation/volvulus, or appendicitis)
  - ▶ **Neurologic:** not arousable, abnormal primitive reflexes, meningeal signs

- ► **Genitourinary:** non-descended testis; penile or vaginal discharge
- ► **Musculoskeletal:** cold, limp extremities; swollen or warm joints
- Workup and Treatments
  - ► Full septic workups include a CBC, blood culture, catheterized urinalysis, urine culture, and lumbar puncture.
  - ► Include a chest radiograph if respiratory signs or symptoms are present (focal findings, tachypnea, SaO2 <95%).
  - ► Include rapid RSV/influenza and viral cultures, if suspected.
  - ► Antipyretic (acetaminophen 15 mg/kg)
  - ► Hospital admission versus outpatient management (see *Figure 1*)

Figure 1. Suggested Algorithm for Children up to 24 Months with Fever and No Localizing Source for Infection

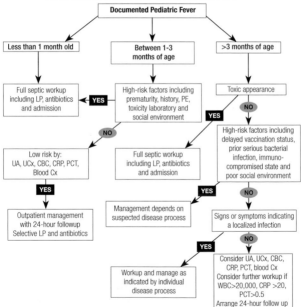

- **Antibiotics:** (Do not delay administration in ill-appearing patients.)
  - ▶ Age 0-28 days (neonates) – Ampicillin 100 mg/kg IV **AND** cefotaxime 50 mg/kg IV **OR** gentamicin (aged-based loading dose)
  - ▶ Age 29-56 days – Children ill enough to be admitted should be treated as neonates. Low-risk children who are well enough to be discharged home do not require antibiotics, but consider a dose of ceftriaxone.
  - ▶ Age 2-24 months – No antibiotic therapy is indicated for well-appearing children who do not have a defined bacterial source and who will be discharged.

Neonatal Fever Workup (birth-1 month of age)

- During the neonatal period, children are at particularly high risk of developing emergent infections that require acute treatment.
- Because of this, a complete septic workup – including a lumbar puncture (LP) – is indicated.
- A full septic workup should be performed, even if there are signs of bronchiolitis.
- The timely initiation of antibiotics also is a top priority.
- Consider evaluation for herpes simplex in febrile neonates with the following risk factors: age <3 weeks, vesicles, seizure, toxic, CSF pleocytosis, or RBCs, maternal history of herpes.

Febrile Child Workup (4-8 weeks of age)

- If the infant appears ill, a full septic workup (including LP) and conservative treatment should be initiated, including antibiotics and admission.
- If the infant is well-appearing, workup should include CBC, blood culture, UA with culture, and LP.
- Procalcitonin (PCT) can be useful in assessing risk of SBI (PCT <0.5 ng/mL decreased risk; >2.0 ng/mL increased risk).
- CRP can be useful in assessing risk of SBI (CRP <20 decreased risk; >40 increased risk).
- Stool cultures should be performed selectively.
- Chest radiographs are only indicated when signs of respiratory disease are present.
- In select cases, an LP and hospital admission may be omitted in well-appearing infants who have the following: negative workup, reliable follow-up in 12-24 hours, competent parents who can comply with care and follow-up instructions, no initiation of antibiotic therapy (*Figure 1*).

Febrile Child Workup (age 2-24 months)

- For children in this age group, management is based on the localizing signs and symptoms and the height of the temperature.
- The incidence of occult bacteremia has dramatically decreased since the introduction of the Hib (*H. influenzae* type b) and conjugated pneumococcal vaccines.
- Children with a source of fever (pneumonia, urinary tract infection, etc.) should be treated accordingly; disposition depends on the severity of illness, ability to maintain hydration and tolerate oral medications, and availability of close follow up.
- Workup, including CBC, PCT, CRP, UA/culture, and blood culture, may be helpful in distinguishing mild from severe bacterial illness (SBI).
- Children with the clinical syndrome of bronchiolitis in this age group rarely have concomitant bacteremia or UTIs; routine blood and urine cultures are often unnecessary.
- CSF analysis and blood cultures should be reserved for ill children who are irritable, toxic-appearing, or have had a seizure.
- Avoid presumptive use of broad-spectrum antibiotics.

Febrile Child Workup (older than 24 months)

- History and physical exam are both more reliable in fully immunized children older than 24 months.
- Evaluation requires obtaining a careful history and physical examination.
- Workup and treatment depends largely on clinical findings and suspected disease.

Disposition

- All febrile neonates should be hospitalized and treated with antibiotics for suspected sepsis until cultures of CSF, blood, and urine are all negative for 48 hours.
- The decision to admit older infants and children for presumptive sepsis depends on the following factors:
  - ▶ Ability to arrange close follow up
  - ▶ Presence of toxicity
  - ▶ Need for monitoring
  - ▶ Need for hydration or other supportive care
  - ▶ Social circumstances

Review Questions

1. A 4-week-old female is brought in by her parents for fever at home and decreased PO intake. There are no other associated symptoms (cough, vomiting, diarrhea, or rash). Heart rate is 160; blood pressure is 75/58; and temperature is 39.1° C. Physical exam is grossly normal. Urine catheterization reveals positive leukocyte esterase and nitrates, with bacteria seen. What is the most appropriate next step?

   A. Full sepsis workup with blood cultures, urine culture, chest x-ray, and lumbar puncture.

   B. Discharge home with PO antibiotics and close follow up.

   C. Single dose of IV ceftriaxone with discharge home on PO antibiotics.

2. A 12-week-old male is brought in by his parents for fever at home with associated cough. There has been no vomiting, diarrhea, or other associated symptoms. Heart rate is 150, blood pressure is 72/53, respiratory rate 28, pulse ox 98% on room air, and temperature is 38.5°. Physical exam is normal, with the exception of the pulmonary exam, which shows diffuse wheezing. Chest x-ray is normal, and rapid RSV is positive. Symptoms improve in the emergency department with nebulized albuterol and acetaminophen. What is the most appropriate next step in management?

   A. Full sepsis workup with blood cultures, urine culture, chest x-ray, and lumbar puncture.

   B. Discharge home with PO antibiotics.

   C. Single dose of IM ceftriaxone with discharge home on PO antibiotics.

   D. Outpatient treatment with close follow up.

3. If a 3-week-old female has a fever and evidence of acute otitis media, the most appropriate management is oral antibiotics and next-day outpatient follow up with the primary care provider.

   True or False?

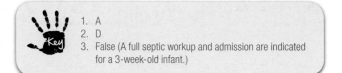

1. A
2. D
3. False (A full septic workup and admission are indicated for a 3-week-old infant.)

Acute Otitis Media

Brian Clothier MD, MS

Background

- Acute otitis media (AOM) is commonly overdiagnosed and unnecessarily treated with antibiotics in the ED for febrile or fussy children.
- Guidelines published in 2013 by the American Academy of Pediatrics (AAP) apply to healthy children between the ages of 6 months and 12 years.[1]
- Growing concerns over antibiotic resistance, medication side effects, and simply practicing good medicine make it essential to get the diagnosis and need for treatment right the first time.
- The lofty goal of the pediatric emergency provider is to provide antibiotic therapy only to the subset of those who will actually benefit from it. This requires the exclusion of those with chronic otitis media, simple middle ear effusions, or red tympanic membranes without acute infection.

Critical Knowledge

- **Make the right diagnosis**. While purulent drainage from a perforated tympanic membrane represents obvious otitis media, the diagnosis often is not that simple. AOM is characterized by the following findings: acute onset <48 hours, middle ear effusion, and middle ear inflammation with otalgia.

  - ▶ **Acute onset <48 hours**
    - Otitis media with effusion lasting longer than 2 days is a different diagnostic entity and does not require treatment with antihistamines, antimicrobials, corticosteroids, or decongestants.[2] Instead, a PCP should follow these chronic cases.

  - ▶ **Middle ear inflammation**
    - Middle ear inflammation is indicated by erythema of the TM or otalgia; this is a requirement for the diagnosis, but does not by itself necessitate antibiotic therapy.

  - ▶ **Middle ear effusion (MEE)**
    - MEE is indicated by a bulging TM, otorrhea, an air fluid level behind the TM, or limited or absent TM mobility.

- Pneumatic otoscopy is the diagnostic modality of choice, as it is the most practical for the ED physician. Expect a normal tympanic membrane to be more mobile under negative pressure than under positive. Clinical observance of an immobile tympanic membrane indicates an effusion is present and has been shown to dramatically improve the accuracy of the diagnosis AOM.[3]

Diagnostic Strategies

Current guidelines allow for some flexibility in making the diagnosis. In some children, pain and fever may be present with TM erythema even though no effusion has developed. In others, an immotile or poorly motile TM associated with fever and pain may be the best clue to the emergency physician that AOM exists. Taking the time to make the child feel as safe and comfortable as possible prior to otoscopy will result in a better examination. Cerumen should be cautiously removed, as necessary, and may be facilitated using a curette or a 1:1 solution of peroxide and water. Take care not to introduce anything into the middle ear through a perforated tympanic membrane, including water, peroxide solutions, or benzocaine.

Severe symptoms

Treatment guidelines take into account the severity of signs and symptoms. These must be considered as you determine a treatment strategy. Severe symptoms include:
- Temperature of 39°C (102.2°F) or higher
- Severe otalgia
- Otalgia lasting more than 48 hours

Treatment
All children need pain control!
- Acetaminophen and topical benzocaine are appropriate for both infants and older children.
- Ibuprofen is not indicated in children less than 6 months of age because there is no evidence to support its safe use.
- Narcotic/codeine preparations are not recommended in the infant population because of the risk of respiratory depression and altered mental status,[2] and are generally not indicated in the treatment of AOM at any age, barring exceptional circumstances.
- Home remedies such as warm oil in the ear canal (if otorrhea is absent and the tympanic membrane is intact) or application of heat over the ear offer little or no risk and may provide additional comfort.

Treatment guidelines are stratified by age, severity of illness/pain, the presence of bilateral symptoms, and whether antibiotics have been administered in the last 30 days.

Age

- All children with confirmed AOM and severe symptoms should be treated with antibiotic therapy.
- Infants less than 6 months of age are considered higher risk and should be treated with antibiotics even if the clinician is uncertain of the diagnosis.
- Children 6 to 23 months with bilateral AOM should be treated even if they do not have severe symptoms.
- Children aged 6 to 23 months with unilateral AOM or those over 2 years of age are candidates for observation without antibiotics, ensuring close follow up as described below

Some may be observed without antibiotics.

- Meta-analysis of multiple previous studies has shown that 7 to 20 children must be treated with antibiotics for AOM in order for one to receive benefit.[4,5,6] Observation without antibiotics is an acceptable treatment for patients over the age of 6 months with unilateral AOM without fever of 39°C or higher, without significant pain, and with guaranteed reassessment in 48-72 hours, should the child not improve or worsen. Children over 24 months are allowed the same liberty with unilateral symptoms.

Antibiotic choices

A variety of factors, including the routine use of the heptavalent pneumococcal vaccine, have changed the causative agent profile for AOM. 35-50% of cases of AOM are caused by nontypable *H influenzae*, 25-40% by *Streptococcus pneumonae,* and 5-10% by *Moraxella caterallis*. Viruses are the sole causative agent in 5–15% of cases, but may play a role in up to 75% of cases.[2]

- For reasons of susceptibility profile, low side effects, price and palatability, initiate antibiotic therapy with "high-dose" amoxicillin at 80-90 mg/kg/day for most children.
- Amoxicillin-clavulanate dosed at 90 mg/kg/day (calculations based on the amoxicillin component) should be initiated for children with failed response to amoxicillin alone (see below), fever of 39°C or higher, moderate to severe otalgia, purulent conjunctivitis, or in cases where coverage for beta lactamase-positive *Haemophilus influenza* or *Moraxella catarrhalis* is desired.

- Children allergic to penicillin, in whom the reaction is not a type I hyper-sensitivity, may be treated with a cephalosporin such as cefdinir (the most palatable), cefuroxime, or cefpodoxime. Those who do have a history of urticaria or anaphylaxis with penicillin may be treated with azithromycin, clarithromycin, or trimethoprim-sulfamethoxazole.
- Parenteral (IV or IM) ceftriaxone may be given as a one-time dose to those who cannot tolerate oral medications.[2]

Duration of therapy

Current recommendations are for 10 days of therapy for all children under 6 years and for all seriously ill children. Older children with mild disease may be treated for 5-7 days.

Treatment failures

Children who present to the ED after 48-72 hours of therapy without improvement should be thoroughly re-evaluated for other etiologies of symptoms. If the diagnosis of AOM is confirmed, the patient's treatment should be "upgraded" by switching to high-dose amoxicillin-clavulanate 90 mg/kg/day (calculations based on the amoxicillin component) or to one of the aforementioned cephalosporins. Those who present to the ED after failure of these treatment modalities should be treated with parenteral cephalosporins. Treatment with clindamycin should be reserved for those who fail the aforementioned regimens and for whom tympanocentesis is desired, but not immediately available.[2]

Prevention

Take the opportunity to teach parents about preventative measures such as avoiding exposure to second-hand tobacco smoke, bottle propping, and having their child immunized with the pneumococcal and annual influenza vaccines.

Review Questions

1. The diagnostic triad of AOM includes all the below EXCEPT?

   A. Onset <48 hours

   B. Middle ear effusion

   C. Bilateral conjunctivitis

   D. Middle ear inflammation

2. What is the most common causative agent of AOM?

   A. Viruses

   B. Nontypable *H influenzae*

   C. *Moraxella caterallis*

   D. *Streptococcus pneumonae*

3. What is the treatment strategy for an otherwise healthy 18-month-old with a unilateral case of AOM who is only mildly ill?

   A. Oral amoxicillin – low dose

   B. Oral amoxicillin – high dose

   C. Oral azithromycin

   D. Observe with prompt follow up

The Crying Infant

Brian Clothier MD, MS

Critical Concept

Evaluation of the fussy or crying infant requires a certain amount of finesse. Paroxysms of crying are common in the second to third week of life and many bewildered parents will present seeking reassurance. However, many serious or even life-threatening diseases will present during the infant period as crying and inconsolability.

Quick tips

- Take a *complete* history. In the newborn period, this should include a prenatal history, including maternal gravity and parity, prenatal care, and infection risks. The birth history should include gestational age and weight and complications of pregnancy and delivery. The nature and onset of the crying, as well as associated symptoms, are particularly important. This information will help you determine if the infant is at risk for infection, congenital anomaly, abuse, or neglect.

- *All* fussy infants are presumed ill until proven otherwise. Most are not critically ill, but to presume the worst will force you to be thorough in your history, physical examination, and thought process.

- Use time to your advantage. Consider observing the patient in the ED over several hours. It is easier to make subtle diagnoses when the patient is re-examined over time; this will provide you and the parent reassurance. Benign causes of crying will cease over short time periods.

Background

Infants and children presenting with "crying" or "fussiness" are extremely common. Parents may describe these children as "just not acting right." Etiologies range from benign to life-threatening. As always in medicine, a broad differential is the key to making the correct diagnosis.

Remember

- Establish the pattern of crying, exacerbating factors, and other signs of illness. Parents will define "fussy" differently based on their frame of reference, which varies based on their culture, socioeconomic status, and parenting experience.

- Benign etiologies are diagnoses of *exclusion*!
- **Consider child abuse.** Any sign of trauma in an infant must raise your suspicion for abuse. Also consider the abuse you may prevent by identifying at-risk situations.
- **5% will have multiple causes that contribute to their illness.**

Differential Diagnosis

The single most important action in the evaluation of the fussy infant is to build an appropriate differential diagnosis and then – either by history, physical exam, or testing – rule out each diagnosis. The following table contains common causes of infant fussiness.

Table 1.

Conditions Associated with Crying or Fussy Infants and Young Children Adapted from Fleisher[1]	
Head and neck	• Encephalitis/meningitis • Skull fracture/subdural hematoma • Glaucoma • Eye foreign body/corneal abrasion • Acute otitis media • Pseudotumor cerebri
Respiratory	• Upper respiratory infections • Viral prodromes: myalgia/arthralgia
Cardiovascular	• Coarctation of the aorta • Congestive heart failure • SVT • Anomalous origin of left coronary artery from pulmonary artery
Gastrointestinal	• Gastroesophageal reflux/esophagitis • Gastritis/gastroenteritis • Appendicitis • Intussusception • Volvulus • Cow's milk protein intolerance • Excess gastrointestinal air • Anal fissure

Genitourinary	• Testicular torsion • Incarcerated hernia • UTI
Integumentary	• Burn • Strangulated finger, toe, penis (hair tourniquet)
Toxic/Metabolic	• Drugs: antihistamines, atropinics, adrenergics, cocaine (including passive inhalation), aspirin • Toxic ingestions/overdose • Metabolic acidosis, hypernatremia, hypocalcemia, hypoglycemia
Musculoskeletal	• Extremity fracture from fall or child abuse
Trauma	• Falls • Physical abuse/neglect
Behavioral	• Colic • Parental anxiety

Treatment Strategy

For all crying or fussy children, a systematic approach to the history and physical will lead you in the right direction.

- **Observe the interaction between the parent and child.** A child who will not console even momentarily while eating or sleeping is potentially ill.
- **Physical examination.** Scrutinize the vital signs, including HR and BP. Thorough physical evaluation includes examination of the corneas and retinas, otoscopy with pneumatic insufflation, auscultation of heart and lungs, palpation of abdomen, palpation of long bones, genital exam, anal exam with/without rectal exam, and complete skin exam (head to toe) for bruising or other lesions. Examine the extremities, including the penis, fingers, and toes for signs of trauma, hair tourniquet, and perfusion.
- **Take off the diaper.** Critical diagnoses such as anal fissure, testicular torsion, hair tourniquet, inguinal hernia, or intussusception will be missed without this key portion of the physical exam.
- **There is no "fussy infant" workup.** Order lab work, imaging studies, and consultation based on your thorough history and physical examination.
- **It is dangerous to discharge a child who is not consolable and for whom you do not have a firm diagnosis.**

Pearls for specific pathologies not covered elsewhere in this text

Benign Intracranial Hypertension

Consider this diagnosis in a crying infant with a bulging fontanel in whom you have ruled out intracranial infection, mass, bleeding, and hydrocephalus. Opening pressure at lumbar puncture will be elevated.

Corneal Abrasion

Start by looking at the hands for long nails. Look for a unilateral red eye without discharge in an otherwise well-appearing infant. Make certain to fluorescein stain the eyes of any crying infant with unknown etiology.

Supraventricular Tachycardia (SVT)

Obtain an ECG on any infant with a significantly elevated heart rate, and certainly if greater than 200 beats per minute. SVT in infants will have a rate >220. The history will be incompatible with sinus tachycardia, p waves will be absent, and the heart rate may change dramatically. Hemodynamically unstable infants should be cardioverted.

Anal Fissure

More common at ages when infants transition to solid foods (4-6 months), cow's milk (12 months), or associated with toilet training. History will describe hard bowel movements associated with straining. The diagnosis can often be made by history before confirmation of fissure on physical exam.

Urinary Tract Infection (UTI)

Recent studies on crying infants support obtaining urinalysis to rule out UTI as a serious underlying etiology.[2,3]

Colic

Critical Knowledge

Colic defined. Most authors agree on the Wessel criteria of crying: more than 3 hours per day, for more than 3 days per week, and for more than 3 weeks in an infant that is well-fed and otherwise healthy.[1]

- Additional characteristics that distinguish colic from mere crying include a **paroxysmal** nature, qualitatively **different** from normal crying, associated with **hypertonia** and **inconsolability.**

- Understand that this definition is limited, as many parents will not wait 3 weeks before seeking assistance, while others will not seek medical attention at all. This illustrates the difficulties with diagnosis and treatment: Some parents find it insufferable; others do not perceive it as a problem.

- Colic is perhaps best defined by what it is *not*. It isn't a surgical cause of abdominal pain. It is not bad parenting, child abuse, or neglect. It is a diagnosis of exclusion after serious pain, infection, and abuse have been excluded, usually by history and physical examination.

Colic is perhaps best understood as the final common pathway for a variety of medical, environmental, biological, and psychosocial factors.

- No single underlying cause has been identified, and much of the literature on the topic is inconclusive and conflicting.

Background

- As the name implies, colic was first thought to be abdominal pain related to the colon. This theory has all but been disproven.

- Symptoms begin as early as 2 weeks of age and usually resolve by 4 months.

- Symptoms tend to occur in the late afternoon or early evening.

- The symptoms vary, but can include high-pitched cries, grimaces, or knees pulled to the chest.

- By definition, the colicky infant is difficult to console and, as such, can be very stressful to inexperienced or overwhelmed parents.

Etiology

- While a cause has never been identified, many factors are thought to play a role.
- A popular theory has been that colic is caused by cow's milk protein intolerance. This hasn't been definitively proven, but it is reasonable to think an allergy to casein or whey may play a role in some infants, as may carbohydrate intolerance from sorbitol-containing fruit juices with a high ratio of fructose.
- Aberrations in the microflora of the gut have been identified and support the use of probiotics.[2]
- Feeding methods, nicotine exposure, serotonin levels, and parental stress/anxiety have all been implicated.

Differential Diagnosis

Any of the conditions listed in *Table 1* can cause abrupt onset of crying in a young infant and should be considered and ruled out prior to diagnosing colic.

Key Concepts

- Ascertain the length and frequency of crying, as well as associated signs and symptoms.
- A thorough physical examination is paramount and should include gastrointestinal and neurological examination.
- Radiographic imaging and lab studies are unnecessary in an otherwise healthy-appearing infant.[3]

Treatment

- Various strategies exist for managing colic, but there are few evidence-based guidelines.
- **Diet**
  - ▶ No evidence exists for changing the diet.
  - ▶ Breastfeeding mothers must be encouraged to continue to nurse.
  - ▶ Infants taking cow milk-based formulas should only be switched to hypoallergenic formulas such as casein or whey hydrolysate if there is suspicion for milk-protein allergy as evidenced by loose-bloody stools or other signs of atopy (rhinitis, wheezing, atopic dermatitis) or a family history of atopy. 30% of children with cow-milk protein allergy will also be allergic to soy protein; therefore, switching to soy formula is without basis and is not recommended in the management of colic.[4]

- **Medications**
  - ▶ Probiotics, specifically *Lactobacillus reuteri,* have been shown to significantly reduce crying time.[2]
  - ▶ Anticholinergics have been described to aid in the resolution of colic.[5] In rare cases, however, they have been associated with apnea, seizures, and syncope; as such, they cannot be recommended. Dicyclomine (Bentyl) should be avoided in children younger than 6 months because of an association with apnea.
  - ▶ Simethicone drops are purported to break up gas bubbles but have not been shown more effective than placebo.[6]
  - ▶ Various herbal remedies are widely available without prescription. Some may be helpful in the treatment of colic. There are no randomized, controlled trials of these products; parents should be educated and must understand the potential risks of their use.
- **Behavioral Modification**
  - ▶ Taking the infant for a ride in the car is near universally believed to help with colic, but is an unproven technique.
  - ▶ Evidence does not support expensive and potentially dangerous interventions, including car ride simulators, crib vibrators, and buckling the infant in a car seat placed atop a running clothes dryer.[1]
  - ▶ Parents should be supported. Caring for a child who cries more than anticipated can be quite stressful, and that stress may contribute to the child's crying — or worse, provoke caregivers to abuse. Teach techniques to soothe the baby such as the 4 Ss: **s**hushing (white noise), **s**waddling (simulates intrauterine environment), **s**winging (produces soothing motion), and **s**ucking (on a breast or pacifier). While these may not be directly effective, they provide parents a sense of empowerment, which may reduce parental stress, ultimately resulting in a better outcome for the child.

Review Questions

1. Which of the following is *not* one of the characteristics of colic?
   A. Paroxysmal, hypotonic, and inconsolable
   B. Three hours a day, three days a week for three weeks
   C. Multifactorial, and likely with biological and psychosocial components
   D. Different from mere crying as there is a different quality of the cry, often sounding as though the child is in pain

2. When should the diet of a colicky infant be changed?
   A. Never
   B. To appease the parents so they feel something is being done
   C. When there is evidence of a milk protein allergy
   D. Excessive gas noted by parents

3. Which medication has been proven safe and effective in the treatment of colic?
   A. Dicyclomine (Bentyl)
   B. Simethicone
   C. Anticholinergics
   D. None of the above

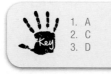
1. A
2. C
3. D

Closed Head Injury

Mary Thiessen, MD

Critical Knowledge/Action

- ABCDs first; immobilize C-spine.
- The aim when treating traumatic brain injury (TBI) is to identify treatable mass lesions, to prevent secondary injury (hypoxia, hypoperfusion, ischemia, and neuronal damage), and to identify any other life-threatening injuries.
- Maintain a broad differential and do not prematurely rule out a diagnosis since the situation leading to the TBI may have been a medical event (seizure, hypoglycemia, arrhythmia, etc).
- Establish a neurologic baseline, and evaluate for any change (pupil reactivity and serial GCS).
- Physical findings suggestive of TBI include location and size of scalp hematoma, signs of basilar skull fracture, fontanel fullness, pupil size, and low or decreasing GCS.
- Infants with significant intracranial hemorrhage may not have apparent external injuries; instead, they may present with vomiting, irritability, apnea or seizures.
- Many children with mild head injuries have stable vitals and appear alert and interactive; therefore, you need to be attentive to the patient's history, mechanism, and physical exam.

Table 1. Pediatric GCS

Response	Children >4 to Adult	Infant/Children <4	Score
Eye opening	Spontaneous	Spontaneous	4
	To verbal stimuli	To verbal stimuli	3
	To pain	To pain	2
	No response	No response	1
Verbal	Alert and oriented conversation	Coos, babbles/ appropriate words; oriented	5
	Disoriented conversation	Irritable; cries, but consolable; confused	4

	Speaking, but inappropriate words and nonsensical	Cries to pain and not consolable/inappropriate words	3
	Incomprehensible or moans	Moans or grunts to pain/incomprehensible	2
	No response	No response	1
Motor	Obeys commands	Spontaneous movement	6
	Localizes to pain	Withdraws to touch/localizes to pain	5
	Withdraws to pain	Withdraws to pain	4
	Decorticate posture	Decorticate posture	3
	Decerebrate posture	Decerebrate posture	2
	No response	No response	1

Adapted from Wright, D., & Merck, L. (2011). Head trauma in adults and children. In J. Tintinalli (Ed.), *Tintinalli's Emergency Medicine* (7th ed., pp. 1692-1709). New York: McGraw Hill Medical.

Epidemiology/Physiology

- 85% of pediatric head injuries are classified as "mild."[1]

- Minor head injury represents almost 400,000 ED visits each year, with children from 0-4 years of age most commonly affected.

- Fewer than 5% of minor head-injured children have intracranial injury,[2] and fewer than 1% require neurosurgical intervention.[3,4]

- Younger age, particularly 2 years and under, can be a strong criterion for identifying risk of intracranial injury.[5]

- Primary injury occurs at the moment of insult when mechanical forces (impact, acceleration-deceleration, and rotational) generate direct trauma to the head.

- Primary injuries include cerebral contusions; subdural, epidural, subarachnoid, and intraparenchymal hematomas; diffuse axonal injury; direct cellular damage; tearing/shearing of tissue; and loss of blood-brain barrier.

- Secondary injury occurs hours to days after the initial traumatic injury and involves impaired cerebral blood flow, edema, and increased intracranial pressure.

- Subdural hematoma is the most common intracranial injury.

- Parietal bone is the most commonly fractured skull bone; basilar skull fractures involve parietal or temporal bones.

Differential Diagnosis/Critical Concepts

- **Mild TBI:** GCS 14-15
- **Moderate TBI:** GCS 9-13
- **Severe TBI:** GCS ≤8
- Concussion (also referred to as mild TBI) has been defined by the American Academy of Neurology as "a trauma-induced alteration in mental status that may or may not involve loss of consciousness." Confusion and amnesia are hallmarks of concussion.[6]
- Concussion recently has been redefined as "a complex pathophysiologic process affecting the brain, induced by biomechanical forces."[7]
- Postconcussive symptoms refer to the constellation of acute symptoms after head injury: **somatic** (headache, dizziness, blurriness); **emotional** (anxiety, irritability); and **cognitive** (concentration and memory).[8]
- The severity of concussion can be determined only after resolution of concussive symptoms, the normalization of neurologic exam findings, and a return to baseline cognitive function.[7]
- Any athlete who is suspected of having suffered a concussion should be removed from participation until he or she is evaluated by a physician with training in the management of sports concussions.[9]
- No athlete should be allowed to participate in sports if he or she is still experiencing symptoms from a concussion.[9]
- Most studies have shown almost complete resolution of concussive symptoms by the sixth week in 80% of patients, but some patients may have symptoms for months to years.[10]
- Clinicians should discuss concussive symptoms with patients and appropriate follow up with a primary care provider or concussion clinic; neuropsychiatric testing should be considered.
- Second-impact syndrome is a form of re-injury that happens before the previous concussion has completely resolved. The brain is vulnerable to even minor impact during the post-concussive period, and a re-injury can lead to devastating complications or death.[11]

Abusive Head Trauma

- Approximately 80% of deaths caused by TBI in children <2 years can be attributed to abusive head trauma.[12]

- Multiple terms have been used to describe abusive head trauma, including "shaken baby syndrome" or "shaken impact syndrome"; however, the terms "nonaccidental head trauma" or "inflicted head injury" are preferred, since they do not suggest shaking as the only mechanism.[13]

- Victims of inflicted head injury tend to be younger in age, with the majority in their first year of life; have a history of prematurity and pre-injury medical problems; no mechanism offered by the caregiver; worse outcomes; higher severity of injuries; and higher mortality rates. Boys are more commonly affected than girls.

- Children with missed inflicted head injury are younger and more commonly misdiagnosed with accidental head injury or viral gastroenteritis.[14]

- Most children with abusive head trauma are less than 2 years old. A head CT should be performed for the following: changes in mental status; physical findings of head injuries, such as bruising around eyes, ears, and face; scalp hematomas; and underlying skull fracture, or when abuse is suspected.[13]

- In addition to the head CT, a fundoscopic exam should be done with ophthalmologist consultation, a skeletal survey, screening for blunt abdominal trauma (LFTs and pancreatic enzymes), and labs (CBC and coagulation panel).[13]

Neuroimaging

- CT scan is the current imaging study of choice.

- Many signs and symptoms (vomiting, headache, behavioral changes, etc.) may accompany a head injury, but they are not pathognomonic for intracranial injury.

- Researchers have derived decision rules to help physicians identify those head-injured children who are at risk of intracranial hemorrhage. The goal is to identify and diagnose patients who have serious head injury, and those who have neurosurgical pathology.

- The CHALICE[15] study is a large, prospective cohort study that derived a highly sensitive clinical decision rule for identifying which children need CT scanning after head injury. The study identified 14 high-risk variables seen in *Table 2*. The study has a sensitivity of 98% and specificity of 87% for predicting clinically significant head injury in children.

- In 2009, PECARN[16] derived and validated a prediction rule in a large multicenter study that aimed to identify children who are at very low risk of clinically important TBI for whom CT is not needed. Two prediction rules were developed: one for children <2 years old (sensitivity 100%, NPV 100%) and one for children >2 years old (sensitivity 97% and NPV 99.9%). The authors concluded that they identified a low-risk population for whom CT scanning is not needed *(Table 3)*.

Table 2. CHALICE Study

*The children's head injury algorithm for the prediction of important clinical events rule**

A CT scan is required if any of the following criteria are present. If none of the variables are present, then the patient is at low risk of intracranial pathology.

History

- Witness LOC >5 min
- History of amnesia (either anterograde or retrograde) >5 min
- Abnormal drowsiness
- ≥ 3 vomits after head injury
- Suspicion of non-accidental injury
- Seizure after head injury in a patient with no history of epilepsy

Examination

- GCS <14, or GCS <15 if <1 year old
- Suspicion of penetrating or depressed skull injury or tense fontanel
- Signs of basilar skull fracture
- Positive focal neurology (defined as any focal neurology, including motor, sensory, coordination, or reflex abnormality)
- Presence of bruise, swelling, or laceration >5 cm if <1 year old

Mechanism

- High-speed accident as pedestrian, cyclist, or occupant (speed >40 mph)
- Fall >3 meters (9 ft)
- High-speed injury from a projective or an object

*Dunning J, Patrick Daly J, Lomas JP, et al: Derivation of the children's head injury algorithm for the prediction of important clinical events decision rule for head injury in children. *Arch Dis Child* 91: 885, 2006.

Table 3. Pediatric Emergency Care Applied Research Network (PECARN) Low-Risk Criteria for Infants and Children with Minor Head Injury*

Children <2 years old
• Normal mental status
• No scalp hematoma except frontal
• LOC <5 seconds
• Non-severe mechanism*
• No palpable skull fracture
• Normal behavior per parents

Children >2 years old
• Normal mental status
• No LOC
• No vomiting
• Non-severe mechanism
• No sign of basilar skull fracture
• No severe headache

*Severe mechanism: motor vehicle collision with ejection, rollover, or death of passenger; pedestrian or bicyclist without helmet struck by motorized vehicle; fall >3 ft (age <2 yrs) or >5 ft (age >2 yrs); head struck by high-impact object.

*Kupperman N, Holmes JF, Dayan PS, et al: Identification of children at very low risk of clinically-important brain injuries after head trauma: a prospective cohort study. *Lancet* 374 (9696): 1160, 2009.

Treatment

- Supplemental O2 to prevent hypoxemia
- Airway protection with orotracheal intubation
- C-spine immobilization
- RSI induction with etomidate or propofol; paralysis with succinylcholine or rocuronium; atropine only if symptomatic bradycardia occurs
- Appropriate neurosurgical involvement
- IVF resuscitation with NS or LR
- Target ventilation to $PaCO_2$ 35-40 mmHg and O2 sat >95%
- Hyperventilation ($PaCO_2$ 30-35 mmHg) only as a temporizing measure to reduce elevated ICP (level 3 recommendation)
- Mannitol 0.25-1 mg/kg to reduce ICP (hypotension may result)

- Hypertonic saline 3% or higher may be used for hyperosmolar therapy to reduce ICP; also has management potential for hypotension; may cause central pontine myelinolysis.
- Ventriculostomy for elevated ICP or signs of herniation
- Sedation decreases ICP and helps optimize cerebral perfusion pressure.
- Phenytoin or fosphenytoin has been shown to be helpful in preventing early post-traumatic seizures (<1 week), but not late post-traumatic seizures.[17]

Disposition

- Asymptomatic, low-risk infants and children who are at least 2-4 hours post-injury can be safely discharged without imaging. Careful instructions and return precautions (lethargy, irritability, focal deficits, and vomiting) should be thoroughly discussed with reliable caregivers.[18]
- Children <2 years old and thought to be at intermediate risk should be observed for 4-6 hours, or a head CT should be performed. If the patient remains stable or improves, the child may be safely discharged to reliable caregivers with primary care follow up.
- A patient with a normal head CT and normal neurologic assessment after minor head trauma may be safely discharged to a competent caregiver.
- Head-injured children at moderate to high risk should be admitted.[18]

Review Questions

1. Which is the most commonly fractured skull bone?
    A. Frontal
    B. Parietal
    C. Temporal
    D. Occipital

2. The American Academy of Neurology recommends an athlete may return to play if he/she has a normal neurologic evaluation and:
    A. Concussive symptoms are improving
    B. After one week of rest
    C. A normal CT scan
    D. Concussive symptoms have resolved

3. All of the following tests should be ordered to rule out non-accidental head injury EXCEPT:

   A. CT and/or MRI
   B. Skeletal survey
   C. Skull radiographs
   D. Ophthalmologic evaluation
   E. Coagulation studies

4. Which of the following is a true statement about identifying risk of intracranial injury in minor head-injured children?

   A. The same criteria should be used for children <2 years as older children.
   B. Location and size of a scalp hematoma doesn't indicate risk of underlying head injury.
   C. According to PECARN, children with altered mental status and/or skull fractures are at high risk of traumatic brain injury.
   D. According to the CHALICE study, if a child has only one of the variables, then no CT scan is necessary.

5. Which of the following treatment measures is appropriate when stabilizing a head-injured child?

   A. Target the ventilation to PaCO2 35-40 mmHg.
   B. No supplemental oxygen is needed unless patient is hypoxemic.
   C. If RSI is indicated, then atropine is also indicated for pretreatment.
   D. Mannitol is a good choice for lowering ICP in a hypotensive patient.
   E. Phenytoin has been shown to prevent early and late post-traumatic seizures.

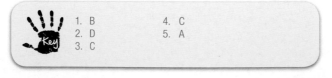

1. B		4. C	
2. D		5. A	
3. C			

Blunt Abdominal Trauma

Josh Ennis, MD

Critical Knowledge

- **Have a high index of suspicion for internal injury.**
- Children with no outward signs of injury may have serious intra-abdominal pathology.
- Half of children with blunt intestinal injuries have no peritoneal signs.
- ABCs, IV, O2, monitor
- **Establish IV access quickly.** An intraosseous line is indicated if access can't be established after two tries or 60 seconds (medial proximal tibia, distal femur, proximal humerus).
- Administer two 20-ml/kg boluses, repeat once more and/or give blood products if continued hypotension or tachycardia.
- Perform abdominal exam, plain films, and FAST as soon as possible, and then determine the next branch point.
  - ▶ **Observation and serial exams:** stable patient with benign exam
  - ▶ **CT scan:** stable patient with questionable exam, severe mechanism, or continued high index of suspicion
  - ▶ **Immediate surgical intervention:** positive FAST with or without Cullen's sign (periumbilical ecchymosis) or Grey Turner's sign (flank ecchymosis), free air, or unstable patient

FAST Exam Pearls

- Positioning: patient supine or Trendelenburg, threshold of 300-500 mL free fluid (extrapolated from adult data)
- Sensitivity improves with experience (i.e., >100 exams, can diagnose smaller volumes)
- In *pediatric* population with blunt abdominal trauma:
  - ▶ **Poor sensitivity** 65-80%
  - ▶ **High specificity** >95-98%
- FAST exam screens for intraperitoneal fluid. It can also detect intrathoracic fluid if included in the study (i.e., evaluating the costophrenic angle). It does NOT diagnose injury.

- **PEARL**
  - ▶ Can develop greater volume of free fluid over time. Consider repeat FAST exam if clinically indicated (especially in patients not undergoing CT).
- **LIMITATIONS**
  - ▶ Injuries not causing free fluid (i.e., hollow viscus injuries)
  - ▶ Injuries causing free intraperitoneal fluid in volumes less than detected by FAST exam
  - ▶ Retroperitoneal injuries: ureteral, pancreatic, duodenal, IVC/aorta, pelvic
  - ▶ Pelvis view: empty bladder, bowel gas scatter, extraperitoneal pelvic fluid accumulation

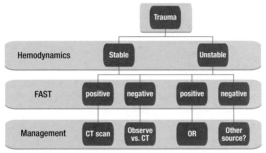

Decision for Further Imaging

- A recent prospective, multicenter, observational cohort consisting of the Pediatric Emergency Care Applied Research Network (PECARN), derived a 7-point clinical prediction rule to aid in identifying children at very low risk of intra-abdominal injury requiring acute intervention after blunt abdominal trauma.
- This consisted of seven history and physical exam criteria with a sensitivity of 97%.
- Of those injuries not captured by the prediction rule, clinicians identified all but one requiring acute intervention.
- Patient characteristics of those missed by the prediction rule presumably would have been identified by positive FAST, hematuria, lab abnormalities, or clinical suspicion on account of painful/distracting injury, intoxication, or gestalt.

- Of all abdominal CT exams performed, 23% were in this very low-risk population. Although this study awaits external validation, this rule suggests potential for substantial reduction in number of unnecessary abdominal CT scans by providing evidence to aid clinical decision-making.

Figure 5. Clinical Risk Stratification of Children with Blunt Torso Trauma

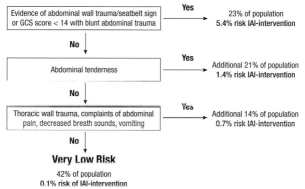

Reprinted from *Annals of Emerg Med*, EPub, Holmes J et al. "Identifying Children at Very Low Risk of Clinically Important Blunt Abdominal Injuries." ©2012, with permission from lead author, Elsevier, and *Annals of Emergency Medicine*.

Epidemiology/Anatomy

- Trauma is the leading cause of morbidity and mortality in the pediatric population.
- Following head and extremities, abdomen is third most commonly injured region.
- Abdomen is the most common fatal traumatic injury that goes initially unrecognized.
- Anatomical differences in children make them more vulnerable to major abdominal injuries with very minor forces. In children, the abdomen begins at the level of the nipple. Children's small, pliable rib cages and undeveloped abdominal muscles provide little protection of major organs. Solid organs (e.g., spleen, liver, kidneys) are vulnerable to injury.

Differential/Critical Concepts

- **Abdominal wall bruising:** Bruising of the abdominal wall after motor vehicle collision is an important finding. The sensitivity and specificity for a significant intra-abdominal injury are 73.5% and 98.8%, respectively. About 1 in 9 children with abdominal wall bruising will be diagnosed with a significant intra-abdominal injury.

- **Stomach injuries:** Blunt injuries to the stomach occur more frequently in children than in adults. The injury is usually a blowout or perforation of the greater curvature. Children who are struck by a vehicle or who fall across bicycle handlebars shortly after eating a meal are at greater risk. Consider injury to the stomach if the child has peritoneal signs and/or bloody nasogastric drainage. Abdominal x-ray films may show pneumoperitoneum.

- **Small intestinal injury:** The most common intra-abdominal organ injured in restrained children involved in MVCs. Rapid deceleration may cause the lap belt to compress the intestines against the spine. An increase in intraluminal pressure may lead to rupture or tear. Duodenal injuries are rare; a coiled spring appearance on contrasted CT is suggestive. Occurs in the areas of fixation at the Treitz ligament or at the ileocecal valve. Up to 50% of children with lap seat belt injuries have associated retroperitoneal injuries. Flexion-distraction lumbar spine injury may also occur. **Beware: It is common for these to present as a delayed finding in children** (24-48 hours post trauma).

- **Rectal injuries:** Except for the occasional straddle injury, child abuse or sexual activity causes most isolated rectal injuries in children.

- **Splenic injuries:** Relatively common in pediatric trauma. After CT categorization of injury, most patients with splenic injuries respond to nonoperative management.

- **Hepatic injury:** Most are managed nonoperatively, after CT classification and surgical consultation. The exception, of course, is children with massive hepatic injuries or with perihepatic vascular involvement who are not hemodynamically stable and have transfusion requirements of greater than 25-40 mL/kg/d.

- **Pancreatic injury:** Blunt trauma causes most pancreatic injuries. A frequently cited mechanism involves falling into bicycle handlebars. CT scanning is a useful diagnostic modality in evaluating most pancreatic trauma. Operative exploration or ERCP may be needed to diagnose and treat ductal injury. Amylase and lipase are neither sensitive nor specific in the diagnosis of pancreatic injury, however, a high level of either is suggestive.

- **Renal injury:** Blunt abdominal trauma involves renal injury in 10%-20% of cases. The pediatric kidney is more susceptible to blunt injury due to the relative lack of perirenal fat and decreased protection from incompletely ossified ribs. Contusion is the most common renal injury encountered in children. Conservative management is standard for low-grade renal injury (grades I-III), including bed rest for 24 hours, serial hematocrit, heart rate monitoring, and frequent physical examinations. Management of high-grade renal injury is more controversial (grades IV-V). Absolute indications for renal exploration are an expanding or pulsatile renal hematoma. Relative indications include urinary extravasation, nonviable tissue, arterial injury, and the need for complete staging. The presence or absence of hematuria and the amount thereof do not correlate with the severity of renal injury. There are reports of successful nonoperative management of grade IV injuries. All grade V injuries required operative management, and only 30% achieve long-term renal salvage.

- **Diaphragmatic injury/thoracic injury:** Mechanisms significant enough to cause intra-abdominal injury may also cause concomitant intrathoracic injury and/or rarely diaphragmatic injury. The astute clinician must be cognizant of these entities. FAST exam may reveal hemothorax at the costophrenic angle. Chest radiograph may reveal abdominal contents within the thorax.

Treatment

- **Solid organ injury management:** Nonoperative management is considered the standard of care for most children with blunt solid organ injury who are clinically stable. This is successful in more than 95% of appropriately selected cases. A five-year, multi-institutional review of 1,818 pediatric patients who sustained splenic, hepatic, pancreatic, or renal trauma found a nonoperative management failure rate of 5%. The reasons for failure were shock, peritonitis, persistent hemorrhage, pancreatic injury, hollow viscus injury, and ruptured diaphragm. Overall mortality for this cohort was 0.8%, with those patients in the failure group. Time to failure was 59% by 4 hours and 87% by 24 hours. A significantly increased risk of failure was associated with bicycle-related mechanism of injury, isolated pancreatic injury, and isolated grade V injury. Multiple solid organ injuries were associated with a higher risk of failure, as well. The data emphasize the importance of early vigilance in the care of the child with a solid organ injury.

Those who will fail nonoperative management will likely do so early, within the first 12 hours. Pancreatic injuries do not behave as other solid organ injuries and are associated with a higher need for operative intervention. For isolated liver or spleen injury, current recommendations are based on CT grade of injury. **Grade I:** no ICU stay, 2 total hospital days, and 3 weeks activity restriction. **Grade II:** no ICU stay, 3 total hospital days, and 4 weeks activity restriction. **Grade III:** no ICU stay, 4 total hospital days, and 5 weeks activity restriction. **Grade IV:** 1 day of ICU stay, 5 total hospital days, and 6 weeks of activity restriction. These guidelines have been prospectively evaluated and demonstrate significant reduction in length of stay without adverse sequelae.

- **Management of hollow viscus injuries:** These injuries are often missed on the initial assessment of children involved in blunt trauma. Have a high index of suspicion, especially if there is a significant mechanism. If there is any question after serial exams and labs, obtain a surgical consult.

Review Questions

1. Can a FAST exam reliably rule out solid organ injury in pediatric patients?
2. Is abdominal wall bruising sensitive for intra-abdominal injury in pediatric patients?
3. What is the most frequently missed injury in children with blunt abdominal trauma?
4. Is CT sensitive for hollow viscus injury in children?
5. When should an intraosseous line be considered?

1. No
2. Yes
3. Hollow viscus
4. No
5. After two peripheral attempts and/or 60 seconds

Orthopedic Trauma

Drew Watters, MD

Introduction
Critical Knowledge

- Understand the differences that age imparts on anatomy, physiology, and pathology.
- Preverbal children cannot describe the bones that are injured.
- In general, children will not use an injured limb. Look for a limb that the child does not move, or "self-splints" by holding.
- Look for overlying signs associated with fractures. Fully move all joints to ensure there are no dislocations or areas of tenderness. Be sure to assess femurs and pelvis, as these fractures may be rapidly life-threatening.
- Treat pain appropriately; it is appropriate to use narcotics.

Background and Anatomy

- Pediatric orthopedic injuries are commonly seen in urgent care centers, emergency departments, and outpatient clinics.
- Children have relatively more pliability, which means a lot more damage can be done to soft tissue without associated fracture.
- Children have growth plates and ossification centers that fuse as they age, and their smaller muscle mass can increase risks for ligament injuries and dislocations.
- Pliable bones lead to different fractures than those seen in adults.
- Pain is often poorly addressed in children. Narcotics are but one tool physicians may use to alleviate pain.

Differential Diagnosis

- Contusion
- Sprain
- Hematoma
- Ligamentous injury
- Dislocation
- Fracture
- Non-traumatic injury/metabolic disease (see Chapter 9)

Critical Concepts
Open vs. Closed Fractures
- One must immediately determine if a fracture is open in order to quickly treat it with irrigation, antibiotics, and orthopedic consultation.

Referred Pain
- Pain may be felt away from the site of injury, especially in children with limited verbal skills. Complaint of knee pain may stem from hip injury, and vice versa. Shoulder pain can be due to underlying spleen or liver injuries.

Nonorthopedic (False) Pain
- Medical illnesses can present with apparent inability to ambulate – pain in an extremity that leads to non-use. Examples include nutritional deficiencies, myofascial sources of pain, or inflammatory diseases.

Injury Type
- A good history of the mechanism can make the differential diagnosis much smaller. For example, a fall onto an outstretched hand ("FOOSH") can cause scaphoid, radius, or supracondylar fractures, or elbow dislocations.
- Falls with a twisting motion may cause spiral fractures. A fall onto a bent elbow can cause an olecranon fracture.
- Being tackled from the side can cause the "unhappy triad" of ACL, medial meniscus, and MCL tears.
- Fractures in athletes, especially runners, are often due to chronic, repetitive stress. Consider imaging for repetitive stress, even without acute significant mechanism.

Treatment
- Pain is poorly addressed in pediatric trauma and fractures.
- Treatment will vary by injury, but should always include pain control.
- Pain control includes splinting, ice, comfort measures, and medications.
- Ibuprofen is first line in simple, uncomplicated fractures (e.g., nondisplaced radius buckle fracture). Its efficacy is equivalent to acetaminophen, codeine, or oxycodone with fewer adverse effects.
- Acetaminophen is an acceptable alternative and provides similar pain relief.
- Short-term (less than one week) NSAIDS do NOT impair healing.
- Narcotics should be used for major fractures, or if pain is unimproved with NSAIDs.

- Splinting should immobilize the joint above and below the injury.
- Splints must be checked after placement to ensure adequacy and appropriate fit.
- Disposition planning should include consideration of:
  - The child's safety
  - The need for a wheelchair, crutches, assistance, and limitations
  - A follow-up plan to see an orthopedist or PCP, if necessary
  - Instructions to return with worsening signs or symptoms
  - Instructions on fracture care at home
- Serious injuries or multiple injuries may warrant admission for observation.

Nursemald's Elbow

Critical Concepts
- A subluxation of the radial head under the annular ligament
- Often mistaken for a true fracture
- Classically caused by pulling or lifting a toddler by an outstretched hand
- Usually presents with a child unwilling to use the affected arm

Diagnosis
- Anxiety is often greater than pain.
- Arm is held in 15-20 degrees of flexion, often supported by the other arm.
- Bruising, redness, or signs of trauma are absent.

Treatment
- Easily treated without radiographs, if there is no concern for coexisting injury.
- Reduced by hyperpronation of the hand, followed by extension and then flexion at the elbow (hyperpronate, extend, then flex all the way; all in one smooth motion). The thumb of one hand can be placed on the radial head to palpate and guide the reduction.
- Hyperpronation vs. supination: (95% vs. 77% reduction on first attempt)
  - If two tries fail, attempt the other technique.
- If unable to reduce the dislocation after 2-3 attempts, x-rays should be obtained.
- Families should be counseled that recurrence is common, and educated to avoid axial traction.

Dislocations
Critical Concepts
- Separation of a bone from the joint in which it normally rests
- May be associated with fractures or neurovascular injuries
- May include ligament or tendon damage
- Require manipulation and reduction to restore function
- If unreduced, may cause permanent injury to joint, nerves, and bones
- Always assess nerve and vascular function before and after reduction.

Diagnosis
- Differential includes ligamentous injury, muscle injury, or fracture.
- Abnormal contours of the joint may be seen or felt.
- Extremity may be rotated, of irregular length, or nonfunctional.
- Range of motion will by limited due to joint disruption.
- Radiographs are warranted to evaluate for associated fractures.
- Assess nerve and vascular function to ensure no compromise.

Treatment
- After initial assessment, pain should be managed, and muscle relaxers may aid reduction. Successful reduction may require sedation.
- Specific reduction varies by affected joint, and there are myriad techniques.
- Reduction often requires a large force, but avoid sudden motions that may cause injury.
- In general, the joint should be realigned with gentle traction, rotating the joint to free the dislocated bone from entrapment.
- After reduction, the joint should be splinted or placed in a sling.
- Obtain post-reduction x-rays to ensure reduction and reassess for fractures.
- Reassess the extremity for neurovascular function after splinting.

Fractures
Critical Concepts
- Generally the result of trauma, and are often associated with other injuries
- If one fracture is found, assess for others.
- Combination fractures of note include:
    - Lumbar fractures associated with calcaneous fractures

- ► Maisonneuve fracture (medial malleolus fracture with a proximal tibial fracture)
- ► Lisfranc fractures (fracture and dislocation of the midfoot)
- If history is unusual for injury, raises concern for underlying pathology or abuse
  - ► Consider bone cysts, cancer, or osteogenesis imperfect.
  - ► Assess safety of child and report if there is concern for abuse.
- Fractures may be of varying severity, with little or no radiographic evidence.

Diagnosis

- Conduct physical exam to localize areas of injury and look for coexistent injuries.
- Generally, x-rays are needed for complete diagnosis
- X-ray may show obvious deformity, cortical irregularities, or irregularity in comparison of growth plates.
- Subtle findings may include a prominent fat pad. Articular injury can cause lucency between the cortex and surrounding soft tissue; therefore, any obvious lucency along the cortex should be concerning for occult fracture.
- Pediatric fractures may have unique patterns (see *Figure 1*).
  - ► **Torus:** buckling of the cortex
  - ► **Greenstick:** bending of the bone with unilateral cortex irregularity
  - ► **Plastic deformities:** bending of the bone with no cortical irregularities

Figure 1. Pediatric Fracture Patterns

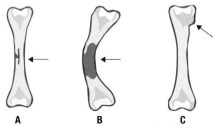

A　　　　**B**　　　　**C**

A. **Greenstick fracture** – arrow demonstrates the direction of force causing the fracture.
   (Note the fracture line opposite to the side of force along with a vertical fracture component.)

B. **Plastic deformity** – arrow demonstrates the direction of force causing the fracture.

C. **Torus fracture** – arrow demonstrates the buckle deformity in the bony cortex.

Treatment

- Femur and pelvic fractures must be diagnosed and treated emergently, as they can cause significant blood loss and shock.
- Pain should be treated appropriately.
- Fractures should be elevated, splinted, and cooled as quickly as possible for stability and pain control.
- Reduction and splinting should be done as indicated, once definitive diagnosis is made.

Pelvic Fracture

Critical Concepts

- Often the result of large forces, and can be fatal
- Often associated with other orthopedic and intra-abdominal injuries
- May be unstable and require immediate treatment

Diagnosis

- Portable x-rays should be obtained immediately if there is concern for fracture.
- Be sure to fully palpate and stress the pelvis.
- Place your hands on the lateral pelvic wall and compress; press also on the pubic symphysis.
- Any instability or deformity requires emergent evaluation and care.
- If fracture is found, CT of the abdomen/pelvis is indicated to rule out additional bleeding or injuries.
- If the patient is unstable, emergent evaluation by surgery and interventional radiology (if available) is indicated.

Treatment

- IV access, pain control, and fluid resuscitation should be initiated.
- If instability is felt during primary exam, a pelvic binder should be placed.
- If a binder is unavailable, a sheet may be folded, placed around the pelvis, and then tied tightly across the anterior pelvis to hold the fracture.
- After binder placement, reassess the pelvis and lower extremities.
- Emergent consultation by orthopedic surgery should be made.
- If patient is unstable or there is active bleeding, interventional radiology may need to perform embolization.

Compartment Syndrome

Critical Concepts

- Neurovascular compromise of tissue due to increasing pressure in a contained space, such as the fascia of an extremity
- Be aware of increasing pain, as it is the first symptom.
- Failure to treat may lead to limb ischemia, nerve damage, and necrosis.

Diagnosis

- Early signs include inordinate pain, or **pain with passive movement** of the associated compartment's muscles (e.g., forearm pain elicited by passive finger flexion). This is the most sensitive clinical finding.
- Late signs include pallor, pulselessness, coldness, and paresthesias. **Do not wait for these signs!**
- The syndrome may be diagnosed by measuring pressures directly in the compartment.
- If there is concern, emergent orthopedic consultation should be obtained.

Treatment

- Elevate and ice the area to reduce swelling and prevent increasing pressure.
- If compartment syndrome is diagnosed, fasciotomy must be performed.
- Incise through the skin and fascia of the affected compartment.

Growth Plate Injuries

Critical Concepts

- Fractures are classified as Salter-Harris (SH) Types I-V (see *Figure 2*) .
  - ▶ **I:** no visible fracture
  - ▶ **II:** fracture through metaphysic only
  - ▶ **III:** fracture through epiphysis only
  - ▶ **IV:** fracture through both meta- and epiphysis
  - ▶ **V:** crush injury in plate
- Growth plate injuries may lead to nonunion healing, unequal extremities, chronic pain, and myositis ossificans (bone formation in surrounding muscle).
- SH Type V is difficult to diagnose, and may have serious sequelae. You must have a high level of suspicion.

- The age of the child affects potential outcome; younger children have higher risk of growth abnormalities.

Figure 2. Salter-Harris (SH) Fracture Types

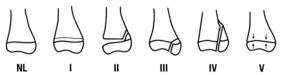

NL: normal physis
Type I SH fracture: fracture through the physis
Type II SH fracture: fracture through the physis and metaphysis
Type III SH fracture: fracture through the physis and epiphysis
Type IV SH fracture: fracture through the physis, metaphysis and epiphysis
Type V SH fracture: crush injury of the physis (arrow demonstrates crush force).

Diagnosis
- Obtain radiographs and assess for evidence and severity of injury.
- Compare the growth plate to the contralateral side.
- Occasionally, CT is required to delineate the extent of injury.

Treatment
- Use ice, elevation, and mild compression. Treat pain accordingly.
- SH Type I and II fractures may often be treated by splinting and orthopedic follow up in 7-10 days.
- SH Types III-V require orthopedic consultation, as they often require surgical fixation.

Spinal Injuries
Critical Concepts
- May be life-threatening, causing respiratory failure, paralysis, or shock
- Spinal cord injury without radiographic abnormality (SCIWORA) is *not* rare.
- Clinical suspicion must be high, especially with neurologic signs or symptoms.
- Younger children have greater pliability and higher risk of SCIWORA.

Diagnosis

- A thorough physical exam is needed to evaluate neurologic function.
- X-rays of the pediatric spine may be useful, but frequently miss serious injuries.
- CT or MRI is warranted if there is a significant clinical concern.
  - ► Long-term radiation risk is greatest under the age of 8, and minimal in older patients.

Treatment

- Initial treatment by EMS or emergency staff should include spinal immobilization.
  - ► May include brace, car seat, foam, or rolled towels.
- Assess and manage the ABCs, with attention to the airway.
- Pain and agitation should be treated appropriately.
- Evidence of injury warrants emergent evaluation by a spinal surgeon.

Review Questions

1. A 16-year-old girl presents after diving into a pool from a 3-meter board; she is complaining of immediate right shoulder pain. She has pain to palpation at the superior, anterior aspect of the shoulder. She cannot abduct the shoulder or range it actively, but it can be (painfully) ranged passively. The best test and most likely diagnosis are:

   A. X-ray and dislocation

   B. X-ray and AC separation

   C. X-ray and fracture

   D. CT and dislocation

   E. CT and fracture

2. A 5-year-old boy presents after a fall with left thigh pain and bruising laterally. X-rays show curvature of the femur with no irregularity of the cortex. The patient ambulates with complaint of pain in the lateral thigh. What is the best next step?

   A. Consult orthopedics.

   B. Place in a posterior leg splint.

   C. If patient is ambulatory, arrange follow up with orthopedics in 3-5 days.

   D. CT the femur.

   E. X-ray the contralateral thigh.

3. A 15-year-old girl is in an MVC and presents intubated and sedated. Primary survey reveals multiple abrasions, contusions, and lacerations. Her pelvis feels stable to examination. She is hypotensive and tachycardic. What is the most appropriate first step?

   A. X-ray pelvis

   B. Ultrasound abdomen and pelvis

   C. Initiate IV fluids

   D. CT abdomen and pelvis

4. A 13-year-old boy fell onto his left elbow and suffered a supracondylar fracture. He has diffuse swelling to the arm and severe pain on palpation. What is the most appropriate initial treatment?

   A. Measure compartment pressures.

   B. Administer lorazepam for pain.

   C. Elevate and ice the arm.

   D. Consult orthopedics.

5. A 7-year-old girl fell 12 ft onto her feet, and now complains of severe pain in the right knee. X-rays of the knee are negative. What is the most appropriate next step?

   A. Place in a posterior splint and follow up with PCP in 7-10 days.

   B. Place in knee immobilizer and follow up with PCP in 7-10 days.

   C. CT of the knee

   D. MRI of the knee

   E. Discharge patient for follow up with orthopedist in 7-10 days.

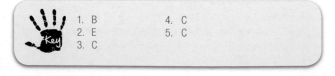

1. B   4. C
2. E   5. C
3. C

Non-Traumatic Orthopedics

Dale P. Woolridge MD, PhD

Osteomyelitis

Critical Knowledge

- Bone infection usually is caused by hematogenous spread.
- S. *aureus* is the most common organism.
- Treatment requires antibiotics and rarely surgery.

Background

- 50% of cases occur in children age 0-5 years.
- Infection occurs in three ways: **1.** Hematogenous spread is most common in children. **2.** Contiguous spread of infection after trauma or surgery is less common. **3.** Infection due to vascular insufficiency is rare in children.
- Any bone may be affected, but the femur and tibia are the most common sites.
- S. *aureus* causes the majority of infections with methicillin-resistant S. *aureus* (MRSA) increasing nationwide. Other organisms include Strep species, Gram negatives and H. *influenzae* (*Table 2*).

Differential Diagnosis/Critical Concepts

- Suspect osteomyelitis in children with fever, malaise, and bone pain. Swelling and point tenderness are often present.
- Differential diagnosis (*Table 1*)
- Workup includes:
  - ▶ Blood culture – positive in 50% of children
  - ▶ CBC – white blood cells normal or elevated
  - ▶ Erythrocyte sedimentation rate (ESR) and C-reactive protein (CRP) is usually increased, although it may be normal, especially in neonates and children with sickle cell disease.
  - ▶ X-rays are often normal for several days after onset of symptoms. Soft tissue swelling may be seen in the first days of illness. Periosteal elevation and bone destruction usually takes 10-21 days to be seen.

- ▶ Bone scan or MRI-bone scan usually shows increased uptake within 48-72 hours of symptoms onset. Advantages of the bone scan include decreased cost, ability to see multiple foci, and no sedation is needed. MRI is preferred if pelvic or vertebral infection is suspected, surgical intervention is necessary, or abscess is suspected.

Treatment

- Orthopedic consultation
- Surgery is rarely needed in cases of osteomyelitis caused by hematogenous spread. Surgery is needed if infection is caused by contiguous spread or infection is not improving on antibiotics.
- Antibiotic treatment
  - ▶ MRSA *not* suspected: Nafcillin or oxacillin **PLUS** cefotaxime or ceftriaxone
  - ▶ MRSA *suspected*: Vancomycin **PLUS** cefotaxime or ceftriaxone

Table 1. Differential Diagnosis for a Limping Child by Age

All Ages	Age 4-10
Septic Arthritis	Legg-Calves-Perthes
Osteomyelitis	Transient synovitis
Cellulitis	Arthritis (JRA, Lyme disease, RF)
Fracture	Neoplasm
Age 1-3	**Age 11-16**
Arthritis (JRA, Lyme disease)	Slipped capital femoral
Developmental dysplasia of the hip	Osgood-Schlatter
Leg-length discrepancy	Arthritis (Lyme disease, SLE, gonococcal)
Foreign body in the foot	

Table 2. Most Common Organisms Causing Septic Arthritis

Age 0-2 Months	Age 2 months to 5 years	Age >5 years
Staph aureus	Staph aureus	Staph aureus
Group B Strep	Strep pyogenes	Strep pyogenes
Gram-negative enterococci	Strep pneumoniae	Neisseria gonorrhoeae
N. gonorrhoeae	Kingella kingae	

Septic Arthritis

Critical Knowledge

- Serious infection of the joint space most commonly is caused by *S. aureus*.
- Can be difficult to distinguish from transient synovitis.
- Requires rapid diagnosis and treatment with antibiotics and often operative drainage.

Background

- Most common in children age 0-3 years.
- Can occur in any joint, but most commonly occurs in knee, hip, and elbow.
- Bacteria invade the joint most often by hematogenous spread, but can also occur by direct extension, or from inoculation (arthrocentesis or venipucture).
- Organisms causing septic arthritis vary with the age of the patient. (*Table 2*)
- Before Hib vaccine, *H. influenzae* was a common pathogen.

Differential Diagnosis/Critical Concepts

- Difficult to diagnose; clinical presentation is subtle, especially in younger children.
- Clinical manifestations include fever, malaise, guarding of a limb, limp, erythema, swelling, warmth, and pain with passive range of motion.
- Differential diagnosis (*Table 1*)
- Workup includes x-ray, CBC, erythrocyte sedimentation rate (ESR), blood cultures, ultrasound, arthrocentesis.
- If *N. gonorrhoeae* is suspected, cultures of blood, joint fluid, pharynx, cervix, and rectum should be obtained.
- Differentiating septic arthritis from transient synovitis (*Table 3*).
- Radiologic imaging
  - ▶ X-rays may show increase in joint space or bulging of soft tissue.
    - Not sensitive for detection of septic arthritis
    - Used to rule out trauma, Legg-Calves-Perthes, slipped capital femoral epiphysis, Osgood Schlatter, or malignancy
  - ▶ Ultrasound is used to diagnose joint effusion and guide needle aspiration.

- Arthrocentesis is the most important diagnostic tool.
- Fluid analysis suggestive of septic arthritis:
  - **Cell count:** >50,000/mm^3 with >80% neutrophils
  - **Gram stain:** diagnostic for infection (Negative Gram stain does not rule out septic arthritis.)
  - **Glucose:** decreased to 30% of serum
  - **Culture:** can be negative in 1/3 of patients with septic arthritis

Treatment

- Antibiotic treatment
  - Base antibiotic choice on Gram stain results if available.
  - If Gram stain results are not available, antibiotic choice is the same as osteomyelitis recommendations.
- Surgical therapy
  - Obtain prompt orthopedic consult.
  - Joint must be adequately drained in order for infection to improve.

Transient Synovitis

Critical Knowledge

- Most common cause of acute hip pain in children ages 3-10
- Uncertain etiology; thought to be related to recent viral illness
- Diagnosis of exclusion

Background

- Benign self-limited condition believed to be related to recent viral illness
- Most common cause of acute hip pain in children ages 3-10
- Male predominance
- Usually unilateral pain involving the hip and occasionally, the knee.

Differential Diagnosis/Critical Concepts

- A diagnosis of exclusion easily confused with septic arthritis
- Clinical manifestations include afebrile or low-grade fever, guarding, refusal to internally rotate or bear weight on affected limb, pain with passive range of motion

- Workup focuses on excluding other causes and includes x-ray, CBC, sedation rate, blood cultures, ultrasound, possibly arthrocentesis. (See differential diagnosis in *Table 2.*)

Evaluation

- X-ray
  - ▶ Normal or may show joint effusion
  - ▶ Used primarily to rule out other causes for joint pain
- Ultrasound
  - ▶ More accurate than x-ray for detecting effusion
  - ▶ Joint effusion seen in 60%-70% of children with transient synovitis, but is not specific
  - ▶ Used to guide aspiration and rule out septic arthritis
- Arthrocentesis
- Should be performed if child has ultrasound evidence of effusion and any one predictor for septic arthritis (*Table 3*).

Treatment

- Supportive care
- NSAIDS
- Close follow up with re-evaluation by primary care provider within 24 hours

Table 3. Differentiating Septic Arthritis from Transient Synovitis

Predictors of Septic Arthritis	Predicted Probability of Septic Arthritis
History of fever	**0 predictors** = 0.1% probability septic arthritis
Non-weight bearing	**1 predictor** = 2.1%-5.3% probability septic arthritis
Sedation rate >40 mm/h	**2 predictors** = 33.8%-62.2% probability septic arthritis
Serum WBC >12,000/mm^3	**3 predictors** = 93%-95.2% probability septic arthritis
	4 predictors = 99.8% probability septic arthritis

Kocher et al., Differentiating Between Septic Arthritis and Transient Synovitis of the Hip in Children: An Evidence Based Clinical Prediction Algorithm. *The Journal of Bone and Joint Surgery* 1999 81: 1662-70.

Slipped Capital Femoral Epiphysis

Critical Knowledge

- Displacement of the femoral head on the femoral neck caused by growth disturbance of the proximal femoral growth plate.
- Should be suspected in an obese adolescent child who complains of hip, thigh, or knee pain.
- Prompt recognition and orthopedic consult are necessary in order to prevent further slipping, which can lead to permanent deformity and arthritis.

Background

- Most common in overweight adolescents during growth spurt (girls age 10-14, boys age 12-15).
- Occurs bilaterally in 25% of children with SCFE.
- Acute slips occur when traumatic force displaces the femoral head; accounts for 25% of cases.
- Chronic slips occur when no trauma is identified and are thought to be caused by genetics, hormones, and increased shear forces.

Differential Diagnosis/Critical Concepts

- Acute slips present with a painful hip held in external rotation and decreased range of motion.
- Chronic slips are harder to diagnose. Patients can present with vague complaints including hip, groin, or knee pain often associated with exercise. External rotation of the hip with flexion is highly suspicious for SCFE.

Diagnosis

- **X-ray:** need AP view of pelvis and frog-leg of the affected hip. Earliest finding on x-ray is widening of the growth plate. On AP look for Klein's line. Draw a line along the border of femoral neck. On normal hip, line intersects a portion of the femoral head. In SCFE, femoral head is below the line. On frog-leg view, femoral head is medial and posterior to the femoral neck.

Treatment

- Non-weight bearing
- Urgent orthopedic referral; pinning in-situ is the treatment of choice.
- If left untreated, slipping continues and results in deformity, arthritis, and avascular necrosis.

Osgood-Schlatter Disease

Critical Knowledge

- A benign knee condition thought to be caused during periods of rapid growth, which consists of pain and edema of the tibial tubercle occurring in adolescents.

- Treatment includes limiting activities that are pain-provoking, and taking NSAIDS. Contraction of the quadriceps causes repetitive stress on the patellar tendon, which is transmitted to tibial tubercle causing micro avulsions and inflammation of the tubercle.

- Occurs most often in athletic adolescents (girls age 10-12) and (boys age 12-14) undergoing rapid growth.

Differential Diagnosis/Critical Concepts

- Usually presents as chronic intermittent knee pain. Pain is worse with activity, especially jumping, running, and squatting; and improved with rest.

- On physical exam, soft-tissue edema and tenderness of the tibial tubercle are present. Pain is reproduced by extension against resistance. Knee exam is otherwise normal with full range of motion.

- Diagnosis is primarily clinical. Lab tests are not needed unless there is concern for other diagnosis. X-rays are recommended to rule out other etiologies. X-rays may be normal or show prominence or calcification of the tibial tuberosity.

Treatment

- Avoid activities that cause pain, especially jumping and running, until pain has been gone for 2-4 months.

- NSAIDS

- Rest, ice, compression, elevation

- Once pain has subsided, exercises that strengthen hamstrings and increase quadricep flexibility may help prevent recurrence.

- If symptoms do not improve with conservative treatment, patient should follow up with orthopedics. Surgery is rarely indicated.

Legg-Calves-Perthes Disease

Critical Knowledge

- Idiopathic osteonecrosis of the femoral head
- Suspect Legg-Calves-Perthes disease (LCPD) in children 3-12 years old presenting with insidious onset of limp, hip, and/or knee pain.
- Children with LCPD should be made non weight-bearing and referred to orthopedist.

Background

- Osteonecrosis of the capital femoral epiphysis is thought to be caused by vascular occlusion of the femoral head, which makes it more vulnerable to subchondral fracture. Ischemia, infarction, and eventual necrosis ensue.
- Occurs most often in boys (5:1 male predominance) age 4-8 years old.
- Seen bilaterally in 10% of children.

Differential Diagnosis/Critical Concepts

- Usually presents with painless limp or intermittent hip and knee pain lasting weeks to months.
- Physical exam reveals decreased range of motion with internal rotation and abduction and atrophy of thigh musculature. Positive roll test is elicited when examiner invokes guarding, or muscle spasm with internal rotation. Leg-length discrepancy is seen in severe disease and suggests total collapse of femoral head.
- Diagnosis includes exclusion of infectious etiologies with CBC, sed rate, CRP, and occasional arthrocentesis.
- Plain radiographs can establish diagnosis, but are often normal early in disease process. Five radiographic stages can be seen on x-ray: **1.** cessation of growth – smaller femoral head epiphysis; **2.** subchondral fracture – linear lucency in femoral head epiphysis; **3.** resorption of bone; **4.** re-ossification of new bone; **5.** healed
- More severe course is expected if >50% of femoral head is involved.
- Bone scan and MRI are useful for early diagnosis of LCPD.

Treatment

- Goal of treatment includes eliminating hip irritability, restoring normal range of motion, containment of femoral head within acetabulum, and maintaining round femoral head.

- Refer child to orthopedist.
- Nonoperative treatment includes physical therapy, crutches, and abduction bracing.
- Surgery is reserved for severe disease.
- Complications of LCPD include femoral head deformity and degenerative joint disease.

Other Causes for Limping in Children

Critical Knowledge

There are several other conditions that can present with limping and joint pain in children. These include, but are not limited to, rheumatic fever (RF), juvenile rheumatoid arthritis (JRA), systemic lupus erythematous (SLE), Lyme disease, and neoplasm.

It is important to have a broad differential, so as not to miss a critical diagnosis.

Background

- RF is a complication from untreated *streptococcal* infection that causes damage to connective tissue of heart, joints, and blood vessels. Morbidity related to cardiac and neurologic complications. Common in school-age children.
- JRA is an autoimmune disease that can cause inflammatory arthritis and is most common in girls age 4-10 years
- SLE involves generation of autoantibodies, which leads to inflammation of microvasculature and multiorgan system involvement. Most common in females of childbearing age.
- Lyme disease is caused by the spirochete, *Borrelia burgdorferi,* which is transmitted by Ixodes ticks and found predominantly in the northeastern United States. Most commonly seen in children 5-9 years old, but can occur at any age.
- Common musculoskeletal tumors in children include rhabdomyosarcoma, osteosarcoma, and Ewing's sarcoma. Rhabdomyosarcoma is most common in children less than 10 years old. Osteosarcoma is most common during adolescence, while Ewing's sarcoma is most common in children 10-20 years old.

Differential Diagnosis/Critical Knowledge

- Joint involvement in RF occurs early in the disease. Symptoms range from mild arthralgia to migratory arthritis with redness, swelling, and extreme pain. Usually associated with fever. Diagnosis based on Jones criteria. No specific confirmatory lab, but a positive *Streptococcal* antibody test helps support the diagnosis. Synovial fluid may have elevated WBC but no organisms.

- JRA presents with acute or insidious joint pain in one or more joints. Intermittent fevers and evanescent rash accompany systemic JRA. Diagnosis depends on clinical findings of arthritis in one or more joints for greater than 6 weeks with other causes excluded. ESR is usually elevated. CBC can reveal lymphopenia and occasional thrombocytopenia. ANA and rheumatoid factor positive, 25% and 20% respectively.

- Acute lymphocytic leukemia often presents with arthritis and can be difficult to distinguish from JRA. The presence of lymphocytosis and neutropenia and thrombocytopenia raises suspicion for leukemia.

- SLE presents most commonly with arthralgia, myalgias, and arthritis. Small joints of hands, wrists, and knees are often involved. Other complaints include fever, malaise, malar rash, renal disease, and many other multisystem complaints. Diagnosis based on a series of clinical and laboratory findings. Screening labs should include CBC, BMP, UA, ANA, anti-dsDNA.

- Suspect Lyme disease in a child who has acute arthritis and has been in an endemic area. Arthritis usually begins as a migratory polyarthritis that develops into monoarticular process involving the knee or ankle. Without treatment, episodes last approximately 1 week and can recur. Chronic arthritis develops in 10% of patients. Lyme disease can affect multiple organ systems. Diagnosis includes an antibody titer and a confirmatory Western blot test.

- Rhabdomyosarcoma should be suspected in a child with painless soft-tissue mass at any site. Osteosarcoma and Ewing's sarcoma most often present with pain or swelling in a bone or joint. Workup for a suspected bone tumor should include x-ray, CBC, ESR, CRP, alkaline phosphatase, electrolytes, and joint aspiration. Children need immediate referral to orthopedics and oncology.

Treatment

- RF prevented by early antibiotic treatment of *Strep* infections. Once diagnosed, give NSAIDS to decrease inflammation and appropriate referral to rheumatology, cardiology, or neurology.

- Treatment of JRA includes referral to rheumatologist. Drug regimens can include NSAIDS, methotrexate, etanercept, and steroids.

- Treatment of SLE involves specialty referrals, NSAIDS, and immunosuppressive drugs. Fever necessitates inpatient admission.

- Antibiotic treatment is recommended for arthritis caused by Lyme disease. Recommended antibiotics include doxycycline for children older than 8 years, and amoxicillin for younger children.

- Treatment for pediatric bone tumors includes a combination of chemotherapy, surgical resection, and radiation.

Review Questions

1. What organism is a common cause of osteomyelitis in children with sickle cell disease?
   A. *Streptococcus species*
   B. *Staphlococcus aureus*
   C. *Staphlococcus epidermidis*
   D. *Salmonella*

2. An 8-month-old male infant presents with increased irritability, low-grade fever and will not move his right leg. No obvious swelling, redness, or warmth is present. X-ray is within normal limits. Laboratory values are as follows WBC = 18,000 mm^3, Sed rate = 50mm/hr, blood culture is pending.
   A. What would be your next step in evaluating this patient?
      a. IV antibiotics/call pediatric consultant for admission
      b. Lumbar puncture
      c. Parenteral antibiotics/next day outpatient follow up
      d. Ultrasound of hip to evaluate for effusion

B. What is the recommended antibiotic treatment for this child?
   a. Ciprofloxacin
   b. Azithromycin + gentamycin
   c. Nafcillin + ceftriaxone
   d. Cephalexin

3. What diagnostic studies should be ordered to differentiate transient synovitis from a septic joint?
   A. CBC, CRP, x-ray
   B. CBC, sedation rate, ultrasound, and possible arthrocentesis
   C. CBC, BMP, MRI
   D. Sedation rate, CRP, bone scan

4. What treatment is recommended for children with transient synovitis?
   A. Supportive care including pain control with NSAIDS and close follow up with pediatrician
   B. Pain control, antibiotics, and close follow up with pediatrician
   C. Casting and outpatient orthopedic referral
   D. Admission with prompt orthopedic referral

5. What is the earliest radiograph change associated with SCFE?
   A. Epiphysis posterior to metaphysic
   B. Widened blurred growth plate
   C. Periosteal proliferation of the epiphysis
   D. Premature fusion of the growth plate

6. Which view is most sensitive for detecting SCFE?
   A. AP
   B. Lateral
   C. Frog leg AP
   D. Frog leg lateral

7. True or false: Osgood-Schlatter can be ruled out clinically if a child presents with bilateral intermittent knee pain?

8. **How long does a child with Osgood-Schlatter disease need to restrict their activity?**
   A. 2-4 weeks
   B. 2-4 weeks after pain is gone
   C. 2-4 months
   D. 2-4 months after pain is gone

9. **Which activities are most likely to cause pain to a patient with Osgood-Schlatter disease?**
   A. Deep knee bends
   B. Descending stairs
   C. Running and jumping
   D. All of the above

10. **Which of the following are associated with poor prognosis following LCPD?**
    A. Age greater than 9 at time of diagnosis
    B. Greater than 50% involvement of the femoral head
    C. Flattened femoral head
    D. All of the above

11. **A 6-year-old boy presents to the emergency department complaining of left hip pain for 3 weeks. Pain is worse with activity and better with rest. Roll sign is positive. A pelvic x-ray is performed, which reveals a subchondral fracture. What is the next step in management of this patient?**
    A. Make non-weight bearing and refer to orthopedist
    B. Inpatient admission
    C. CBC, sedation rate, CRP, blood culture and ultrasound
    D. MRI

12. **A 7-year-old female presents with multiple painful joints. She is otherwise health but does report having sore throat and fever 2 weeks previously. What is the most likely diagnosis?**

Key	1.	B	6.	D
	2a.	D	7.	False
	2b.	C	8.	D
	3.	B	9.	D
	4.	A	10.	D
	5.	B	11.	A
	6.	D	12.	Rheumatic Fever

GI Medical Emergencies

Parisa P. Javedani, MD

Acute Pancreatitis

Critical Knowledge

- Reversible process involving edema, inflammatory cells, necrosis, apoptosis, and hemorrhage.
- Can result in exocrine failure, endocrine failure, or both.
- Incidence is 13.2/100,000 children/year, equating to 11,000 children/year in the U.S.

Epidemiology

- Difficult to estimate true incidence or prevalence.
- Majority of information is based on case reports.

Differential Diagnosis

- Common causes
  - ▶ Gallstones
  - ▶ Medications: valproic acid, L-asparaginase, prednisone, 6-mercaptopurine
  - ▶ Idiopathic
  - ▶ Trauma: MVA, sports injury, falls, abuse
  - ▶ Infectious: mumps, hepatitis A, rotavirus, mycoplasma, adenovirus, coxsackie B4
  - ▶ Metabolic abnormalities: DKA, hypertriglyceridemia, hypercalcemia
  - ▶ Inherited diseases: cystic fibrosis
  - ▶ Toxins: alcohol, venom of some scorpion stings, brown recluse spider, and Gila monster lizard

Symptoms

- Abdominal pain (80%-90% of cases)
- Nausea or vomiting (40%-80% of cases)
- Bilious vomiting
- Ileus

- Abdominal distension
- Less commonly: fever, jaundice, ascites, and pleural effusion

Diagnostic Studies

- Serum lipase is more sensitive and specific than amylase (elevations occur earlier and last longer).
- CBC, electrolytes
- Ultrasound: pancreatic heterogeneity, edema, peripancreatic fluid collection
  - ▶ Helpful in determining if gallstone is the underlying cause
  - ▶ Operator-dependent
- CT is *not* recommended initially, but may be useful several days later if necrosis is suspected.

Management

- Gallstones: endoscopic retrograde cholangiopancreatography, cholecystectomy for patients with cholelithiasis within 2-4 weeks
- Early enteral feeding reduces long-term complications.
- Intravenous fluids
- Pain medication

Complications

- **Early**
  - ▶ Lungs: respiratory distress syndromes, pneumonia, or pulmonary effusions
  - ▶ Renal failure
- **Late**
  - ▶ Pancreatic necrosis or pseudocyst
  - ▶ Recurrent pancreatitis

Gastroesophageal Reflux

Critical Knowledge

- GERD is a common finding in young children.
- Conservative therapies should be attempted first.

Background and Epidemiology

- GERD is caused by:
  ▶ Transient relaxation of the lower esophageal sphincter (LES)
  ▶ Inhibition of peristalsis
- Incidence of childhood GERD is 0.9/1,000 person-years.

Risk Factors

- Immaturity of esophageal and stomach
- Short abdominal esophagus <1 cm
- Increased number of nonpropagated esophageal contractions
- Increased frequency of transient LES relaxation
- Delayed gastric emptying

Symptoms

- Infants
  ▶ Failure to thrive
  ▶ Regurgitation
  ▶ Excessive crying
  ▶ Irritability
  ▶ Arching (Sandifer syndrome)
  ▶ Sleep disturbance
  ▶ Hiccups, sneezing, drooling
  ▶ Respiratory symptoms: cough, wheezing, stridor, apnea
- Children
  ▶ Heartburn
  ▶ Abdominal pain
  ▶ Chest pain (noncardiac)
  ▶ Chronic cough
  ▶ Regurgitation

- ► Nocturnal asthma
- ► Dysphagia
- ► Odynophagia

Differential Diagnosis
- Rule out other potential causes.
  - ► Food allergy
  - ► Pyloric stenosis
  - ► Intestinal obstruction (malrotation with intermittent volvulus)
  - ► Nonesophageal inflammatory disorders
  - ► Infection
  - ► Inborn error of metabolism
  - ► Hydronephrosis
  - ► Increased intracranial pressure
  - ► Rumination
  - ► Bulimia

Diagnostic Studies
- **Upper gastrointestinal study or barium swallow:** rule out pyloric stenosis, intestinal malrotation, duodenal web, vascular ring, hiatal hernia, esophageal stricture.
- **Upper endoscopy and biopsy:** does not exclude esophagitis if normal.
- **Esophageal pH monitoring:** variability of results (type of equipment or probe, placement of probe, patient factors including diet, activity, and position).
- **Radionucleotide scintigraphy with technetium:** rule out aspiration and delayed gastric emptying.
- **Laryngotracheobronchoscopy:** visualize airway abnormalities that may predispose patients to aspiration or findings suggestive of acid reflux-mediated damage.
- **Esophageal manometry:** evaluate for reduced LES tone, frequent transient LES reflux, and abnormalities in esophageal peristalsis.

Treatment of Pediatric GERD

- Start with conservative therapies:
  - ► Prone positioning
  - ► Thickening of infant feeds
  - ► Small volume foods
- If conservative management fails, try pharmacologic management:
  - ► Antacids neutralize or reduce gastric acid.
  - ► H2 receptor antagonists (cimetidine, ranitidine, and famotidine): block H2 receptors of parietal cells to decrease gastric acid secretions
  - ► Proton pump inhibitors (omeprazole) inhibit the H+/K+ ATPase system to suppress gastric acid secretion.
  - ► Prokinetic agents (metoclopramide) inhibit dopamine release, increase LES pressure, and promote gastric emptying.
- If intractable symptoms, consider surgical management:
  - ► Fundoplication: most effective for refractory esophagitis or strictures

Gastroenteritis

Critical Knowledge

- The term "gastroenteritis" only applies to children with nausea, vomiting, AND diarrhea.
- Avoid diagnosing a child who has only nausea and vomiting with gastroenteritis without looking further for a cause of illness.
- Dehydration is the main concern.
- Gastroenteritis is a diagnosis of exclusion in infants under 3 months of age.

Background and Epidemiology

- 75%-90% of gastroenteritis is caused by self-limited viral infections (Norwalk virus, rotavirus, enteric adenovirus), and remainder is largely bacterial, particularly *Escheria coli*.
- Most etiologic agents that cause gastroenteritis are highly contagious via fecal-oral transmission. The major exception is *Staphylococcal* food poisoning.
- Contaminated food (*Shigella*, *Staphylococcus*, Norwalk virus, *Vibrio* species), contaminated water (*Giardia*, *Shigella*, Norwalk virus, *Vibrio* species), and undercooked meat (*Campylobacter jejuni*, *E. coli*, *Salmonella*) are other sources of exposure.

- Regardless of the infectious agent, acute gastroenteritis causes inflammatory changes to the bowel mucosa, which decrease the absorptive capacity of the GI tract. This leads to significant fluid loss in the stool.
- Fasting due to nausea and vomiting worsens the ability of the inflamed bowel to absorb fluid.

Differential Diagnosis

- Viral gastroenteritis is a clinical diagnosis.
  - ▶ Symptoms include nausea, vomiting, watery diarrhea, and fever.
  - ▶ Severe abdominal pain is not typically seen in acute gastroenteritis.
  - ▶ Be sure to evaluate for an acute surgical cause of the patient's symptoms (i.e., appendicitis).
- **Gastrointestinal conditions:** inflammatory bowel disease, intussusception, pseudomembranous enterocolitis, appendicitis, food allergy, lactase deficiency
- **Extraintestinal condition:** *Strep* pharyngitis, bacterial sepsis, otitis media, pneumonia, meningitis, urinary tract infection
- The most common causes of bloody stool (either gross or occult) are *Shigella* and *E. coli* 0157:H7. This is the variant associated with hemolytic uremic syndrome.
- Check immediately for hypoglycemia in a child with altered mental status.

History and Physical

- Consider the following:
  - ▶ Skin turgor: Pinch a small fold of skin at the umbilical level or lateral abdominal wall, release it, and measure how long it takes for skin to return to normal form.
  - ▶ Capillary refill time
  - ▶ Tearing
  - ▶ Fluid intake
  - ▶ Weight *before* illness and *during* illness
  - ▶ Urine output and stool output
  - ▶ Has oral rehydration been attempted?

- Dehydration determination
  - ▶ 5% dehydration if 2↑ of the following: overall ill-appearing, capillary refill time >2 seconds, absent tears, dry mucous membranes
  - ▶ The three best examination signs of dehydration are: abnormal respiratory pattern, abnormal skin turgor, and prolonged capillary refill time.

Laboratory Testing

- Obtaining labs
  - ▶ Recommended only if patient is severely dehydrated (>10%), requiring IV fluids and electrolytes.
  - ▶ Obtain stool cultures if diarrhea >5 days, bloody stool, toxic appearance, or if diagnosing an outbreak.

Treatment

- Rehydration fluids
  - ▶ Goal is early rehydration.
  - ▶ Replace the fluid loss over 4 hours.
  - ▶ Oral rehydration solution (ORS) with sodium:glucose ratio of 1:1; the ratio of sodium, dextrose, and bicarbonate replaces the electrolyte loss.
  - ▶ Clear liquids (water, soda, chicken broth, apple juice) are NOT recommended; hyperosmolarity and lack of potassium, bicarbonate, and sodium can lead to hyponatremia.
  - ▶ Rehydrate with normal saline or lactated Ringer's at a rate of up to 40 mL/kg in the first 1-2 hours. Then convert to oral rehydration or an IV solution containing dextrose.
- Antiemetics
  - ▶ Ondansetron is the only recommended antiemetic in dehydrated children (0.15 mg/kg PO/IV; max 4 mg).
  - ▶ Use the fluid deficit in the first 4 hours.
  - ▶ Do not use antidiarrheal medications if acute gastroenteritis is suspected.

Estimation of Dehydration Severity

	Mild (3%-5%)	Moderate (6%-9%)	Severe (>10%)
Symptoms	Well-appearing, normal vital signs (slightly increased heart rate), normal to slightly decreased urine output	Ill-appearing, tachycardic, tachypneic, normal blood pressure, capillary refill <4 seconds, cool skin, sunken eyes, prolonged skin turgor, decreased tears, tacky mucous membranes, decreased urine output	Toxic-appearing, tachycardic, tachypneic, hypotensive, decreased pulses, capillary refill >4 seconds, mottled skin, absent tears, dry mucous membranes, minimal urine output
Treatment	Goal: restore fluid deficit and maintain hydration. ORS: 50 mEq/L of sodium, 25 g/L of dextrose, and 30 mEq/L of bicarbonate. Replacement at 50 mL/kg; **ADD** 10 mL/kg for every loose stool or episode of vomiting.		Usually requires hospitalization, esp. if caregiver unable to rehydrate adequately, poor ORS intake, profuse diarrhea, intractable vomiting, irritable or drowsy, lack of symptomatic improvement after 24 hrs **Infants:** 30 mL/hr, **Toddlers:** 60 mL/hr, **Children:** 90 mL/hr; **ADD** 10 mL/kg for every loose stool or episode of vomiting

% Dehydration = (pre-illness weight − current weight/pre-illness weight) × 100

Oral Rehydration Solution (ORS) options

World Health Organization ORS	Recommended for all ages
Commercial ORS (Pedialyte)	Recommended or all ages
Sports Drink (Gatorade)	Not recommended for kids <2 years
Soda	Not recommended
Water	Not recommended
Juice*	Not recommended due to high osmotic load from glucose

*Dilution with ½ water, ½ juice yields a more acceptable glucose concentration.

Intravenous Rehydration Rules

- Hemodynamically unstable patients should receive one or more 20-ml/kg boluses of isotonic crystalloid or colloid irrespective of the type of dehydration.
- IV fluids must be tailored to any electrolyte abnormalities that may be present.

- Daily requirements: Na^+ (3-4 mEq/kg/day); K^+ (1-2 mEq/kg/day)
- Maintenance fluids = daily requirement + deficit + ongoing losses.
  - ▶ Use the 4:2:1 rule to calculate hourly maintenance.
  - ▶ Daily maintenance: 100 mL/kg for the first 10 kg, 50 mL/kg for next 10 kg, and 20 mL/kg for the next 10 kg
- For maintenance fluids, consider starting with D5 1/2NS for children >2 years; D5 1/4NS for children <2 years.
- Add potassium to maintenance fluids only after urine output is confirmed.
- Adding additional base (bicarbonate or acetate) to the IVF is usually not necessary unless high ongoing losses (stool) or renal dysfunction exists.
- Do not adjust the serum Na^+ >10-15 mEq/L/day. If abnormality is greater than this, the patient must be admitted for volume and electrolyte correction over 24-48 hours.

Review Questions

1. Which of the following is *not* a common cause of pancreatitis in children?
   - A. Cystic fibrosis
   - B. Trauma
   - C. Idiopathic
   - D. Gallstones
   - E. Norovirus

2. A child presents with mid-epigastric abdominal pain, nausea, and vomiting. You suspect pancreatitis. Which of the following is most helpful in making your diagnosis?
   - A. Lipase
   - B. Transaminases
   - C. CT scan of the abdomen
   - D. CBC and electrolytes

3. An infant presents with cough and wheezing associated with feeds. You evaluate the infant and are concerned for failure to thrive secondary to gastroesophageal reflux disease. Which of the following therapies should you not recommend to the parents?
   - A. Thicken feeds
   - B. Start proton pump inhibitors
   - C. Decrease the volume of each feed
   - D. Ensure the patient is prone when feeding

4. A 6-week-old infant arrives with her first-time parents at 1:00 a.m. after several episodes of non-bilous emesis. She has a heart rate of 200 bpm, a fever of 39.0°C, and seems listless. What is the appropriate course of action?

A. Try oral hydration and an antipyretic to resolve the tachycardia. Arrange follow up with the pediatrician in the morning for gastroenteritis.

B. Start an IV, give 10 mL/kg of normal saline, and discharge the patient when she can tolerate oral feeding. Diagnosis of gastroenteritis.

C. Check her glucose immediately.

D. Initiate a workup for a septic infant.

E. C and D

5. A 4-year-old child arrives with his family. They ate at the family reunion yesterday and all had vomiting and diarrhea for about 12 hours. The patient has persistent nausea and vomiting, but the diarrhea has stopped. He feels thirsty, but vomits after chugging his bottle of juice. He looks well with normal vital signs and a benign abdominal exam. How can you help?

A. Initiate an IV and give repeated 20 mL/kg boluses.

B. Reassure parents that he will be OK, continue pushing fluids, follow up with PCP as needed.

C. Slow down his intake to 30 mL every 15 minutes. Use a diluted sports drink or juice. Slowly increase the frequency of the feeding.

D. Use an antiemetic such as ondansetron to aid in your oral rehydration.

E. C and D

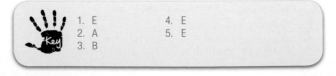

Key

1. E
2. A
3. B
4. E
5. E

GI Surgical Emergencies

Emily Grover, MD
Alice Min, MD

Malrotation/Volvulus

Critical Knowledge

Infants often present in the first 3 weeks of life with bilious vomiting or signs of acute bowel obstruction. Patients may also present with signs of peritonitis or in shock. Symptoms include vomiting, which will ultimately become bilious and abdominal pain that is constant, not colicky. Patients may often have blood streaks in their stool. They may or may not have abdominal distention.

Background

- **Malrotation** = incomplete or abnormal rotation of the midgut during the 5th to 8th week of embryologic development
- **Volvulus** = twisting of midgut around the vascular stalk, causing obstruction and compromise of vascular supply
- Occurs 1 in 500 live births; symptomatic in 1/6,000 live births.
- Malrotation accounts for 10% of neonatal intestinal obstruction.
- Diagnosed in 75% of patients by 1 year of age.

Differential Diagnoses

- Pyloric stenosis – emesis is always nonbilious; child usually appears well
- Intussusception
- Duodenal stenosis or atresia
- Incarcerated hernia
- Hirschsprung's disease

Diagnostics

- Flat and upright abdominal x-rays
    - "Double bubble" sign = gas in stomach and duodenum, otherwise airless abdomen
    - May also see distended loops of bowel overriding the liver.
- If stable, upper GI series can be done.

- ► Failure of duodenojejunal junction to cross midline; will be seen on the right side of the spine.
- ► Can also see abrupt ending or corkscrew tapering appearance of contrast.
- ► Specificity is 100%, but sensitivity is only 54%.
- Ultrasound
  - ► Inversion of superior mesenteric artery and superior mesenteric vein is very indicative of malrotation and possibly volvulus.
  - ► Other ultrasound findings suggestive of volvulus include duodenal dilatation with tapering, fixed midline bowel, whirlpool sign, and dilation of distal superior mesenteric vein.
  - ► Normal ultrasound findings do not exclude malrotation/volvulus.

Treatment
- Prompt surgical consultation
- IV fluid resuscitation
- Nasogastric tube placement if signs of obstruction
- Labs – CBC, electrolytes, blood cultures, etc.

Pyloric Stenosis

Critical Knowledge
Usually presents with nonbilious projectile vomiting in 2nd or 3rd week of life. Vomiting occurs just after or near end of feeding. Emesis often becomes projectile within one week of onset. Classically, patient is a hungry infant, who feeds avidly after vomiting and has failed to gain weight or lost weight. Patients also may present with severe dehydration and constipation. Classic electrolyte abnormality is hypochloremic, hypokalemic, and metabolic alkalosis. Peristaltic waves may be seen traveling left to right over the abdomen during feeding. In 60%-80% of cases, the mobile hard pylorus, or "olive," may be palpated in the epigastrium.

Background
- Affects 1 in 150 males, and 1 in 750 females.
- More frequent in first-born males.
- Also known as infantile hypertrophic pyloric stenosis (IHPS).

- Defined as diffuse hypertrophy and hypoplasia of the smooth muscle causes narrowing of the antrum of the stomach that is easily obstructed.
- Vomiting starts at birth in about 10% of cases.

Differential Diagnoses
- GERD – Vomiting is usually nonforceful, nonprojectile regurgitation.
- Malrotation/volvulus

Diagnostics
- Ultrasound
  - High sensitivity (90%-99%) and specificity (97% 100%)
  - Hypoechoic muscle ring greater than 4 mm with a hyperdense center
- Upper GI series if ultrasound negative
  - Retention of contrast in stomach
  - Long narrow pyloric channel with double track of barium

Treatment
- IV fluid resuscitation
- Correction of electrolyte abnormalities
- Surgical consult – pyloromyotomy is curative

Intussusception

Critical Knowledge
Intussusception is the most frequent cause of intestinal obstruction in the first 2 years of life. A portion of the intestine telescopes into another segment, most commonly at the ileocolic junction. The classic patient is a thriving infant between the ages of 3 and 12 months who develops recurring paroxysms of abdominal pain. Patients will be in severe pain, often drawing up their knees. Colicky pain often lasts a few minutes at a time, 10-20 minutes apart. Vomiting and diarrhea occurs soon after onset of pain in about 90% of cases. Classic "currant jelly stools," which are bloody bowel movements with mucus, are only seen in about 50% of cases. However, guaiac-positive stools are almost always present. Physical exam may reveal a palpable sausage-shaped mass over the right side of the abdomen. Patients may also present with fever, lethargy, shallow respirations, and may need a septic workup. Complications of intussusception include intestinal hemorrhage, incarceration, necrosis, and perforation.

Background

- The male to female ratio is 3:2.
- Cause is unknown in approximately 85% of cases.
  - ▶ Meckel's diverticulum, intestinal polyp, lymphoma, and complications of HSP have all been found to be lead points for intussusception.
  - ▶ There may also be an association with viral illnesses, possibly related to hypertrophied lymphoid tissue.

Differential Diagnoses

- Gastroenteritis – usually will have more diarrhea, ill contacts
- Meckel's diverticulum – bleeding is usually painless
- Incarcerated hernia
- Testicular or ovarian torsion
- Malrotation with volvulus
- Henoch-Schonlein purpura may coincide with or be a cause of intussusception.

Diagnostics

- Air contrast enema may be diagnostic and curative.
  - ▶ Barium and air enemas can both be diagnostic and therapeutic.
  - ▶ Air enemas are thought to be safer, due to the risk of perforation and contaminating abdominal cavity with barium.
  - ▶ Enema is contraindicated in patients with obvious surgical abdomen or patients suspected to have strangulated bowel, perforation, or presence of severe toxicity.
- Ultrasound has been shown to diagnose up to 92% of intussusception.
- Ultrasound may show a "bulls-eye" or target lesion; a lead point may be identified.

Treatment

- Obtain surgical consult before performing diagnostic procedures.
- If reduction is successful, admit patient for observation.
- There is a 3%-4% recurrence rate after hydrostatic or pneumatic reduction (usually within 24 hours).

Appendicitis

Critical Knowledge

Pediatric patients often do not present with classic symptoms of appendicitis (abdominal pain localizing to the right lower quadrant, and anorexia). Children may present with a variety of symptoms and with varied progression of symptoms, including fever, diffuse abdominal tenderness, irritability, constipation, diarrhea, vomiting, and refusal to walk. Because of these vague indicators, the incidence of perforation at the time of presentation is high (40%). Because other conditions may mimic appendicitis and physical findings may be inconclusive, it is important to perform repeated abdominal exams over several hours. Walking, jumping up and down, and climbing onto the stretcher may all cause pain. Temperature and white blood cell count may be normal.

Background

- Most common nontraumatic pediatric surgical emergency
- More common over age of 2 years
- Peak incidence 9-12 years

Differential Diagnoses

- Gastroenteritis
- UTI
- Intussusception
- PID
- Constipation
- Ovarian pathology

Diagnostics

- **Ultrasound:** With experienced sonographers, ultrasound has sensitivity of 85% and specificity of 94%. Ultrasound findings that suggest appendicitis include noncompressible tubular structure in the RLQ, free fluid in the RLQ, and thick appendix wall >2 mm. If the appendix is not visualized, consider serial exams or other diagnostic options.
- **CT scan:** One study showed sensitivity and specificity of CT to be 94% and 95%, respectively, which was superior to ultrasound.
- **MRI:** MRI without contrast has shown sensitivity and specificity of 98% and 97% respectively; in addition, it does not carry the radiation risks of CT.

Treatment

- Surgical consultation
- Resuscitate with IV fluids
- Labs – CBC, urinalysis, pregnancy test
- Broad-spectrum antibiotics if perforation is suspected

Meckel's Diverticulum

Critical Knowledge

Most commonly presents with painless acute lower GI bleeding in children younger than 5 years. Intestinal obstruction is also present in 25%-40% of pediatric patients. Heterotopic mucosa in diverticulum is most commonly gastric (80%), but may also be pancreatic, ileal, jejunal, or colonic. Bleeding often results from ulceration of gastric mucosa. Meckel's diverticulum may also be lead point causing intussusception. Acute inflammation of diverticulum may mimic appendicitis.

Background

- Incidence is approximately 2%; is often asymptomatic.
- Classically presents in patients younger than 2 years.
- Results from incomplete obliteration of the omphalomesenteric duct, connecting the midgut to the yolk sac.
- A *true* diverticulum contains all layers of intestinal walls.

Differential Diagnoses

- Appendicitis
- Intussusception
- Malrotation with volvulus
- Anal fissure
- Bacterial enteritis

Diagnostics

- Plain abdominal x-ray
  - ▶ May show signs of obstruction or perforation.
  - ▶ May be normal.

- Meckel's scan
  - ▶ Radionuclide imaging technique using technetium-99m-pertechnetate, which is taken up by heterotopic gastric mucosa in the diverticulum
  - ▶ Noninvasive
  - ▶ Involves less radiation exposure than that from an upper GI series and small bowel follow-through study
  - ▶ Sensitivity ranges from 75%-100%
  - ▶ Specificity more than 80%
  - ▶ False-positive results in up to 15%
  - ▶ False-negative results in up to 25%
  - ▶ Meckel's diverticulum must be actively bleeding at a minimum rate of 0.1 mL per minute in order to be visualized.

Treatment

- Resuscitate with IV fluids.
- Transfuse with blood products if needed.
- Place nasogastric tube if bowel obstruction is present.
- Obtain surgical consultation.

Necrotizing Enterocolitis

Critical Knowledge

Necrotizing enterocolitis primarily affects the GI tract, but also may have serious systemic effects. Typically, this condition is seen in the NICU in premature infants within the first few weeks of life. Occasionally, term infants may be affected, with the average age of onset within the first week of life. Term neonates with NEC are usually systemically ill with other predisposing conditions, such as birth asphyxia, respiratory distress, congenital heart disease, metabolic abnormalities, or a history of abnormal fetal growth pattern. Initial symptoms may be subtle and can include feeding intolerance, delayed gastric emptying, abdominal distention, ileus, decreased bowel sounds, abdominal wall erythema (late finding), and hematochezia. Systemic signs may be nonspecific and can include apnea, lethargy, decreased peripheral perfusion, shock, and cardiovascular collapse.

Background

- Necrotizing enterocolitis is the most common gastrointestinal medical and/or surgical emergency occurring in neonates.
- Incidence is inversely related to birth weight and gestational age.
- Mortality is higher in premature infants.
- Cause is unknown.
- No single organism has been identified as the trigger.
- It also has been associated with an anoxic episode.
- Ischemia and/or reperfusion also may play a role in development of condition.

Differential Diagnoses

- Hirschsprung's disease
- Malrotation with volvulus
- Sepsis

Diagnostics

- Plain abdominal x-ray: supine and left lateral decubitus
  - Pneumatosis intestinalis (air within bowel wall) is pathognomonic.
  - Hepatic portal air
  - Intra-abdominal free air if perforation has already occurred
  - Dilated loops of bowel in early disease

Treatment

- IV fluid resuscitation
- Broad-spectrum antibiotics
- NPO
- Surgical consultation

Hirschsprung's Disease

Critical Knowledge

In neonates, disease history often includes delayed passage of meconium (greater than 48 hours), abdominal distention, and repeated vomiting. Older children often present with symptoms of chronic constipation. Patients may be malnourished, resulting from abdominal distention, early satiety, and discomfort due to chronic constipation. Hirschsprung's enterocolitis is a fatal complication of Hirschsprung's disease and typically presents with abdominal pain, fever, foul-smelling and/or bloody diarrhea, as well as vomiting. Enterocolitis may progress to sepsis, transmural intestinal necrosis, and perforation if not recognized early. Physical exam often reveals tympanitic abdominal distention and symptoms of intestinal obstruction. Rectal exam often reveals an empty rectal vault.

Background

- Occurs in approximately 1 in 5000 live births.
- Four times more common in males than females.
- Nearly all children with Hirschsprung's disease are diagnosed by 2 years of age.
- Results from the absence of parasympathetic ganglion cells in the myenteric and submucosal plexus of the rectum and/or colon.
- Ganglion cells are derived from the neural crest. They migrate caudally with the vagal nerve fibers along the intestine and arrive in the proximal colon by 8 weeks of gestational age, and in the rectum by 12 weeks of gestational age. Failure of complete migration leads to an aganglionic segment.
- Overall mortality of Hirschsprung enterocolitis is 25%-30%.
- Family history of this condition may be present.
- Strongly associated with Down syndrome.

Differential Diagnoses

- Constipation from other cause
- Malrotation with volvulus
- Gastroenteritis
- Meconium plug syndrome

Diagnostics

- Plain abdominal x-ray
  - ▶ May show signs of obstruction.
- Barium enema
  - ▶ May show a transition zone between a narrowed aganglionic segment and a dilated and normally innervated segment.
  - ▶ May also reveal a nondistensible rectum (classic sign of Hirschsprung disease).
- Rectal biopsy provides a definitive diagnosis.

Treatment

- IV fluid resuscitation
- Nasogastric tube placement if suspected obstruction
- NPO
- Broad-spectrum antibiotics for patient with enterocolitis
- Surgical consultation

Review Questions

1. **Which of the following is true regarding malrotation/volvulus?**
   A. Symptoms of abdominal pain and vomiting are rare.
   B. Vascular supply to the midgut is never in danger when this condition occurs.
   C. A "double bubble" sign may be seen on plain films.
   D. Blood in the stool is necessary to make this diagnosis.

2. **Which is the most likely presentation of volvulus?**
   A. 1-month-old with colicky abdominal pain, feeding well
   B. 3-week-old born at 39 weeks, non-bilious vomiting, but seems hungry and appears well
   C. 3-week-old born at 34 weeks with bloody stool, fever, distended abdomen, and irritability
   D. 2-week-old born at 38 weeks with bilious vomiting, poor feeding, and constant irritability

3. **All of the following are commonly seen in patients with pyloric stenosis, EXCEPT:**
   A. Dehydration
   B. Projectile emesis
   C. Non-bilious vomiting
   D. Normal weight gain

4. **Which of the following is true regarding pyloric stenosis?**
   A. A palpable "olive" is always present on physical exam.
   B. Hypochloremic, hypokalemic, metabolic alkalosis is common.
   C. Abdominal plain films are diagnostic.
   D. This condition classically presents after 6 months of age.

5. Which of the following has been associated with intussusception?
   A. Meckel's diverticulum
   B. Polyp
   C. Lymphoma
   D. All of the above

6. All of the following are true regarding intussusception, EXCEPT:
   A. The classic "currant jelly" stools are seen in a majority of cases.
   B. The ileocolic junction is the most common site.
   C. Barium and air enemas can be both diagnostic and therapeutic.
   D. Complications include intestinal hemorrhage, incarceration, necrosis, and perforation.

7. Which of the following is true regarding appendicitis?
   A. Pediatric patients often present with classic symptoms of appendicitis, similar to adults.
   B. Fever and elevated white blood cell counts are always present.
   C. Perforation at the time of presentation is very rare.
   D. Walking, jumping up and down, and climbing onto the stretcher may all cause pain.

8. Which of the following is appropriate in the management of appendicitis?
   A. IV fluid resuscitation
   B. Surgical consultation
   C. Urinalysis and CBC
   D. All of the above

9. Which of the following is true regarding Meckel's diverticulum?
   A. Commonly presents with painful lower GI bleeding
   B. Heterotopic mucosa in diverticulum is most commonly gastric
   C. Does not contain all layers of the intestinal wall
   D. Rarely seen as lead point in intussusception

10. **Which of the following is true regarding necrotizing enterocolitis?**
    A. Pneumatosis intestinalis is pathognomonic.
    B. It most commonly affects term infants.
    C. Systemic effects like shock are rarely seen.
    D. Antibiotics are not indicated.

11. **All of the following are associated with necrotizing enterocolitis, EXCEPT:**
    A. Prematurity
    B. Anoxic episode
    C. Feeding intolerance
    D. All are associated with NEC

12. **Which of the following is true regarding Hirschsprung's disease?**
    A. Definitive diagnosis is made by plain abdominal x-ray.
    B. Results from embryologic failure to develop intestinal smooth muscle.
    C. Constipation is a rare symptom.
    D. History may include delayed passage of meconium.

Key			
1.	C	7.	D
2.	D	8.	D
3.	D	9.	B
4.	B	10.	A
5.	D	11.	D
6.	A	12.	D

Foreign Body Aspiration

Katherine Hiller, MD, MPH

Critical Knowledge

- Symptoms vary significantly depending on the location of the foreign body (FB) in the airway.
- If the patient can cough and make sounds, the foreign body airway obstruction is partial; no immediate intervention is needed.
- If the victim cannot cough or make any sound, the obstruction is severe; immediate intervention is necessary.
  - ► For a child, perform subdiaphragmatic abdominal thrusts (Heimlich maneuver) until the object is expelled or the victim becomes unresponsive.
  - ► For an infant, deliver five back blows (slaps) with the infant in head down position followed by five chest thrusts repeatedly until the object is expelled or the victim becomes unresponsive.
  - ► If the victim becomes unresponsive, lay rescuers and health care providers should perform CPR, but should look into the mouth before giving breaths, removing a foreign body if it is seen.
  - ► If the obstruction persists, perform direct laryngoscopy to visualize and remove any foreign bodies; perform endotracheal intubation as needed.
  - ► If the foreign body cannot be removed and the patient cannot be ventilated, possible measures include pushing the foreign body into a main stem bronchus, emergent consultation with anesthesia or a surgical service, needle cricothyroidotomy, or emergent tracheostomy.
- **Maintain a high index of suspicion for foreign body aspiration.**
  - ► Delayed diagnosis may lead to severe and potentially irreversible complications.
  - ► History suggestive of foreign body aspiration mandates endoscopic evaluation, regardless of radiological findings.
    - Common signs and symptoms include choking, coughing, stridor, wheezing, respiratory distress, or airway obstruction.

- Lower airway symptoms may mimic asthma, croup, or URI, leading to frequent missed diagnoses.
- Diagnostic studies include neck and chest radiographs, fluoroscopy, computed tomography, and flexible bronchoscopy.[1]
- Definitive diagnosis and treatment is rigid bronchoscopy performed by highly skilled personnel under general anesthesia.

Epidemiology and Anatomy

- Foreign body obstruction of the upper airway can be immediately life-threatening.
- Causes 300 childhood deaths per year in the U.S., with 65% of victims less than 2 years old.[2]
- 60-80% of tracheobronchial foreign bodies occur in children less than 3 years.[2]
- Peak incidence occurs between ages 10 and 24 months.[1]
- 7% of all lethal accidents occur in children aged 1-3.[3]
- Male to female ratio is 2:1.
- Serious complications from aspirated foreign bodies tend to occur in infants and younger children because of their small airway size.[4]

Types of foreign bodies aspirated

- Peanuts (87%), beans (6%), and other FBs (6%) are common.[5]
- The severity of the foreign body aspiration is, in part, determined by the nature of the foreign body.
- The majority of fatal accidents caused by food-based foreign bodies are due to cylindrical or round foreign bodies that fit perfectly against the wall of the respiratory tract and cause asphyxia.[6]
- Oil content in peanuts, seeds, and nuts may cause intense inflammatory responses.[3]

Location of foreign body in the respiratory tree

- Foreign bodies have the potential for migration from one location to another.
- Tracheal foreign bodies are uncommon (3%-12% of foreign body aspirations); however, when the FB is located in the larynx or trachea, respiratory distress and stridor are highly suggestive.[1]

- Foreign bodies are usually aspirated into one of the main bronchi, with the right slightly more frequently involved than the left (55% vs. 40%).[5]
- The majority of FBs (75%-94%) migrate to the bronchi and clinical signs are less constant, making the diagnosis difficult.[1]

Differential Diagnosis and Critical Concepts

- Differential diagnosis
  - ▶ Asthma/reactive airway disease
  - ▶ Pneumonia
  - ▶ Croup
  - ▶ Bronchiolitis
  - ▶ Epiglottitis
  - ▶ Laryngitis
  - ▶ Pulmonary lesions/disease
  - ▶ Upper respiratory infection
- High index of suspicion is essential.
- Most predictive variables for a FB retrieved on bronchoscopy:[7]
  - ▶ Age 10-24 months
  - ▶ FB in the mouth
  - ▶ Severe respiratory complaints
  - ▶ Hypoxemia
  - ▶ Stridor following the acute event
  - ▶ Unilateral abnormal lung sounds
  - ▶ Abnormal trachea on radiograph
  - ▶ Unilateral infiltrate, atelectasis, or hyperinflation on radiograph
  - ▶ A sudden episode of coughing and choking or chronic, unexplained pulmonary infections should raise suspicion for foreign body aspiration.
  - ▶ Wheezing (especially unilateral) in a patient without a history of asthma or other pulmonary disease should strongly suggest foreign body aspiration until proven otherwise.
- Early diagnosis prevents complications.

Signs and Symptoms, Three Stages[4]

- Initial stage
  - ▶ History of a choking episode – especially while eating or playing, followed by paroxysms of coughing or gagging.
  - ▶ Initial symptoms include acute respiratory distress, stridor, increased respiratory effort, or complete obstruction.
  - ▶ Physical exam findings include diminished breath sounds or wheezes from affected lung, but may be normal.
  - ▶ A history of choking while holding or eating an object in the mouth is very predictive of foreign body aspiration.[7]
- The **second stage** is an asymptomatic interval.
- The **third stage** is characterized by symptoms of delayed complications.
  - ▶ Repeated or prolonged respiratory infections, wheezing refractory to conventional therapy, CXR findings
- No single sign, symptom, or combination has been shown to reliably confirm or exclude FB (besides bronchoscopy).

Diagnostic Testing

- 80%-96% of cases are radiolucent; however, radiographs may show indirect signs of bronchial obstruction.[1]
- PA and lateral CXR, soft tissue neck (AP, lateral)
  - ▶ CXR findings[13]
    - Hyperinflation or obstructive emphysema (range, 44%-64%)
    - Mediastinal shift (range, 4%-71%)
    - Pneumonia (range, 4%-23%)
    - Atelectasis (range, 9%-22%)
    - Radiopaque foreign body (range, 3%-16%)
    - Unilateral whole-lung opacification (2%)
    - Normal (12%-25%)
- Inspiratory and expiratory views may show unilateral air trapping.
  - ▶ Lateral decubitus can be used in place of inspiration/expiration when patient cooperation is an issue.
- Sensitivity and specificity of chest radiographs are increased when performed 24 hours after aspiration.[8]

- CT scan has a high sensitivity (up to 100%), but a variable specificity (67%-100%); it may reduce bronchoscopy time by providing surgeon information about the site and size of the FB.[1]
- Virtual bronchoscopy may be available at some institutions.[9]
- Flexible bronchoscopy has a high sensitivity and specificity, and has been suggested as a first step when radiographic signs are inconclusive. Advantages include that it may be performed with procedural sedation rather than general anesthesia.[10]
- Diagnostic sensitivity of various signs or symptoms.[1]
  - ▶ **Choking crisis:** sensitivity of 75%-91% and a specificity of 10%-92%
  - ▶ **CXR:** sensitivity of 62%-88% and a specificity of 30%-97%
  - ▶ **Clinical examination:** sensitivity of 56%-86% and a specificity of 26%-65%
  - ▶ **Chest CT:** sensitivity 100%; specificity 67%-100%
- The diagnosis of foreign-body aspiration is often delayed.
  - ▶ Diagnosis within a day is made in only 60%-70% of patients.[2]
  - ▶ Diagnosis is delayed by one week in 8%-33% of cases.[6]
  - ▶ Many delayed diagnoses are related to reliance on a negative x-ray and are diagnosed as asthma or URI.[4]
  - ▶ 75% of complications occur in cases where diagnosis is delayed.[6]
  - ▶ Potential complications of foreign body aspiration include pneumomediastinum, pneumothorax, hydropneumothorax, bronchial stenosis, abscess, atelectasis, pneumonia, bronchiectasis, foreign body dislodgment, and bronchospasm.[11]
    - ▪ When there is a clinical index of suspicion (choking history with typically aspirated foods), bronchoscopy is indicated despite normal radiographic studies.
    - ▪ Obtain inspiratory and expiratory (or lateral decubitus) chest radiographs in all patients.
    - ▪ With normal chest radiographs, a poor history for aspiration, and mild or no symptoms without focal findings on physical examination, the patient may be discharged with follow up in a few days.
    - ▪ If diagnosis remains unclear after plain films and there is a historical or clinical suspicion of aspiration, CT, flexible bronchoscopy, or fluoroscopy may be obtained.

Treatment

- Initial first aid (pediatric basic life support)
  - ▶ If the patient can cough and make some sounds, the airway obstruction is mild.
    - Do not interfere; allow the patient to maintain a position of comfort.
    - Allow the victim to clear the airway by coughing while you observe for signs of severe foreign body airway obstruction.
  - ▶ If the victim cannot cough or make any sound, the airway obstruction is severe.
    - For a child, perform subdiaphragmatic abdominal thrusts (Heimlich maneuver) until the object is expelled or the victim becomes unresponsive.
    - For an infant, deliver five back blows (slaps) with the infant in head-down position followed by five chest thrusts repeatedly until the object is expelled or the victim becomes unresponsive.
    - Abdominal thrusts are not recommended for infants because they may damage the relatively large and unprotected liver.
    - If the victim becomes unresponsive, lay rescuers and health care providers should perform CPR, but should look into the mouth before giving breaths.
    - If a foreign body is seen, it should be removed.
    - Health care providers should not perform blind finger sweeps because they may push obstructing objects further into the pharynx and may damage the oropharynx.
    - If an object can be seen in the pharynx, health care providers should attempt to remove it, and then rescuers should attempt ventilation, followed by chest compressions.
- **Advanced Interventions**[12]
  - ▶ If foreign body airway obstruction is not relieved with thrusts or compressions and the condition deteriorates to respiratory failure or cardiopulmonary arrest, more aggressive interventions are necessary.
  - ▶ Obtain neutral, in-line positioning of the head, neck, and shoulders and anterior displacement of the chin or jaw to facilitate an open mouth.
  - ▶ Perform direct laryngoscopy to visualize and remove the foreign object.

- Performance of bag mask ventilation prior to attempting to remove the foreign body may worsen the obstruction.
- If the foreign body cannot be seen in the pharynx or larynx, it may be in the esophagus, compressing the trachea.
- BLS maneuvers may dislodge the foreign body into the oropharynx, where it can be removed.
- If the foreign body is visualized in the subglottic space or trachea and cannot be removed, BLS maneuvers may dislodge it into the oropharynx.
- Alternatively, pushing the foreign body into a main stem bronchus with an endotracheal tube may allow ventilation of the other lung, but carries the risk of causing irreversible airway obstruction.
- Emergent consultation with ENT, anesthesiology, or general surgery should be obtained.
- If above measures fail to clear the airway and the patient cannot be intubated or ventilated, emergency needle cricothyroidotomy is the procedure of last resort to provide oxygenation.
- Perform temporizing measures until definitive airway is established.
- True complete airway obstruction is a relative contraindication to needle cricothyroidotomy, as air cannot escape from the lungs; an emergent tracheostomy may be more appropriate.

- **Bronchoscopy**
  - Flexible bronchoscopy is generally used for diagnostic, not therapeutic purposes; however, it may be more useful in retrieving FBs that have migrated deeper into the subsegmental bronchi than rigid bronchoscopy can reach.[10]
  - Rigid bronchoscopy under general anesthesia is necessary for removal and is the treatment of choice.
  - Requires consultation with pediatric pulmonologist or surgeon.
  - Most pulmonologists are not trained in rigid bronchoscopy or FB removal with flexible bronchoscopy.
  - If only personnel trained in diagnostic flexible bronchoscopy are available, consider flexible bronchoscopy with a plan for transfer to facility with rigid bronchoscopy capability.

- ► May be performed on outpatient basis if there is no concern for respiratory status.
- ► A history strongly suggestive of foreign body aspiration dictates rigid bronchoscopy, regardless of results of radiographic studies.
- ► Should also be considered in cases with persistent respiratory signs and symptoms to diagnose delayed presentations.
- ► Potential complications of bronchoscopy
  - Pneumomediastinum, tracheal laceration, vocal cords laceration, subglottic edema, bronchospasm and necessity for thoracotomy, bronchotomy, or lobectomy (overall rate of complication low, 6%-8%).[11]
- ► Complications are more likely in patients with delayed diagnosis (>1 week since aspiration).[3]
- ► Education and prevention are important.
  - Increase diagnostic acumen of treating physicians and heighten public awareness to reduce morbidity and mortality.
  - Parents should be instructed to abstain from feeding nuts and seeds to young children and to keep small, potentially ingestible objects out of reach.

Review Questions

1. **Which is true regarding the treatment of FB aspiration?**
   A. Bronchoscopy is only indicated when a foreign body is confirmed on radiographic testing.
   B. As soon as a patient starts choking after a suspected foreign body aspiration, abdominal thrusts should be performed to remove the foreign body.
   C. The rate of complications from bronchoscopy increases when the diagnosis is delayed more than one week.
   D. Blind finger sweeps should be made to retrieve a foreign body.
   E. Flexible bronchoscopy is the procedure of choice for removal of aspirated foreign bodies.

2. You are evaluating a 2-year-old patient who presents with sudden onset of coughing and mild respiratory distress. The child has no history of reactive airway disease. Which of the following is true regarding the diagnostic workup?

    A. Foreign body aspiration is rare in this age group.

    B. Inspiratory and expiratory chest radiographs are indicated.

    C. Foreign body aspiration is ruled out with a normal CXR and a normal physical exam.

    D. A radiopaque foreign body is likely to be found on CXR.

    E. A delay in diagnosis of FB aspiration does not increase complication rates.

3. All of the following are true, EXCEPT:

    A. Foreign body aspirations are more common in males.

    B. Aspirated foreign bodies are most commonly organic food matter.

    C. Foreign body aspirations are often misdiagnosed as asthma or respiratory infections.

    D. Most aspirated foreign bodies are retrieved from the left main stem bronchus.

    E. Foreign bodies in the lower respiratory tree are more likely to result in a delayed diagnosis.

4. Which has the highest diagnostic sensitivity and specificity?

    A. Plain chest radiograph

    B. Inspiratory/expiratory chest radiograph

    C. Computed tomography

    D. Physical exam

    E. History suggestive of aspiration

Foreign Body Ingestion

Katherine Hiller, MD, MPH

Critical Knowledge

- Very common pediatric problem, especially in children ages 6 months to 3 years.
- Usually not immediately life-threatening compared to foreign body (FB) *aspiration*; many ingestions are asymptomatic and resolve without complications.
- Keep a high index of suspicion for foreign body ingestion with symptoms such as gagging, vomiting, dysphagia, refusal to eat, wheezing, or foreign body sensation.
- The longer foreign bodies are retained, the more likely complications become.
- Retained ingested FBs may lead to potentially serious complications, including respiratory distress, perforation, obstruction, and death.
- FBs lodged in the esophagus should be treated with immediate removal.
- Disc batteries lodged in the esophagus should be removed emergently because of the potential for damage to the esophagus.
- Once FBs advance past the esophagus, they usually pass spontaneously, but long and sharp objects may need to be removed from the stomach.
- Ingestion of multiple magnets or a magnet and a metal object can cause obstruction and/or perforation.
- Helpful diagnostic tests include plain radiographs and contrast esophagrams.
- In asymptomatic patients with acute (<24 hrs) ingestion, observation for 24 hours may be appropriate.

Epidemiology and Anatomy

- Foreign body ingestions are extremely common.
  - ▶ 82,197 incidents of ingestion in 2011 in patients younger than 5 years were reported by the American Association of Poison Control Centers.[1]

- ► 5%-10% of children have swallowed a coin.[2]
- Typical age of presentation is 6 months to 3 years; boys are more likely than girls.
- 98% of cases are accidental; rarely, prisoners, psychiatric patients, and victims of gang initiation rituals may present with FB ingestion.[3]
- Most childhood esophageal foreign bodies are round or spherical.
- Coins are the most common foreign body ingested and make up 50%-75% of childhood esophageal foreign bodies.
  - ► Pennies are the most common coin ingested.
  - ► Other objects include toys/toy parts, needles and pins, batteries, bones, and food.
- Children are less likely than adults to have foodstuff foreign bodies lodge in the esophagus.
- Fish bone ingestions are more common in Asian communities.
- Children with anatomic esophageal or GI tract abnormalities or physiologic abnormalities (eosinophilic esophagitis) are more likely to suffer FB impaction.
- Of FBs that come to medical attention, 80%-90% pass spontaneously, 10%-20% require endoscopic removal, and <1% require surgical removal.[3]
- Ingested foreign bodies may lodge in the esophagus or more distal portions of the GI tract, including the pylorus, duodenum, cecum, appendix, or rectum.
  - ► Impaction in the esophagus is the most common, and potentially, the most serious.
    - 70% of esophageal FBs become lodged at the thoracic inlet.
      - — The narrowest portion of the pediatric GI tract
      - — The level of the circopharyngeus sling (C6)
    - 15% become impacted at the level of the aortic arch.
    - 15% become impacted at the gastroesophageal junction.
  - ► Foreign bodies that reach the stomach safely will usually traverse the remainder of the GI tract without complications.
    - A variety of foreign bodies, including screws, tacks, and staples, have been documented to traverse the entire GI tract safely.

- Objects longer than 5 cm or greater than 2 cm in diameter may not pass through the tight turns of the duodenum and other portions of the lower GI tract.
  - ► Very sharp objects, such as sewing needles or toothpicks, have a higher risk of perforating hollow viscera.
    - Bowel perforation from sharp objects has resulted in peritonitis, abscess formation, inflammatory tumors, hemorrhage, and death.
  - ► Magnets, when more than one is ingested, or a magnet and a metal object have been known to cause obstruction and perforation.[4]

Differential Diagnosis and Critical Concepts

- Differential Diagnosis
  - ► Foreign body aspiration
  - ► Esophageal stricture
  - ► Esophagitis
  - ► GERD/gastritis/peptic ulcer disease
  - ► Reactive airway disease
  - ► Pharyngitis
  - ► Gastroenteritis
  - ► Munchausen syndrome
  - ► Obstruction, large or small bowel
  - ► Intussusception
  - ► Pyloric stenosis
  - ► Aspiration pneumonia
  - ► Pneumomediastinum
  - ► Acute appendicitis
  - ► Psychiatric diseases – autism, bulimia, mental retardation, personality disorders
- History/presentation
  - ► A history of swallowing a FB with consistent symptoms makes the diagnosis straightforward.
  - ► When there is no definite history of FB ingestion, the diagnosis of a FB can be difficult as the symptoms may mimic other common childhood conditions.

- ► May be asymptomatic (30%-40% of patients with esophageal coins)
- Adverse effects and symptoms usually result from esophageal impaction.
- Symptoms of esophageal impaction can include:
  - ► Gagging, vomiting, drooling, (possibly coughing) dysphagia, refusal to eat, foreign body sensation, pain, localization, wheezing, or generalized irritability
  - ► Impacted esophageal foreign bodies may also cause secondary airway symptoms due to the softer cartilage of the trachea.
- Symptoms suggestive of other potentially serious complications include:
  - ► Ingestion of button batteries or magnets
  - ► Esophageal perforation: neck swelling, crepitus, and pneumo-mediastinum
  - ► Stomach or GI perforation: fever, abdominal pain and tenderness
  - ► Bowel obstruction: abdominal distension, pain, and tenderness
- Diagnostic approach[5]
  - ► If history is suggestive of FB ingestion, perform radiographic evaluation (CXR, soft tissue neck, abdominal XR).
    - ▪ Asymptomatic patients who have ingested a small (less than 1 cm in maximum diameter), nonsharp object may not require any imaging studies.
    - ▪ Radiopaque foreign bodies are found in approximately 65% of cases.
  - ► If the foreign body is not radiopaque but is large enough to become impacted (i.e., a large food bolus) and the symptoms suggest esophageal impaction, obtain either a contrast esophagram or immediate endoscopy.
    - ▪ Esophagrams pose risk of aspiration and make subsequent endoscopy more difficult.
  - ► Handheld metal detectors provide an alternative to radiography as an initial screen when a coin ingestion is suspected.[6]
    - ▪ Compared favorably with radiography in determining presence or absence of a coin and coin location (esophagus vs distal GI tract)
    - ▪ Follow up is suggested because esophageal coins may be missed (especially in obese children).

- ▶ A compass may be used to determine whether FBs are magnetic.[4]
- ▶ Missed foreign body ingestion with retained FB can occasionally lead to serious sequelae, including bronchoesophageal fistula, mediastinitis, esophageal diverticulum, lobar atelectasis, aortoesophageal fistula, and need for thoracotomy for FB removal.

Treatment

- *Prevention* of FB ingestion is the best treatment, with efforts regarding education of supervision of play and appropriate toys in the toddler and preschool groups.
- **Oropharyngeal foreign bodies**
  - ▶ Multiple methods have been used successfully for removal, including forceps and tongue depressor, transnasal flexible endoscopy, direct laryngoscopy, and indirect laryngoscopy.[7]
- **Esophageal foreign bodies**
  - ▶ Objects causing acute airway compromise or obstruction should be removed emergently.
  - ▶ Symptomatic patients who are able to swallow their secretions may undergo endoscopy within 12-24 hours, allowing for fasting and age appropriate anesthesia.[8]
  - ▶ Sharp esophageal foreign bodies and disc batteries should be removed emergently.
    - ▪ Disc batteries may cause esophageal injury within hours, leading to permanent sequelae and should be removed immediately.
  - ▶ Coins throughout the esophagus have been shown to have good spontaneous passage rate in a 12- to 24-hour observation period.[9]
    - ▪ 22% of proximal, 33% middle, 37% distal coins
  - ▶ No serious complications have been documented from an esophageal coin that was impacted for less than a few days; however, the esophageal mucosa may grow around a coin after several days, making removal more difficult.
  - ▶ Observation for spontaneous passage is a possible option.[9]
    - ▪ Most favorable when the object is lodged at the gastroesophageal junction, but can also work with coins in proximal or mid esophagus
    - ▪ Avoids costs and potential complications of removal techniques

- Randomized prospective study of immediate endoscopic removal of esophageal coins compared to 16-hour observation in 60 patients.[10]
    - Spontaneous passage occurred equally in observation group and surgical group (25%).
    - Spontaneous passage is more likely in older patients (66 vs. 46 months), male patients, and coins in distal 1/3 of esophagus.
    - No complications were found in either group.
- Allow a period of 12 to 24 hours for spontaneous passage with general criteria for observation:
    - Round, noncorrosive (e.g., coins) foreign bodies
    - Asymptomatic patient (i.e., no respiratory distress)
    - No history of esophageal disease
    - Ingestion occurred less than 24 hours prior
    - Good follow up
    - Consultation with physician who would be involved in potential removal
- Esophageal removal techniques
  - Removal techniques vary regionally and depend on the duration of impaction, associated symptoms, and the nature of the foreign body.
  - Medications such as glucagon or diazepam have been unsuccessfully used to facilitate the passage of foreign bodies from the esophagus.[11]
  - Traditional removal methods include rigid esophagoscopy under general anesthesia, and flexible endoscopy under sedation.
  - Esophagoscopy under general anesthesia has been the method of choice for many years.
    - Essential in patients not meeting criteria for observation or alternative removal techniques
    - Safe and efficacious
    - Applicable to all types of foreign bodies
    - Allows for direct examination of the esophageal lumen
    - Can be used in patients with respiratory distress
    - Possible, but rare, complications of endoscopy or esophagoscopy include pharyngeal bleeding, bronchospasm, accidental extubation, stridor, hypoxia, esophageal perforation, and mediastinitis.[10]

Alternative Treatments

- Direct laryngoscopy with or without sedation can be diagnostic and therapeutic for coins in the upper esophagus and nonmetallic small objects (such as bones)
- Alternative methods for coins and similar round, smooth objects have been developed. Strict selection criteria for alternative techniques include a single "serious complication."
- Balloon-tipped catheter under fluoroscopic guidance to extract or advance the coin
  - ▶ Success rate of approximately 90% (extraction or advancing FB into stomach).
  - ▶ Higher failure rates in younger children (<2 years).
  - ▶ Significant cost savings compared to rigid esophagoscopy.
  - ▶ Criticized due to lack of airway control, poor control of the foreign body during extraction, and inadequate visualization of the esophagus.
  - ▶ Complications are rare (~2%) and include epistaxis, vomiting, respiratory distress, and esophageal perforation.
- Bougienage to advance the coin into the stomach
  - ▶ When used selectively, has a high success rate at several institutions and very safe with few complications.
  - ▶ Much less costly than esophagoscopy with general anesthesia.
  - ▶ Has been used by trained emergency physicians safely and effectively.[12]
- Fluoroscopic-guided grasping endoscopic forceps covered by a soft rubber catheter
  - ▶ Takes only 1 minute, but experience is limited.

Stomach and Lower GI Foreign Bodies

- Most round objects (e.g., coins) will traverse the GI tract in 3 to 8 days without any complication, but some may take up to 4 weeks.
- Management recommendations for sharp objects are varied, but conservative; watchful waiting is usually safe.
  - ▶ Some objects remain in the stomach for a long duration.
  - ▶ Weekly radiographs for progression
  - ▶ 3 to 4 weeks should be allowed for passage out of the stomach before surgical or endoscopic removal is necessary.

- ► Removal should be considered for objects in same position for more than 1 week or with any fever, vomiting, abdominal pain, or other significant symptoms.
- Surgical/endoscopic removal in certain circumstances
  - ► Sewing needles have increased propensity for perforation and should be removed.
  - ► Long objects (greater than 3-5 cm in children >1 year, 2 cm <1 year) and sharp objects should be removed from the stomach before they have passed beyond the duodenal curve because they are more likely to cause complications or require surgical removal.[13]
  - ► If object cannot be removed, perform daily radiographs with surgical removal if no progression in 3 days.
- **Disc battery ingestion**
  - ► Disc batteries that pass the esophagus spontaneously can be observed.
  - ► Disc batteries that lodge in the esophagus should be removed emergently because of the potential to injure the esophagus rapidly from corrosive effects.
  - ► Batteries should be removed endoscopically from the stomach if they have been retained for more than 48 hours or are larger than 2 cm in diameter.
  - ► Once batteries are past the duodenal sweep, 85% pass in less than 72 hours.
  - ► Radiographs should be obtained every 3-4 days to follow the progress until it has passed, unless symptoms develop.
  - ► Only sporadic cases of systemic absorption of battery contents have been suggested in the literature, and no serious toxicities have been reported.
- **Magnet ingestion**
  - ► When more than one magnet, or a magnet and a piece of metal is ingested, they may attach across intestinal walls, causing volvulus, bowel necrosis, fistula, perforation, obstruction, and peritonitis.
  - ► Bowel perforation is common (75%) and fatalities have been reported.[4]
  - ► A compass may be used to determine whether a radio-opaque FB is magnetic.
  - ► If more than one magnet is present and within endoscopic reach, early endoscopy is warranted.

▶ If the magnets are not large and are beyond endoscopic reach, careful monitoring vs. surgical consultation should be decided on a case-by-case basis.[3]

Review Questions

1. **Which of the following is true regarding pediatric foreign body ingestions?**

   A. Foreign body ingestions are rare and usually cause immediate life-threatening symptoms.

   B. Most ingested foreign bodies become impacted at the gastroesophageal junction.

   C. Most foreign bodies that reach the stomach safely will traverse the remainder of the GI tract without complications.

   D. Most foreign body impactions are a result of large food boluses.

   E. Girls are more likely to have a foreign body ingestion.

2. **For which of the following cases would expectant observation be appropriate?**

   A. Single, round, noncorrosive esophageal FB on radiograph

   B. Multiple, adherent, magnetic FBs past the duodenum

   C. History of esophageal disease

   D. Button battery lodged in the esophagus

   E. Ingestion occurred two days ago, esophageal FB on radiograph

3. **Which of the following objects should be urgently removed?**

   A. Single magnet in the small bowel

   B. Button battery in the stomach

   C. Button battery in the small bowel

   D. Sewing needle in the stomach

   E. Penny in the esophagus

Dermatology

Mark D. Wright, MD

Dermatologists learn to recognize skin disorders through visual memory. During the course of training they see uncommon and rare diseases often enough to recognize them. Emergency physicians don't have that luxury; by the time they see an uncommon disease for the second time, its name and appearance will likely have been forgotten. A morphology-oriented diagnostic algorithm, which uses a series of descriptive words to describe the disease in question, can help avoid this problem. It can then be cross-referenced to an algorithm[1] or dermatology atlas in order to further narrow the diagnosis.

Background

- Skin is the largest body organ.
- ED visits for rashes occur more frequently in children.
- Pediatric dermatology can seem overwhelming; however, there are a relatively limited number of conditions that present frequently.
- Avoid scanning through an atlas for a rash that "looks similar."
- Learn basic dermatologic terminology to communicate better with dermatology colleagues; a properly described rash can often be diagnosed by a dermatologist over the phone.

Critical Knowledge

- **Most important concept**: Is the patient with a rash acutely ill or not (sick vs. not sick)?
- Priority knowledge acquisition order:
    1. Learn and recognize emergent conditions.
    2. Learn common disorders and their variants.
    3. Learn normal variants (nonpathologic conditions).

Diagnostic Strategies
Skin Lesion Terminology
- Types
  - ► Flat lesions – macule <1 cm <patch
  - ► Raised lesions – papule <1 cm <nodule
  - ► Plaque (raised >1 cm; diameter >height, often scaled surface)
  - ► Vesicle <1 cm <bulla (fluid-filled)
  - ► Pustule <1 cm <abscess or cyst
  - ► Erosion (thin epidermis loss)
  - ► Ulcer (full-thickness loss)
- **Color** – white, brown, pink/red (erythematous), purple (violaceous), yellow
- **Border** – well-defined (circumscribed), ill-defined.
- **Shape** – round, oval, irregular, raised, pedunculated (stalk), annular, linear, serpiginous
- **Distribution** – generalized, acral (extremities), central, focal/discrete, grouped
- **Recommended Diagnostic Approaches**
  - ► Diagnostic algorithm by Peter Lynch, MD[1] – electronic application in development.
  - ► Review each condition then use a print or online dermatology atlas to review multiple images of same condition (review variants).

Categories
- **Emergent/urgent** – Meningococcemia, Kawasaki's disease (KD), Rocky Mountain spotted fever (RMSF, *Rickettsia*), *Staphylococcal* scalded skin syndrome, erythema multiforme major (maximal variant) → Stevens-Johnson syndrome/toxic epidermal necrolysis (TEN), toxic shock syndrome (TSS). Less common: Drug reaction with eosinophilia and systemic symptoms (DRESS), purpura fulminans, melanoma.
- **Newborn skin variants (nonpathologic)** – salmon patch, milia, port-wine stain, Mongolian spots, infantile acne, sucking blisters, hemangiomas of infancy, erythema toxicum. *(See Chapter 1.)*
- **Infectious/viral** – Viral exanthems (multiple; enteroviral; check also for enanthems: Koplick spots, oral ulcers).
  - ► 1st disease (rubeola = measles; "morbilliform" rash)

- ▶ 2nd disease (scarlet fever=strep pyogenes)
- ▶ 5th disease (erythema infectiosum, parvovirus B19)
- ▶ 6th disease (roseola infantum=HHV-6/7), herpes (simplex, zoster), molluscum contagiosum, hand-foot-and-mouth disease (HFMD=Coxsackie A-16). Varicella (chickenpox), Lyme disease, warts (verruca vulgaris), pityriasis rosea, erythema multiforme (EM-viral, drugs, idiopathic); erythema nodosum (multi), smallpox (biologic warfare agent)

- **Bacterial** — Impetigo (common, bullous), cellulitis, subcutaneous abscess/MRSA, hidradenitis supperativa, scarlet fever (scarlatiniform rash: red "sandpaper"), folliculitis, acne, pilonidal abscess

- **Fungal** — Tinea(s): pedis, capitis, corporis, cruris; candidiasis, pityriasis (tinea) versicolor

- **Environmental/other** — sunburn, insect bites (insect, fleas, bed bugs), scabies, coin-rubbing lesions (cultural), drug reactions, pityriasis rosea

- **Vascular** — urticaria, pyogenic granuloma, vasculitis (Henoch-Schonlein purpura)

- **Immunologic** — idiopathic thrombocytopenic purpura

- **Pigmented lesions** — acanthosis nigrans (metabolic syndrome), melanoma, café-au-lait (neurofibromatosis, check for axillary freckling), cloasma/melasma (pregnancy), vitiligo, blue nevus

- **Eczematous disorders** — eczema + variants (dishydrotic, atopic dermatitis) seborrheic dermatitis, perioral dermatitis, contact dermatoses (metal, allergic, poison ivy/oak), keratosis pilaris, pityriasis alba

- **Mass-like lesions** — lipoma, epidermoid (sebaceous) cyst, ganglion cyst, pyogenic granuloma

- **Oral lesions** — aphthous ulcers, herpes simplex (cold sores), hand-foot-mouth disease (HFMD), angular kelitis, thrush, gingivostomatitis

- **Genital** — pearly penile papules, genital warts, balanitis, phimosis/paraphimosis

- **STIs** — genital warts, molluscum contagiosum

- **Scalp/hair/nails** — alopecia areata, trichotillomania, pediculosis capitis (head lice)

- **Nails** — paronychia, ingrown toenail, subungual hematoma, onychomycosis (nail fungus), kerion

Review Questions

1. Which should be considered first in an acutely ill-appearing child presenting with a petechial rash?
   A. Idiopathic thrombocytic purpura
   B. Meningococcemia
   C. Henoch-Schonlein purpura
   D. Erythema infectiosum

2. A 10-year-old obese female presents with a darkened band of skin around her neck near her shirt collar. This is most likely related to:
   A. Erythema multiforme
   B. Pityriasis alba
   C. Metabolic syndrome
   D. Scabies

3. An 11-year-old female presents with symmetric redness of her cheeks. She is otherwise well-appearing. What is the most likely etiologic agent?
   A. Coxsackie A-16
   B. Parvovirus B-19
   C. *Candida albicans*
   D. 1-Adam-12

4. A 15-year-old Caucasian male presents with a rash on his chest and back with a few lesions on his neck and proximal arms. All of the lesions are slightly erythematous, appear approximately the same size except for a larger one, which he thinks appeared first. The lesions are slightly itchy with some fine scale at the center. What is the most likely diagnosis?
   A. Pityriasis alba
   B. Pityriasis (tinea) versicolor
   C. Pityriasis rosea
   D. Hidradenitis superativa

1. B
2. C
3. B
4. C

Urinary Tract Infections

Nicholas B. Hurst, MD
Abby Massey, MD

15

Critical Knowledge

- Urinary tract infection (UTI) is the single most common serious bacterial infection in infants.
- UTIs account for approximately 5% of fevers in children under 1 year of age.[1]
- Diagnosis and treatment of urinary tract infection in infants is important to prevent renal scarring, hypertension, and renal insufficiency.
- Infections in this age group may be the result of anatomical abnormalities.[2]

Background/Epidemiology/Anatomy

- Overall prevalence of UTI is 7% in those presenting with fever.
- UTIs account for 5%-14% of pediatric ED visits in the U.S.[3]
- In general, girls have a higher prevalence of urinary tract infections than boys due to anatomical differences[1] (i.e., shorter urethra and proximity to contaminants).
- Boys are more likely to have urinary tract infections during the first 3 months of life.
- The body's natural defense against urinary tract infections is to empty the bladder regularly and completely.
- Any abnormality in the urinary tract that limits or inhibits this function leads to a greater likelihood of urinary tract infections.
- Vesicoureteral reflux may be present in up to 30%-50% of children diagnosed with urinary tract infections.[4]

Diagnosis/Differential

- The first step in evaluation is "sick or not sick."
- A toxic-appearing or severely ill-appearing child with suspected UTI should be promptly treated with appropriate antimicrobial therapy.[6]
- Fever may be the only presenting symptom in infants with UTIs.
- In young infants (≤ 3 months) presenting with a fever (temperature greater than 38°C or 100.4°F), considerations for evaluation include the presence

of a serious bacterial infection, including meningitis, bacteremia, cellulitis, osteomyelitis, and urinary tract infection.

- Certain subgroups of older infants (>3 months) and toddlers should be evaluated for urinary tract infections, even in the absence of urinary symptoms (as urinary symptoms may be difficult or impossible to illicit in this age group). These include highly febrile (temperature greater than 102.2°F) in girls less than 1 year old, circumcised boys less than 6 months old, and uncircumcised boys less than 1 year old.[4]

- In older children with complaints of abdominal pain and dysuria, the differential of renal calculi, vulvovaginitis, and urethritis from STIs should be considered. If fever is also present, appendicitis should be added to the list.

- Culture is the "gold-standard" to diagnosis. Diagnosis of a urinary tract infection should be made through urinalysis and urine culture, where the former can be negative at the time of evaluation.

- For infants, toddlers, and children who are not yet potty-trained, catheterized urine samples are ideal. However, bagged urine samples can serve as a last resort evaluation due to parental refusal, but these cultures are not reliable.

- A suprapubic aspiration (SPA) should not be obtained routinely because of the degree of invasiveness, and should only be used in situations where a catheterized urine is not possible (i.e., hypospadias, adhesions).

- Urine may be obtained from a potty-trained infant/toddler via clean catch; the parents should be instructed on the proper method of cleaning prior to retrieval.

- A screening macroscopic urinalysis should be evaluated for the presence of nitrites and leukocyte esterase (an indirect test for bacteria and leukocytes, respectively).

- Microscopic analysis should be performed routinely in infants irrespective of the macroscopic analysis. Microscopic analysis allows the identification of leukocytes, bacteria, and epithelial cells (an indication of contamination) that may be present.

- Diagnosis is made when a UA shows pyuria/bacteriuria **AND** culture of a specimen obtained through cath **OR** SPA shows ≥ 50,000 CFU/mL of a uropathogen.[6]

Treatment

- Treatment of urinary tract infections is dependent on the age of the child.
- For infants 2-24 months, PO and IV routes for antibiotic treatment are equally effective.[6]
- Duration of antibiotic therapy should be at least 7 days. 10- and 14-day courses are also acceptable.[6]
- Infants less than 2 months of age with a UTI should be admitted and treated with IV antibiotics (ampicillin and cefotaxime **OR** ampicillin and gentamicin) initially. Patients may be transitioned to an outpatient oral course of antibiotics at the discretion of the admitting physician. This is usually after sepsis has been completely ruled out, and the patient has remained afebrile. Oral therapy should be tailored to the culture and sensitivity of the urine. The total duration of therapy should be 2 weeks.
- Infants between 1 and 3 months who appear acutely ill should be admitted and treated similarly to infants less than 1 month. (Their antibiotic therapy should include a third-generation cephalosporin and gentamicin.)
- With *E. coli* being a significant cause of CNS infection in neonates, consider a lumbar puncture in all children under 1 month and ill children under 2 months.
- Infants between 1 and 3 months who are not acutely ill may be managed as outpatients under the discretion of the emergency physician.
- Pyelonephritis may be treated either as an inpatient or outpatient, depending on certain patient-related factors. To be a candidate for outpatient management, the child must be nontoxic-appearing, able to tolerate oral medications without vomiting, be free of severe obstructing or refluxing uropathy, and compliant with treatment. These patients may be treated with a 10- to 14-day course of an oral third-generation cephalosporin. Children with persistent fever after the third day of treatment, or those who can no longer tolerate oral therapy (i.e., vomiting) should be reassessed for inpatient admission.

Imaging

- Renal and bladder ultrasound (RBUS)
  - ▶ Evaluate for anatomic abnormalities (i.e., cystic/dysplastic kidneys, duplicating collecting systems, renal scarring).
  - ▶ Should be performed for children <2 years with first UTIs; any age with recurrent UTIs or family history of renal/urologic disorders; or those who do not respond to appropriate antimicrobial therapy.
  - ▶ Timing of ultrasound is guided by clinical severity (within 2 days in severely ill or when improvement is not substantial).
  - ▶ May be done as an outpatient for infants discharged home from the ED.
- Voiding cystourethrogram (VCUG)
  - ▶ This test determines the presence of vesicoureteral reflux and the severity of the reflux if present (Grade 1-5).
  - ▶ Recommended for children when RBUS shows hydronephrosis, scarring, or other signs of obstruction; any age with two or more UTIs; family history of renal/urologic disorders; poor growth; or hypertension.
  - ▶ VCUG should be performed once the acute episode is over and the urine has been cleared of bacteria.
- It is the responsibility of the ED physician to inform the parents of the importance and need for follow-up imaging when a UTI is diagnosed.

Take-Home Points

- Consider UTI in a febrile infant with no apparent source.
- Diagnosis requires a UA ideally obtained through cath, clean catch, or SPA AND culture.
- Treat based on local regional sensitivities.
- Oral and IV regimens are equally effective.
- Duration of treatment should be 7, 10, or 14 days.
- RBUS for all first-time UTIs with VCUG considerations.

Algorithm for Suspected UTI in a Febrile Child from 2-24 Months[6]

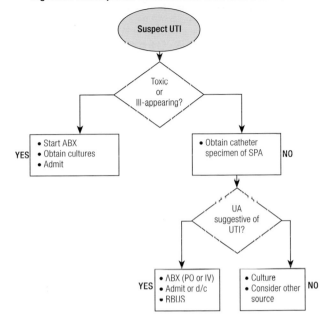

Review Questions

1. You have diagnosed an 18-month-old child in the emergency department with an uncomplicated UTI. She is tolerating PO. All of the following are acceptable treatment regimens EXCEPT:

   A. Cefixime 8 mg/kg PO daily for 7 days

   B. Amoxicillin/clavulanic acid 25 mg/kg PO BID for 14 days

   C. Ceftriaxone 75 mg/kg IV daily until afebrile

   D. Cefdinir 14 mg/kg PO daily for 3 days

2. A 6-month-old infant boy presents to the ED with his mother for complaint of a 2-day fever. Otherwise healthy, he has no significant past medical, birth, or family history. Mother reports decreased PO intake but no other symptoms. Initial vital signs include temperature 39.1°C and HR 140. Exam reveals a toxic-appearing, circumcised, Hispanic infant. Which is the next best step in management?

   A. Obtain a catheterized urine specimen for UA and culture.
   B. Acetaminophen 15 mg/kg
   C. Cefepime 75 mg/kg IV
   D. Normal saline fluid bolus at 20 mg/kg

3. You have diagnosed a 4-month-old infant girl with her first incidence of UTI in the ED. She is no longer febrile after antipyretics and is tolerating PO and has an appointment with her pediatrician for follow up in 1 week. What is the appropriate imaging strategy?

   A. No imaging necessary
   B. Renal and bladder ultrasound (RBUS) before discharge
   C. Renal and bladder ultrasound (RBUS) as an outpatient
   D. Voiding cystourethrogram (VCUG)
   E. CT abdomen/pelvis with contrast
   F. CT urography

4. A urine culture should be obtained on all urine specimens regardless of urinalysis results. True or False?

   A. True   B. False

5. What is the most common causative microorganism in pediatric UTIs?

   A. *Enterococcus*
   B. *Staphylococcus saprophyticus*
   C. *Escherichia coli*
   D. *Proteus*
   E. *Staphylococcus aureus*

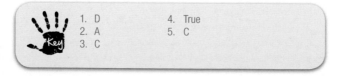

1. D	4. True
2. A	5. C
3. C	

Bronchiolitis

Hans Bradshaw, MD
Dale P. Woolridge, MD, PhD

Definition

Bronchiolitis is a constellation of clinical symptoms and signs, including a viral or bacterial lower respiratory tract infection (LRTI) prodrome in children <2 years of age. It is characterized by increased respiratory effort and wheezing not explained by pneumonia or atopy.[1,2]

Diagnosis

Bronchiolitis is diagnosed clinically based upon history of viral upper respiratory illness and physical examination finding of increased respiratory effort and wheezing in children younger than 2 years. Typical virologic causes are RSV (respiratory syncytial virus), parainfluenza, adenovirus, and influenza viruses. Radiographic or laboratory studies, including tests for specific viral agents, may support the diagnosis, but are not necessary. Radiographs of patients with bronchiolitis typically demonstrate hyperinflation and peribronchial thickening. Per the American Academy of Pediatrics (AAP), virologic tests for RSV rarely alter management decisions or outcomes; however, testing may decrease utilization of antibiotic treatment. An etiologic diagnosis also may be useful if specific antiviral therapy is considered, such as for influenza.[3,4] When an etiologic diagnosis is necessary, the recommended approach is screening by antigen detection or immunofluorescence of respiratory secretions obtained by nasal wash or nasal aspirate (rather than nasopharyngeal swabs).[5] Rapid antigen tests are available for RSV, parainfluenza, adenovirus, and influenza viruses. Culture and polymerase chain reaction (PCR) are additional methods used for viral identification. Differential diagnosis includes viral-triggered asthma or wheezing, pneumonia, chronic lung disease, foreign body aspiration, gastroesophageal reflux disease, aspiration, congenital heart disease, heart failure, and vascular rings.[7]

Clinical Presentation

Patients with bronchiolitis often have a 1-3 day history of upper respiratory tract symptoms, including rhinorrhea, mild cough, fever, and mild respiratory distress. Physical examination findings include tachypnea (respiratory rate >60–80), retractions (intercostal and subcostal), prolonged expiratory phase wheezing, coarse lung sounds or crackles, and mild hypoxemia (oxygen saturation SaO_2

<95%). Patients who are severely affected may have poor feeding, nasal flaring, expiratory grunting, cyanotic appearance, apnea, and poor peripheral perfusion. Other associated findings may include mild conjunctivitis, pharyngitis, otitis media, and urinary tract infections.[6]

Pathophysiology

Bronchiolitis typically is caused by a viral infection that affects infants younger than 2 years during the winter. The most common cause is respiratory syncytial virus (RSV) followed by *parainfluenza* virus, human *metapneumovirus*, *influenza* virus, *parainfluenza*, *adenovirus*, *rhinovirus*, *coronavirus*, human *bocavirus*, and *Mycoplasma pneumoniae*.[8] Viruses penetrate the epithelial cells in terminal bronchioles, resulting in acute inflammation, edema, increased mucus production, and bronchospasm; necrosis of epithelial cells leads to obstruction of small airways and atelectasis. Bronchiolitis is usually self-limited, with respiratory status typically improving over 2-5 days.

Emergency Department Management
Initial Assessment

- Obtain past medical history, including birth history, prior respiratory illnesses, and course.
- Conduct physical examination (auscultation, accessory muscle use, chest retractions, heart rate, respiratory rate, wheezing, inspiratory to expiratory ratio), oxygen saturation (SaO2).
- Perform chest x-ray to look for findings consistent with bronchiolitis and to exclude pneumonia or foreign bodies.
- Consider a white blood cell count, arterial blood gas, and/or electrolytes if patient is in severe respiratory distress or has altered mental status.

Treatment

- Infants whose SaO2 <92% should be treated with supplemental oxygen.
- Antipyretics are indicated for fever (acetaminophen 15 mg/kg every 4-6 hours).
- Children with tachycardia, copious nasal secretions, dry mucous membranes, and difficulty feeding safely secondary to respiratory distress should be given intravenous fluids. Rehydrate patients with 20-mL/kg boluses of normal saline up to 2-3 times, followed by maintenance intravenous fluids.

- Nasal suctioning should be performed on a routine basis if clinically obvious nasal congestion or hypoxic episodes occur. Deep suctioning of the lower pharynx or larynx is not recommended. Chest physiotherapy is also not recommended, unless obvious lobar atelectasis is present.

- Corticosteroids are not recommended in infants with RSV bronchiolitis or pneumonia. In older children, corticosteroids may be beneficial in patients with a RSV infection that may have triggered an asthma exacerbation.

- Antiviral ribavirin (a nucleoside analog that inhibits RSV) use in infants and children with RSV bronchiolitis is not routinely recommended. Ribavirin is expensive and must be given early in the course to be effective. The American Academy of Pediatrics (AAP) recommends that decisions regarding the use of ribavirin administration should be made on the basis of particular clinical circumstances (i.e., underlying congenital heart disease, lung disease, immunosuppression, the need for mechanical ventilation, and clinician experience.[3]

- Antibacterial medications should be used only in children with bronchiolitis who have indications of a co-existing bacterial infection, including pneumonia, urinary tract infections, or otitis media.

- Palivizumab (a humanized monoclonal antibody against the RSV F glycoprotein) may be administered to selected infants and children. The AAP recommends that immunoprophylaxis be considered for certain groups of children who are at risk for severe RSV infection. These include infants and young children with bronchopulmonary dysplasia, prematurity, and hemodynamically significant congenital heart disease,[1] In addition to these conditions, factors that may influence the decision to administer immunoprophylaxis include the presence of other conditions that predispose to respiratory illness (e.g., neurologic disease), distance to and availability of hospital care for severe respiratory illness, logistical difficulties of monthly administration, and cost. The dose of palivizumab is 15 mg/kg intramuscularly once per month for a total of 5 doses. The first dose is administered before the RSV season begins.

- Prevention of RSV infection includes decreasing exposure to RSV and decreasing the risk of acquisition if exposure occurs. Strategies include hand decontamination in medical and home settings, utilizing alcohol-based rubs or washing; avoiding exposure to tobacco smoke; and restricting participation in child care during RSV season for high-risk infants. Families should be educated on the importance of hand sanitation.

- Risk factors for severe disease and/or complications include gestational age <37 weeks, age <12 weeks, chronic pulmonary disease, congenital heart disease, immunodeficiency, congenital/anatomical defects of the airways, and neurologic disease.

Impending or Actual Respiratory Arrest

- These patients require intubation and mechanical ventilation with 100% oxygen and continuous nebulized albuterol (0.5 mg/kg/hr if <12 years old and 10-15 mg/hr if >12 years old).
- Admit to hospital intensive care.

Mild Respiratory Distress

- Inhaled albuterol by metered dose inhaler (MDI) or small-volume nebulizer (SVN) every 20 minutes for 3 doses:
  - ▶ Albuterol MDI with a valved spacer (1/4 to 1/3 puff/kg of 90 mcg/act, maximum 8 puffs)
  - ▶ Albuterol nebulized (0.05-0.15 mg/kg for <1 year; 1.25-2.5 mg for 1-5 years; 2.5 mg/dose for 5-12 years; 5 mg/dose for over 12 years)
- If no response to albuterol, try epinephrine SVN (0.05 mL/kg of 2.25% epinephrine diluted to 3 mL with normal saline given over 15 minutes with maximum dose of 0.5 mL/dose repeated every 2-4 hours).
- Therapy should be discontinued in patients who fail to improve rapidly.[9]

Adjunct Therapies

- 3% hypertonic saline: may reduce length of hospital stay with nonsevere viral bronchiolitis with no significant adverse effects, but not routinely recommended.[11]
- Heliox: Efficacy has been demonstrated. Not routinely recommended.[12]

Criteria for Admission

- Criteria for admission is based on a poor response to rehydration therapy, or albuterol or epinephrine therapy; a persistently elevated work of breathing; hypoxia (oxygen requirement secondary to SaO2 <92%); and history of a complicating illness, such as lung or congenital heart disease, or prematurity.[10]

Discharge Plan

- The decision for inpatient versus outpatient therapy is based on clinical judgment. Discharging to outpatient follow up is appropriate if the child has a good response to rehydration therapy and albuterol therapy via MDI or SVN every 4-6 hours or 1 2 days, tolerates feeding, requires no supplemental oxygen, and is in no respiratory distress.
- Give instructions on using a bulb syringe and demonstrate in the ED.
- Discharged patients must be seen by a primary care physician within 1-2 days.

Review Questions

1. Which of the following is NOT a risk factor for severe disease in pediatric patients with bronchiolitis?

    A. Acquired disease at ages less than 12 months

    B. History of prematurity

    C. Gestational age at birth of less than 37 weeks

    D. Underlying cardiopulmonary disease

    E. Immunodeficiency

2. Which of the following is NOT a typical treatment option for children with bronchiolitis presenting to the ED in respiratory distress?

    A. ABCs

    B. SaO2 monitoring with oxygen therapy to keep >92%

    C. Oral steroids

    D. Rehydration with intravenous fluids if indicated

    E. Trial of inhaled bronchodilators and/or epinephrine

3. Risk factors for severe disease and/or complications include:

    A. Gestational age <40 weeks

    B. Age <24 weeks, chronic pulmonary disease

    C. Congenital heart disease

    D. Immunodeficiency

    E. Gastroesophageal reflux disease

4. **Antibacterial medications should be used only in children with bronchiolitis who have indications of a co-existing bacterial infection, including:**

A. Pneumonia

B. Urinary tract infections

C. Otitis media

D. Cellulitis

E. All of the above

1. A
2. C
3. C
4. E

Asthma (Reactive Airway Disease)

Hans Bradshaw, MD
Dale P. Woolridge, MD, PhD

Definition

Asthma is a chronic inflammatory lung disease associated with repeated episodes of airway obstruction and intermittent symptoms of increased airway responsiveness.[1,2]

Diagnosis

Increased work of breathing, cough, expiratory wheeze, hypoxia, and clinical signs of respiratory distress. Key clinical signs suggesting a diagnosis of atopy associated with asthma include presence of eczema or dermatitis, seasonal allergies, and a family history of asthma. Differential diagnosis includes gastroesophageal reflux, rhinitis, aspiration of a foreign body, cystic fibrosis, or structural abnormalities of the upper and lower airways.[2]

Clinical Picture

Symptoms initially manifest as reversible airway narrowing resulting in cough, wheezing, dyspnea, and poor air exchange. Increased airway response to various triggering factors such as viral upper respiratory infections; exercise; or environmental stimuli, such as cold air, allergens, or air pollutants often precede exacerbations.[2]

Pathophysiology

Airway smooth muscle constriction, wall edema, luminal mucus accumulation, submucosal inflammatory cell infiltration, and basement membrane thickening cause airway obstruction symptoms associated with asthma. Bronchoconstriction results in decreased expiratory airflow and is typically reversible with short-acting inhaled beta-2 agonists (SABA). Asthma causes ventilation perfusion (V/Q) mismatch, resulting in hypoxemia. Beta-2 agonists may increase this mismatch due to increased blood flow in areas of the lung that are poorly ventilated. Supplemental oxygen should be utilized to keep saturations of 92% or greater to prevent long-term detrimental developmental effects.[4,5] Chronic inflammation is present in asthmatic lungs, making anti-inflammatory therapy – such as systemic glucocorticoids – essential. Treating or avoiding the underlying triggers for airway hyper-responsiveness can lessen the severity of the exacerbations.

Emergency Department Management

Guidelines of the National Asthma Education and Prevention Program and the American Academy of Allergy, Asthma, and Immunology, and the European Academy of Allergology and Clinical Immunology[1,2,3]

Initial Assessment

- ABCs
- Obtain:
    - ▶ Brief history, including past medical history, prior asthma hospitalization, and severity of events
    - ▶ Physical examination (auscultation, accessory muscle use, chest retractions, heart rate, respiratory rate, wheezing, inspiratory to expiratory ratio)
    - ▶ Peak expiratory flow rate (PEFR) in compliant children >6 years or not severely ill (see *Table 1*)[6]
    - ▶ Otherwise use pulmonary index score (PIS) based on *five* of following: respiratory rate, wheezing, inspiratory:expiratory ratio, accessory muscle use, and oxygen saturation (see *Table 2*).[7,8]
- Chest x-rays rarely alter management in acute asthma exacerbations, and are only indicated if treatment failure or acute worsening of clinical status in ED, requiring admission to rule out pneumonia, foreign bodies, vascular rings, or pneumothorax.
- Consider a white blood cell count, arterial blood gas, and/or electrolytes if patient is in severe respiratory distress or has altered mental status.
- Electrolyte disturbances (i.e., decrease in potassium, magnesium, and phosphate) may occur with continuous albuterol therapy, necessitating serum electrolyte monitoring.

Treatment

- Categorize patients with PEFR and/or PIS into either: mild-to-moderate (PEFR ≥ 40% of predicted or personal best), severe asthma exacerbation (PEFR <40%), or impending/actual respiratory arrest.
- Goal: treat hypoxemia/hypercapnia caused by airway obstruction using the following medications/interventions.

Impending or Actual Respiratory Arrest

- Mild to severe exacerbation patients all get humidified oxygen to achieve SaO2 ≥ 90%-92%.

- Intubation and mechanical ventilation if patient is not able to maintain consciousness, or in cases of severe hypoxia.
- Continuous nebulized albuterol (10 mg/hr if 5-10 kg, 15 mg/hr if 10-20 kg, 20 mg/hr if >20 kg) combined with ipratroprium (750 mcg/hr for 1st hour if <20 kg or 1500 mcg/hr for 1st hour it >20 kg) delivered with oxygen at a flow rate of 6 to 8 L/min.
- Intravenous corticosteroids (i.e., methylprednisolone 1-2 mg/kg loading dose **THEN** 0.5 mg/kg every 6 hours; maximum dose 60 mg/day).
- Adjunct therapies:
  - ▸ Magnesium sulfate (25-75 mg/kg; maximum dose of 2.5 g over 20 minutes)
  - ▸ Epinephrine IM/SubQ if no IV line (0.01 mL/kg of 1 mg/mL 1:1000 solution with maximum dose of 0.4-0.5 mg)
  - ▸ Epinephrine IV (0.1 mL/kg of 0.1 mg/mL 1:10,000 solution with maximum dose of 0.5 mg **OR** continuous IV infusion 0.1-1 mcg/kg/minute)
  - ▸ Administer antibiotics if co-morbid infection such as pneumonia exists.
- Nonstandard adjunct therapies:
  - ▸ Heliox = decreases flow resistance
  - ▸ Ketamine = bronchodilator
- Admit to pediatric intensive care unit.

Mild-to-Moderate Exacerbation

- Inhaled albuterol by metered dose inhaler (MDI) or small-volume nebulizer (SVN) every 20 minutes for 3 doses:
  - ▸ Albuterol MDI using a valved spacer (1/4 to 1/3 puff/kg of 90 mcg/act, maximum 8 puffs)
  - ▸ Albuterol nebulized (0.05-0.15 mg/kg for <1 year, 1.25-2.5 mg for 1-5 years, 2.5 mg for 5-12 years old, 5 mg for greater than 12 years)
  - ▸ Ipratropium nebulized (250 mcg/dose <20 kg, 500 mcg >20 kg)
- Oral systemic corticosteroids (i.e., prednisolone or prednisone 1-2 mg/kg with maximum dose of 60-80 mg/day)
- If no immediate response to albuterol or if recently on oral steroids:
  - ▸ Repeat assessment including physical exam, PEFR, and SaO2.
  - ▸ Continue inhaled albuterol every 20 minutes or continuous.

► Make admit decision in <1-2 hours based on symptoms and responsiveness to therapy.

Severe Exacerbation

- Oxygen
- High-dose albuterol and ipratropium by nebulizer or MDI with a valved holding chamber every 20 minutes or continuously for 1 hour
- Systemic corticosteroid treatment
- If no improvement after initial treatment, continue oxygen and nebulized albuterol hourly or continuously.
- Consider adjunct therapies, possible intubation, and mechanical ventilation.
- Admit to hospital if incomplete response with PEFR 40%-69% predicted/personal best and continued symptoms (i.e., oxygen requirement, accessory muscle use, chest retractions).
- Admit to hospital if poor response with PEFR <40% predicted/personal best, partial pressure carbon dioxide (PCO_2) ≥42 Hg, and symptoms including drowsiness and confusion.

Criteria for Admission

- Requires albuterol therapy more than every 3 hours despite steroids
- Requires supplemental oxygen
- Consider if patient has history of rapid respiratory failure with recent/past exacerbations, medication noncompliance, lack of access to medical care, or poor social support at home.

Discharge Plan

- Continue inhaled albuterol treatment every 4-6 hours for 2-3 days until seen by a primary care physician.
- Continue 5-7 day course of oral systemic corticosteroid.
- Provide patient education (i.e., medication review, inhaler/nebulizer technique training, review/initiate asthma action plan, environmental control measures, ensure close medical follow up).
- Consider initiation of an inhaled corticosterioid (i.e., budesonide MDI 200 mcg/act 1 inhalation twice daily if >6 years old with maximum dose 4 inhalations/day; budesonide nebulizer for children 1-8 years old with no prior steroid use 0.5 mg/day maximum dose; and with prior steroid use 1 mg/day maximum dose).

Table 1. Predicted Average Peak Expiratory Flow Rates for Normal Children

Height (cm)	PEFR (LPM)
109	147
112	160
114	178
117	187
119	200
122	214
124	227
127	240
130	254
132	267
135	280
137	293
140	307

Height (cm)	PEFR (LPM)
142	320
145	334
147	347
150	360
152	373
155	387
157	400
160	413
163	427
165	440
168	454
170	467

Table 2. Pulmonary Index Score

Score	Respiratory Rate	Wheezing	Inspiratory/ Expiratory Ratio	Use of Accessory Muscle	SaO2%
0	<30	0	2:1	0	>95
1	31-45	End expiration	1:1	Mild	93-95
2	46-60	Entire expiration	1:2	Moderate	90-92
3	>60	Inspiration and expiration	1:3	Severe	<90

- Score range 0-12
    - ▶ <7 mild asthma attack
    - ▶ 7-11 moderate attack = likely admission
    - ▶ >12 severe attack = admit!
- Consider a severe attack in patients unable to speak words (if age-appropriate).

Review Questions

1. Which of the following is NOT a contributing feature to the pathophysiology of asthma?
   A. Airway smooth-muscle constriction
   B. Alveolar spasm
   C. Bronchial wall edema
   D. Bronchial luminal mucus accumulation
   E. Submucosal inflammatory cell infiltration

2. Medications beneficial in severe exacerbations of asthma include:
   A. High-dose inhaled albuterol
   B. Inhaled ipratropium bromide
   C. Oral systemic corticosteroids
   D. Inhaled corticosteroids
   E. Intravenous magnesium sulfate

3. What is the first critical action in treating a pediatric patient with an asthma exacerbation?
   A. ABCs
   B. SaO_2 monitoring with oxygen therapy to keep >92%
   C. Determine PEFR and categorize patient as mild-to-moderate or severe exacerbation
   D. Initiate appropriate albuterol, ipratroprium, corticosteroid, and adjunct therapies
   E. Chest x-ray

4. Benefits of glucocorticoids include:
   A. Early use prevents 1 of 8 hospital admissions.
   B. Oral administration is effective.
   C. Decreased times to clinical improvement and discharge.
   D. Using a steroid that has a longer half-life has been shown to improve compliance.
   E. Inhaled steroids are another treatment option.
   F. All of the above

1. B
2. D
3. A
4. F

Pediatric Pneumonia

Charles Gillespie, MD

Critical Actions

- ABCs, IV, O_2, monitor, pulse oximetry, CXR, CBC
- Consider septic workup in very young and/or toxic-appearing patients.
- Shortness of breath is NOT always pulmonary in origin; consider cardiac dysrhythmia/dysfunction and congestive heart failure.
- Administer empiric antibiotics based on most likely etiologic agents, age of the child, and underlying risk factors.
- Disposition decisions should be based on illness severity, degree of intervention, age of the child, and reliability for follow up.

Background/Epidemiology

- Pneumonia is inflammation of lung tissue from infectious/noninfectious causes.
- Infection may be spread person-to-person by droplet, or via contaminated objects.
- Pneumonia typically follows upper-respiratory infection with subsequent colonization of the lower respiratory tract or, less commonly, by direct hematogenous spread.
- The World Health Organization (WHO) has documented 150 million cases in children <5 years old worldwide, with 20 million requiring hospitalization.
- The WHO cites pneumonia as a major cause of death of children <5 years:
  ▶ 20% in developing countries (29%, including severe neonatal infections)
  ▶ 2% in the industrialized world (5%, including severe neonatal infections)
- Risk factors that increase incidence:
  ▶ Very young (especially prematurity)
  ▶ Chronically ill or immunosuppressed
  ▶ Low socioeconomic status
  ▶ Malnutrition

- ► Tobacco exposure
- ► Daycare
- Immunizations have dramatically reduced the incidence of specific causes of pneumonia.
  - ► *Haemophilus influenzae* type b (Hib) pneumonia has decreased by 99% to fewer than 3 cases per 100,000 in children <5 years who have completed the primary series of Hib vaccines.
  - ► Radiographically diagnosed pneumococcal pneumonia has been reduced by 20% in children who have received the heptavalent pneumococcal vaccine (PCV7 or Prevnar).

Causes of Pneumonia

- The identification of etiological agents is imprecise.
  - ► Most are identified by sampling upper-airway secretions or serology.
    - Questions remain as to generalizability to lower respiratory tract infections.
  - ► Recent comprehensive investigations have failed to identify a specific microbe in 21% of patients with pneumonia.
- Causative organisms vary with age (*Table 1*).
  - ► Viral (60%-90%)
    - RSV and parainfluenza are most common
    - Others: influenza, adenovirus, enterovirus, rhinovirus, measles, varicella, rubella, herpes simplex virus, cytomegalovirus, Epstein-Barr virus, hantavirus
  - ► Bacterial
    - More common in hospitalized children and in newborns
    - Typicals: *Strep pneumoniae, Staph aureus, Haemophilus influenzae, Pseudomonas aeruginosa*
    - Atypicals: *Mycoplasma, Chlamydophila pneumoniae*
  - ► Fungal, protozoal and tuberculosis
    - Consider in chronic pneumonia
    - TB risk factors: urban, immigrant, exposure, immunosuppressed
    - May exhibit geographical predominance
      - — Histoplasmosis, coccidiomycosis, blastomycosis

Clinical Features

- Symptoms in neonates and young infants
  - ► Lethargy, poor feeding
  - ► Fever or hypothermia
  - ► Apnea, flaring, grunting, tachypnea
  - ► Vomiting, diarrhea
  - ► Bradycardia and shock
- Symptoms in older children
  - ► Malaise, headache
  - ► Fever, chills
  - ► Cough with sputum production
  - ► Dyspnea, pleuritic chest pain
- Physical exam signs
  - ► Fever
    - Ear/forehead/rectal temperature >100.4°F (38°C)
    - Oral temperature >100°F (37.8°C)
    - Axillary temperature >99°F (37.2C)
  - ► Tachypnea
    - RR >60 in infants <2 months
    - RR >50 in infants 2 to 12 months
    - RR >40 in children 1 to 5 years
    - RR >20 in children >5 years
  - ► Tachycardia
    - HR >150 in newborns <1 month
    - HR >130 in infants >6 months
    - HR >100 in children >6 years
  - ► Presence of suprasternal, subcostal, or intercostal retractions
  - ► Grunting
  - ► Nasal flaring
  - ► Tactile fremitus
  - ► Dullness to percussion
  - ► Egophony
  - ► Rales

Diagnostic Evaluation

- Approach to diagnosis may vary.
  - ► Based on epidemiological factors (fever, cough, hypoxia; very *sensitive*)
  - ► Based on treatment guidelines (signs/symptoms associated with radiological/microbiological confirmation; very *specific*)
- CXR
  - ► May be unnecessary for patients with suspected community-acquired pneumonia (CAP), who are well enough for outpatient therapy with antibiotics.
  - ► Posterior-anterior and lateral views are recommended for patients with hypoxemia, respiratory distress, failure to outpatient therapy, concern for pleural effusions, and fever of unknown origin.
  - ► Typical radiological findings
    - Bacterial: lobar/segmental consolidation
    - Viral/atypical bacterial: diffuse, patchy, interstitial infiltrate, hyperinflation, peribronchial thickening/cuffing, and atelectasis
    - Findings may vary and overlap, so are not 100% reliable.
- Laboratory testing
  - ► Should be guided by history and physical exam, severity of illness, and co-morbidities.
  - ► CBC
    - Cannot reliably differentiate bacterial versus viral infection
    - Bacterial: ↑WBC count with a left shift (neutrophils)
    - Viral: ↑WBC count with a right shift (lymphocytes)
  - ► Blood culture
    - Positive in ≤10% cases
    - Incidence of bacteremia is rare outside the neonatal period.
    - Not part of outpatient management strategy for otherwise-healthy, fully-immunized children.
    - Part of inpatient management strategy for patients with moderate to severe pneumonia, those returning with clinical deterioration despite outpatient therapy, and part of the workup of newborns.
    - ► Acute-phase reactants (C-reactive protein, erythrocyte sedimentation rate)

- Cannot discriminate between viral versus bacterial causes.
- C-reactive protein: closer correlation with bacteremia and lobar infiltrates than an elevated WBC count.
- In hospitalized patients, may be used in conjunction with clinical findings to assess response to therapy.

► Sputum culture and gram stain
- May help guide antibiotic therapy, though 50% nondiagnostic.
- Consider in hospitalized children able to produce sputum.
- Difficult to obtain in small children.

► Nasopharyngeal/oropharyngeal culture and gram stain
- May detect chlamydophila, pertussis, mycoplasma.
- Ineffective screen for pneumococcal disease in lower respiratory tract.

► Rapid antigen tests for RSV, influenza are available.
- Positive screens may influence treatment strategies in the absence of clinical, radiological, or laboratory findings suggestive of bacterial co-infection.

► Consider PPD skin test for suspicion of tuberculosis.

► Order urine and CSF cultures for neonates at risk for sepsis/meningitis.

Differential Diagnosis

- Allergic alveolitis
- Aspiration pneumonitis
- Atelectasis
- Bronchopulmonary dysplasia
- Chronic pulmonary disease (cystic fibrosis, asthma)
- Coccidiomycosis
- Congenital heart disease/CHF
- Congenital pulmonary abnormalities
- Empyema
- Foreign body aspiration
- Pneumatocele
- Pneumothorax
- Misinterpreted radiological study

- Neoplasm
- Tuberculosis

Critical Concepts

- With treatment, most uncomplicated bacterial pneumonia improves in 1-2 days.
- Immunizations dramatically decrease the incidence of *Haemophilus influenzae* type b and *Strep pneumoniae.*
- Bacterial pneumonia may be preceded by, or occur concomitantly with, viral upper-respiratory infections.
- RSV pneumonia rarely occurs with bacterial co-infection.
- Investigate underlying causes of recurrent pneumonia, such as:
  - ▶ Abnormal secretions/clearance (CF, asthma, ciliary dyskinesia)
  - ▶ Airway obstruction (foreign body, vascular ring, cysts, malignancy)
  - ▶ Aspiration susceptibility (gastroesophageal reflux, vocal cord paralysis, neuromuscular disease, seizure disorder)
  - ▶ Congenital heart disease (especially those with L→R shunt lesions)
  - ▶ Immunodeficiency (HIV, chronic granulomatous disease, hypogammaglobulnemia)
  - ▶ Persistent parapneumonic effusions/empyema
  - ▶ Pulmonary anomalies (bronchopulmonary dysplasia, pulmonary sequestration, tracheoesophageal fistula, tracheal stenosis)
- Remember that infiltrates on CXR may persist for weeks to months following resolution of illness.

Treatment

- Treat hypoxia with supplemental oxygen.
- Treat dehydration with IVF (tachypnea increases insensible water loss).
- Treat fever with acetaminophen/ibuprofen.
- Consider bronchodilators for significant bronchospasm/wheezing.
- Treat empirically with antibiotics based on age and suspected etiology (*Table 2*).

Disposition

- Most cases can be treated on an outpatient basis with close follow up recommended within 24-48 hours.
- Admission considerations:
  - ▶ Children <3 months
  - ▶ History of apnea, cyanosis, desaturation with crying, feeding, or exertion
  - ▶ Underlying lung disease or prematurity
  - ▶ Significant co-morbidities (cardiac, hematologic, immunologic, metabolic, neuromuscular disorders)
  - ▶ Children who appear toxic, dyspneic, or hypoxic (<90%-93% SaO$_2$ at S.L.)
  - ▶ Children who cannot tolerate PO fluids or medications
  - ▶ Evidence of significant pleural effusion on CXR
  - ▶ Suspected bacterial pneumonia in infants (especially multilobar involvement)
  - ▶ Suspected aspiration pneumonia (higher likelihood of progression)
  - ▶ Suspected *staphlococcal* or Hib pneumonia (e.g., pneumatocele on CXR)
  - ▶ Poor response to outpatient therapy within 24-48 hours
  - ▶ Unsupportive family situation

Table 1. Common Etiologies of Pediatric Pneumonia

Age	Organism	Comments
Neonates (<28 days)	Bacteria Group B strep, *E. coli*, *Klebsiella*, *Listeria* Viruses	Neonates: bacterial >viral causes due to aspiration of maternal flora during birth

2 weeks – 2 months	Viruses
	Bacteria
	  Strep pneumo; *Staph aureus*; *Chlamydia*; *Haemophilus*
	  (Hib and non-type b)
		Chlamydia: afebrile pneumonitis with staccato cough and rales in otherwise well infant occurring between 2-19 weeks after birth

2 months – 3 years	Viruses
	Bacteria
	  Strep pneumo; *Staph aureus*
	  Haemophilus
	  (Hib and non-type b)
		Hib ⇓ 99% after conjugate vaccines introduced; asymptomatic colonization with non-type b is common (40%-80%)

continued on next page

Age	Organism	Comments
3 years – 12 years	Viruses Bacteria *Strep pneumo; Mycoplasma* *Chlamydophila*	*S. pneumo* infections ⇓ 80% after PCV7 vaccines introduced; high-risk patients include those with sickle cell, HIV, asplenia, cochlear implant; *Chlamydophila* presents similarly to mycoplasma; treat with macrolides
13 years – 19 years	Viruses Bacteria *Strep pneumo; Mycoplasma;* *Chlamydophila*	*Mycoplasma* most common etiology in school-aged children, especially 10-15 years

Table 2. Common Therapies for Pediatric Pneumonia

Patient Characteristics	Inpatient Therapy (IV)	Outpatient Therapy (PO)
Neonates (<28 days)	*Ampicillin* 50 mg/kg/dose **PLUS** *cefotaxime* 50 mg/kg/dose **OR** *gentamycin* 2.5 mg/kg/dose	Not recommended Consider *acyclovir* 10 mg/kg/dose
1 – 3 months (symptoms of chlamydia)	*Erythromycin** 10 mg/kg/dose **OR** *azithromycin* 10 mg/kg/dose; if febrile add: *cefotaxime* 50 mg/kg/dose if lobar pneumonia: *ampicillin* 50 mg/kg/dose (to cover *S. Pneumo*)	*Azithromycin* 10 mg/kg on day 1; 5 mg/kg on days 2-5 **OR** *erythromycin* 10 mg/kg/dose (*reports of hypertrophic pyloric stenosis and V-tach in neonates)
1 month – 5 years	*Ampicillin* 50 mg/kg/dose (if fully immunized) **OR** *cefotaxime* 50 mg/kg/dose (if very ill or not fully immunized) **OR** *ceftriaxone* 50 mg/kg/dose IM (if poor POs during first 24 hrs) **ADD** *azithromycin* 10 mg/kg/dose (if atypical infection suspected) **ADD** *vancomycin* 20 mg/kg/dose **OR** *clindamycin* 5 mg/kg/dose (if concern for MRSA)	*Amoxicillin* 45 mg/kg/dose **OR** *azithromycin* 10 mg/kg on day 1 **THEN** 5 mg/kg/day × 4 days (Higher prevalence of macrolide-resistant *S. Pneumo* in patients <5 years, as well reports of macrolide-resistant *Mycoplasma*)

6 – 18 years	*Ceftriaxone* 50 mg/kg/dose **OR** *cefotaxime* 50 mg/kg/dose **PLUS** *azithromycin* 10 mg/kg/dose	*Amoxicillin* 90-100 mg/kg/day divided into 2-3 doses per day (nonsevere cases)
		Otherwise, if non-type 1 hypersensitivity allergic reaction (i.e, rash) to penicillin, a 3rd-generation cephalosporin acceptable alternative: *cefdinir* 14 mg/kg/dose divided into 2 doses per day
		If type 1 hypersensitivity (i.e., anaphylaxis) to penicillin: *clindamycin* 30 mg/kg/dose divided into 3-4 doses per day next reasonable alternative.
Critically ill or suspected resistant S. pneumoniae	To standard therapy **AND** *vancomycin* 20 mg/kg/dose	Not recommended
Vent dependent or multiple hospitalizations • **Suspect Pseudomonas, though frequently polymicrobial** (e.g., *S. aureus, Klebsiella, E. coli*)	*Ceftazidime* 50 mg/kg/dose **OR** *cefepime* 50 mg/kg/dose **OR** *meropenem* 20 mg/kg/dose (MRSA & gram negs) +/- *vancomycin* 20 mg/kg/dose (MRSA)	Not recommended
Viral pneumonia • **Antibiotics not useful** • **Most resolve with supportive care** • **May predispose to bacterial infection**	HIV patients with PCP pneumonia *TMP-SMX* 20 mg/kg/day Influenza A or B: *oseltamivir* (≥1 yo) *zanamivir* (>7 yo) May ⇓ duration of illness by 1 day, but not shown to prevent influenza-related complications (i.e., viral or bacterial PNA)	RSV prophylaxis for infants (<2 years) with CLD, congenital heart disease, or preterm birth (<32 weeks gestation): *palivizumab* 15 mg/kg/dose IM *Amantadine, rimantadine* no longer recommended for influenza due to widespread resistance

Review Questions

1. **Which organism often produces pneumonia without fever?**
   - A. *Streptococcus pneumoniae*
   - B. *Bordatella pertussis*
   - C. *Chlamydia trachomatis*
   - D. *Mycoplasma pneumonia*

2. **In which age group do bacterial organisms produce the most cases of pneumonia?**
   - A. 0 to 3 weeks
   - B. 3 months to 3 years
   - C. 3 to 13 years

3. **Match the presentation to the diagnosis.**
   - A. Abrupt-onset, high fever, productive cough
   - B. Nontoxic, afebrile, dry cough
   - C. Sore throat, abdominal pain, persistent cough
   - D. Rapid deterioration following outpatient therapy

   1. *Mycoplasma PNA*
   2. *Staph PNA*
   3. *Strep PNA*
   4. *Chlamydial PNA*

4. **Match the organism to the patient.**
   - A. *Mycoplasma pneumoniae*
   - B. *Pneumocystis jiroveci*
   - C. Group B Strep
   - D. *Hemophilus influenzae* type b

   1. Newborn, no prenatal care
   2. 8 years, transplant patient
   3. 4 years, non-immunized
   4. 15 years, male smoker

5. **Match the drug to the bug.**
   - A. Azithromycin PO
   - B. Amoxicillin PO
   - C. TMP/SMX PO
   - D. Vancomycin IV

   1. *Pneumocystis jiroveci pneumoniae*
   2. *Staph pneumoniae*
   3. *Mycoplasma pneumoniae*
   4. *Strep pneumoniae*

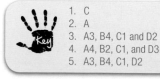

1. C
2. A
3. A3, B4, C1 and D2
4. A4, B2, C1, and D3
5. A3, B4, C1, D2

Sedation

Garrett S. Pacheco, MD
Lisa Doyle, MD

Critical Knowledge

- It is important for the emergency physician to be well-versed in performing procedural sedation.
- The provider needs to be skilled in pediatric resuscitation and management of the pediatric airway.
- The emergency physician should be comfortable with available treatment agents for sedation.
- Providers should be familiar with and able to respond appropriately to adverse reactions to common sedative agents.

Background

- The practice of pediatric sedation has significantly evolved with new pharmacologic agents, improved continuous monitoring, and safety protocols.
- Procedural sedation is a safe, effective, and humane way to facilitate appropriate medical care.
- The emergency physician should identify goals during pre-sedation (i.e., anxiolysis, analgesia, amnesia, sedation, or all of these factors).
- Pre-sedation, intra-sedation, and post-sedation assessment are paramount.
- The emergency physician should have a firm grasp and understanding of the available modalities for providing safe and effective sedation for painful or anxiety-provoking procedures.

Critical Concepts

- Nonpharmacologic measures should be the first option to reduce anxiety and pain in the ED.
- It is important to keep in mind the developmental and cognitive ability of a patient when performing sedation and obtaining analgesia.
- Children between the ages of 2-7 years rarely benefit from a reasoned explanation for a procedure. Children ≥8 years do benefit from an explanation.

- Involvement of a child life specialist can be extremely beneficial in preparing patients for sedation procedures.
- Keep in mind that parents can aid in keeping the patient calm, but they also can be a source of anxiety for the child.

Commonly Used Sedative Agents

Class	Drug	Route	Dose	Onset	Duration	Disadvantages
Anxiolytic	Midazolam	PO, PR, IV, IM, IN	PO/PR 0.5mg/kg IV/ IM 0.1 mg/kg IN 0.2 mg/kg	PO/PR 20-30 min, IV 1 min, IM 5-10 min, IN 5 min	1-4 hrs	No analgesia, paradoxical reaction, respiratory depression, and hypotension
	Lorazepam	PO, IV	0.05	PO 60 min, IV 15-30 min	8-12 hrs	Prolonged duration of action
Hypnotic/ sedative	Propofol	IV	1-2 mg/kg Max unit dose (100 mg) Repeat 0.05 mg/kg	Seconds	Minutes (~6-10 min)	No analgesia, respiratory and CV depression
	Etomidate	IV	0.1-0.3 mg/kg Max unit dose (300 mg)	Seconds	Minutes (15-20 min)	No analgesia, myoclonus, respiratory depression
	Methohexital	IV	1 mg/kg Max unit dose (100 mg)	Seconds	10-90 min	No analgesia, respiratory and CV depressant
	Pentobarbital	IV	2-5 mg/kg Max unit dose (200 mg)	<1 min	30-90 min	No analgesia, respiratory and CV depressant

Dissociative	Ketamine	IV, IM, PO	IV 1-2 mg/kg IM 3-4 mg/kg PO 6-10 mg/kg	IV 1-2 min, IM 3-5 min, PO 30 min	IV 0.5-1 hr, IM 1-2 hrs, PO 2-3 hrs	Increased ICP, intraocular pressure, emetogenesis, hypersalivation, emergence
Combinations	Fentanyl + midazolam	IV	Fentanyl 1-2 mcg/kg, midazolam 0.05-0.1 mg/kg	IV 1-2 min	1-3 hrs	Respiratory depressant increased with combination
	Ketofol (ketamine + propofol)	IV	Propofol 1 mg/kg, ketamine 0.5 mg/kg	1 min	Propofol (minutes); ketamine 15-45 min	Dose regimens vary; modest advantage profile

Derived from the Harriet Lane Handbook, 2012

Treatment

- Ketamine
  - ► Ketamine is the most commonly used agent in the United States for pediatric sedation.
  - ► Can cause a disconnection between the thalamocortical and limbic systems, resulting in amnesia, sedation, and analgesia.
  - ► Minimum dissociative dose is achieved with 1.5 mg/kg IV and 4 to 5 mg/kg IM.
  - ► Should not be used for patients younger than 3 months.
  - ► Not necessary to pretreat with atropine and glycopyrrolate.
  - ► The emetogenic effect of ketamine can be decreased with the use of odansetron.
- Etomidate
  - ► Etomidate is a hypnotic that can safely be used for procedural sedation and analgesia.
  - ► Numerous studies have found it to be efficacious where immobility is desired, such as with diagnostic imaging.
  - ► Has the advantage of having minimal hemodynamic effects compared to other sedating agents.

- For children 10 years and older, the recommended dosing is 0.1-0.3 mg/kg.
- Theoretical risk of adrenal suppression with a one-time dose; providers may want to withhold in patients for whom sepsis is a concern.

- Ketamine and propofol
  - Can be in separate syringes or a single mixed 1:1 syringe (ketofol).
  - The mixing of these agents leads to drug doses lower then the amount required by each agent alone.
  - The emetogenic effect of ketamine is offset by the antiemetic properties of propofol.
  - The emergence reaction seen with ketamine is counterbalanced by the sedative properties of propofol.
  - The hypotension and respiratory depression of propofol are counterbalanced by the sympathomimetic and preservation of the respiratory drive of ketamine.
  - The use of ketofol leads to a shorter recovery time, lower incidence of recovery agitation, and less vomiting.

- Dexmedetomidine
  - Dexmedetomidine is fairly new to pediatric sedation.
  - This agent is useful in painless procedures such as diagnostic imaging, but has the disadvantage of requiring a loading dose over 10 minutes.
  - There is little existing data regarding the optimal dose in pediatrics, but most use 1 mcg/kg over 10 minutes followed by an infusion of 0.5 mcg/kg/hr.

Treatment for the "Ouchless ED"

- Nitrous oxide
  - This agent has been successfully used in the emergency department setting due to its quick onset of action, low incidence of complications, and the rapid return to the patient's baseline level of consciousness.
  - Can be administered without causing pain by not requiring venipuncture.
  - High-concentration continuous flow nitrous oxide (70%) is safe in patients age 1 to 17 years.
  - The most common adverse reactions are vomiting, agitation, and nausea.

- Intranasal midazolam
  - ▶ Is an effective way to obtain sedation without causing pain or discomfort by giving an intramuscular or intravenous injection.
  - ▶ Dosed at 0.2-0.3 mg/kg and will have an onset of 10 minutes.
  - ▶ It has been reported to be irritating to the nasal mucosa.
  - ▶ Oral midazolam can be given in a flavor that is easy for children to take with doses 0.5 mg/kg.

Suggested Checklist for the Essentials of Sedation

Pre-sedation history and physical
Pre-sedation vital signs
PALS resuscitation equipment – SOAP ME
Age-appropriate airway equipment
Continuous cardiac monitoring, noninvasive BP, end tidal CO2 monitoring
Supplemental oxygen
Ability to obtain rapid IV access if using IM sedation

- During the sedation, vital signs should be monitored continuously.
- The most dangerous part of the sedation is AFTER the procedure, when the noxious stimulus is over; this is the time when respiratory depression will most likely occur.
- A child should not be discharged home until the following conditions are met:
  - ▶ Protecting own airway and tolerating PO
  - ▶ Returned to a baseline mental and ambulatory status that is developmentally appropriate
  - ▶ Pain is well-controlled

Review Questions

1. **A 2-year-old arrives in your emergency department after a head injury. She has a boggy right parietal scalp hematoma and needs a brain CT. She is sleepy with purposeful movements and is inconsolable. What are good options for sedation for the CT?**

   A. Midazolam   B. Propofol

   C. Ketamine   D. Etomidate

   E. A or B

2. A 13-year-old asthmatic child arrives with a significantly angulated distal radius fracture. She needs her fracture reduced. She had "some water" at soccer practice 2 hours ago and last ate solids "during lunch at school." She has no allergies and only uses her albuterol inhaler about once a month when she exercises outside. Is she a good candidate for procedural sedation for her fracture reduction?

    A. No! She needs to be NPO for at least 8 hours.

    B. No! She is an asthmatic.

    C. Yes! She meets the ASA NPO guidelines for a safe sedation.

    D. Yes! She is an ASA class II, with a mild systemic disease that is well-controlled on medications.

    E. C and D

3. A healthy 8-year-old male arrives with extensive road rash, multiple lacerations, and embedded gravel after a scooter crash. These are his only injuries. He requires debridement, foreign body removal, and laceration repairs. He weighs 30 kg. What is the best way to proceed?

    A. Scrub away! Haven't you heard of "brutane"?

    B. Apply copious amounts of viscous lidocaine to the road rash and inject the lacerations and foreign bodies with as much local lidocaine as needed to achieve analgesia.

    C. Use ketamine as a dissociative anesthetic, or a combination of an opioid analgesic and a sedative.

    D. Use procedural sedation along with distraction techniques and adjunct local analgesia.

    E. C or D

1. E
2. E
3. E

Analgesia

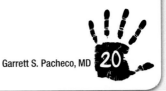

Garrett S. Pacheco, MD 20

Critical Knowledge

- The emergency physician should be aware that analgesia is often underutilized in pediatrics.
- There should be a thorough understanding of the child's developmental level and how this can affect pain assessment.
- The emergency physician should be comfortable with the available analgesia agents and their adverse effects.

Background

- The treatment of pain has often been criticized as being poorly delivered in the pediatric population.
- It is unclear if this is secondary to the lack of experience needed to do so effectively, the inability to quantify pain in young children, or the physician being uncomfortable with the pharmacology in this population.
- There has been stigma attached to the use of opiates in pediatrics due to their side effects, as well as a risk of addiction or dependency that outweighs the need to treat pain.
- Common causes of pain such as constipation, headaches, fractures, lacerations, trauma, sickle cell disease, and otitis media are often addressed in the emergency department.
- It is vital that emergency clinicians be able to manage pain both aggressively and safely.

Critical Concepts

- It is difficult to quantify pain in infants and toddlers.
- Neonates and infants have physiologic responses to pain such as increased blood pressure, respiratory rate, heart rate, crying, flushing, facial expressions, and body movements.
- There are many pediatric pain assessment tools available to help identify pain; emergency practitioners should be aware of which methods are used in their ED.

- There are established and validated self-reported pain scales for children as young as 3 years old, including:
  - ► **N**eonatal **P**ain, **A**gitation and **S**edation **S**cale (N-PASS) and **N**eonatal **I**nfant **P**ain **S**cale (NIPS) are useful in neonates. In addition, the **F**aces, **L**egs, **A**ctivity, **C**ry and **C**onsolability (FLACC) Scale can be used.
  - ► Preschoolers (3-4 years old) benefit from the OUCHER scale.
  - ► Older children can use the FACES scale.
  - ► >12-year-olds can use a numeric scale from 1 to 10.
- The change in the value of the absolute pain score is the most important feature of these scale assessments to gauge the effectiveness of an intervention.
- The *initial* scale used should be the same scale used when *reassessing* a patient's pain.

Treatments

Painless Options to Achieve Analgesia

- Nonpharmacologic measures have been shown to reduce pain, including techniques of distraction and imagery, hypnosis, breathing exercises, and rehearsal.
- High-concentration sucrose solutions are effective in children up to 6 months when 1-2 mL is placed in the cheek with a syringe or pacifier.
- LMX is a topical anesthetic agent composed of 4% lidocaine that has an onset of action of 30 minutes; the effect can last up to 1 hour.
- LET gel (**l**idocaine, **e**pinephrine, **t**etracaine):
  - ► LET is an effective agent used to pretreat and lessen the pain of venipuncture, laceration repair, and lumbar puncture.
  - ► Can be applied painlessly to an open wound.
  - ► Most appropriate for lacerations <5 cm to avoid excess administration and intoxication.
  - ► Onset of action for LET is 20 to 30 minutes.
  - ► Most concerning adverse reaction is methemoglobinemia.
- EMLA cream (**e**utectic **m**ixture of **l**ocal **a**nesthetics) can be used on intact skin and contains both lidocaine and prilocaine.
  - ► 1 g for patients <5 kg
  - ► 2 g for patients >5 kg
  - ► Applied over 10 cm

▶ It takes 1 hour to achieve effect, so plan accordingly.
- The J-tip is a needle-free way of injecting 1% buffered lidocaine with an onset of action of 1-3 minutes.
- Fentanyl administered by nebulizer or intranasally may be a noninvasive way to achieve analgesia.
  ▶ Nebulized fentanyl can be given at a dose of 3 uy/kg.
  ▶ Intranasal fentanyl is dosed 1.5 mcg/kg/dose.
  ▶ Intranasal fentanyl is equivalent to IV morphine for pain relief and is a good option when IV access has not been established or will be difficult.

Local Anesthesia

- Often directed into a wound or laceration by a needle to expedite a procedure.
- Lidocaine is frequently used to achieve local anesthesia rapidly and for a duration of 60 to 90 minutes; maximum dose 4-5 mg/kg *without* epinephrine.
- Lidocaine *with* epinephrine is used to reduce the amount of bleeding (vasoconstrictive effect) and reduces systemic absorption with a maximum dose of 7 mg/kg.
- Bupivacaine is useful for when a longer duration of anesthesia (4-5 hours) is desired; maximum dose 2-3 mg/kg.

Opiate Derivatives

- Emergency physicians should be familiar with pharmacology and the potential adverse reactions of opiate medications.
- Hydrocodone in an elixir combined with acetaminophen is an effective PO medication with the hydrocodone component dosed at 0.15 mg/kg/dose (max 10 mg).
- Morphine sulfate is the most commonly used opiate medication.
  ▶ Onset of action is rapid at 4-6 minutes.
  ▶ Duration of effect for morphine is 2-3 hours when given intravenously.
  ▶ Can be administered PO, IV, IM or subcutaneously.
- Fentanyl is 100 times more potent then morphine.
  ▶ Onset of action is rapid (2-3 minutes).
  ▶ Duration of action is much shorter (30-60 minutes).

- ► One benefit of fentanyl is the lack of the histamine release side effect that occurs with morphine.
- ► Dosing is 1-2 mcg/kg/dose.
- ► Adverse reactions include nausea, vomiting, hypotension, respiratory depression, and pruritus due to histamine release.
- ► With use of fentanyl, one should know how to provide aggressive respiratory support and reversal to rigid chest syndrome with depolarizing or non-depolarizing paralytic agents such succinylcholine or rocuronium, respectively.
- • Hydromorphone can be given by IV or PO with IV dose 0.01-0.02 mg/kg/dose (max 0.2-0.8 mg).
- • Naloxone is the opioid reversal agent of choice; it is dosed at 0.1 mg/kg and can be repeated every 2-3 minutes before setting up an infusion.

Pediatric Analgesic Agents

Analgesics	Dose (mg/kg)	Route	Max Unit Dose (mg/kg)	Duration	Precautions	Comments
Morphine	0.1 - 0.2+	IM/IV/SQ	10	3-4 hrs	Histamine release/ respiratory depression	Better absorbed SQ than IM
Fentanyl	0.001-0.005	IM/IV/IN	0.05	0.5-1 hr	Rigid chest	Decrease dose in infants
Remifentanil	0.001-0.003	IV	0.05	3-4 min	Rigid chest	
Hydromor-phone	0.015	IM/IV		10		
Hydrocodone	0.2	oral	10	4-6 hrs		Combine with acetaminophen
Acetamin-ophen	15	oral/ rectal	1000	4 hrs		
Ibuprofen	10	oral	40	6-8 hrs	Asthma, anticoag-ulated	Only use in patients older than 6 mos.
Ketorolac	0.5-1	IV/IM	15-30	4-6 hrs	Same as ibuprofen	Not to exceed 48 hrs of treatment

Review Questions

1. A 7-year-old boy presents after falling off the monkey bars. He has an obvious deformity to his left wrist. What is the next best step?

   A. Give an oral analgesic such as ibuprofen or acetaminophen.

   B. Send the patient to radiology for x-rays of the left wrist.

   C. Give a dose of intranasal fentanyl while waiting for IV access.

   D. He does not appear that uncomfortable. Wait until you think he needs pain medication.

2. A 12-year-old boy presents with significant right lower quadrant tenderness. Initially his symptoms were diffuse, but over the past day have localized to McBurney's point. You are concerned about appendicitis. A surgeon will not be available for consult for several hours. How do you address this child's pain?

   A. Do nothing because any analgesia will distort the surgeon's exam.

   B. Place warm packs to the abdomen.

   C. Have child life specialist at the bedside to distract the patient.

   D. Give IV morphine immediately.

3. A 4-year-old presents after falling head-first into one of his toys. He has a laceration to his chin. After safely ruling out significant intracranial injury, you decide to anesthetize his wound. What is the best option in doing so?

   A. Lidocaine injected directly into the wound

   B. LET

   C. EMLA

   D. Vapocoolant

4. For the 4-year-old in the previous question, what is a feared complication of this agent?

   A. Tissue necrosis

   B. Dysrhythmia

   C. Seizures

   D. Methemoglobinemia

   E. B, C, and D

1. C
2. D
3. B
4. B, C, and D

Fluid Resuscitation

Larry DeLuca, MD

21

Background

Hypovolemia is the most common cause of shock in children. Hypovolemia can be *absolute* (as in hemorrhage or dehydration from diarrhea or vomiting) or *relative* (as in sepsis, where vasodilation increases the size of the "tank").

Hypovolemia can span a range of severities, from mild dehydration to circulatory collapse. Here are some useful markers to determine the severity of hypovolemia:

Hypovolemic Markers

	Mild Dehydration	Compensated Shock	Decompensated Shock	Circulatory Collapse
Heart rate	Normal or slightly tachycardic	Slight tachycardia	Moderate tachycardia	Severe tachycardia
Blood pressure	Normal	Low-normal	Low	Low or absent
Capillary refill	<2 seconds	>2 seconds	>3 seconds	>5 seconds
Pulses	Strong	Proximal strong, distal weak	Proximal weak, distal absent	Proximal weak or absent
Mental status	Normal	Irritable or confused	Agitated or lethargic	Obtunded or comatose

Adapted from American College of Surgeons' Committee on Trauma, from *Advanced Trauma Life Support for Doctors (ATLS) Student Manual*, 2004, 7th Edition. American College of Surgeons.

Hypovolemia can have many causes, from increased insensible losses during fever to hemorrhage from trauma to vomiting and diarrhea. However, regardless of the cause of the hypovolemia, the most important initial intervention for hypovolemia from *any* cause is crystalloid fluid resuscitation.

Critical Knowledge

- Capillary refill by itself is not always reliable.
- Cold extremities can simulate shock.
- Pay close attention to mental status.

- As shock evolves, blood is shunted to the heart and brain at the expense of the periphery.
- Agitation suggests decreasing cerebral perfusion and impending decompensation.
- Hypotension in children is an ominous sign.
- Unlike adults, children will maintain a near-normal blood pressure until they are close to cardiopulmonary collapse.
- Urinary output is not useful to guide initial resuscitation, but can help assess adequacy of resuscitation over time.
- Normal urinary output is 0.5-1 mL/kg/hr.
- Neonates and infants have less urinary concentrating capability and may not conserve water as readily as older children and adults.
- Be sure to ask parents or caregivers about the number of wet diapers a child has produced compared to normal. Be sure that this represents urinary output and not volume losses from diarrhea.
- One of the most common causes of pulseless electrical activity (PEA) "cardiac arrest" is profound hypovolemia.
- One or more fluid boluses promptly administered can be lifesaving!
- Normal heart rates vary by age
  - **Newborn to 3 months** – mean 140 (awake 85-205; asleep 80-160)
  - **3 months to 2 years** – mean 130 (awake 100-190; asleep 75-160)
  - **2 years to 10 years** – mean 80 (awake 60-140; asleep 60-90)
  - **10 years and over** – mean 75 (awake 60-100; asleep 50-90)
- Normal and low-normal systolic blood pressure varies by age
  - **For children ages 1 to 10:**
    - Normal SBP = 90 mm Hg + (age × 2) mm Hg
    - Low-normal SBP = 70 mm Hg + (age × 2) mm Hg
    - For children 10 years and over, low-normal is approximately 90 mm Hg.

Clinical Presentation

There are many causes of hypovolemia. Fluid resuscitation is not definitive care, but part of patient stabilization. An important part of a successful resuscitation is identifying the factors that led to the need for fluid resuscitation and addressing them. For example, prompt administration of crystalloid fluids and blood products to a trauma patient will do little good if bleeding cannot be stopped. Aggressively search for and treat the causes of hypovolemia.

There are many different IV fluids available; during resuscitation and ongoing therapy, you may change from one fluid to another (for example, from crystalloid to packed red blood cells) as the resuscitation progresses, depending upon the patient's illness and the specifics of the clinical situation. For initial resuscitation, the fluid of choice is isotonic crystalloid (either normal saline [0.9%] or lactated Ringer's solution) given in boluses of 20 mL/kg. Once the patient is stabilized, IV fluid therapy can be adjusted based upon laboratory results (such as hematocrit or electrolyte status) and tailored to the patient's specific needs.

Fluid resuscitation does not need to occur via the IV route. For children who can tolerate oral intake but have lost volume due to fever or diarrhea, oral rehydration may be an acceptable and convenient alternative. It is important to ensure that the child can consume adequate amounts of fluid orally, or dehydration and hypovolemia will worsen. It is also important to use a balanced electrolyte solution (such as Pedialyte) for oral fluid replacement. Replacing fluid losses with water only can result in hyponatremia and other electrolyte disturbances.

In critically ill children, consider intraosseus (IO) access early on. After three unsuccessful attempts or 90 seconds of attempted IV access in a child with shock, place an IO line. The most common place for inserting an IO line is on the flat portion of the tibia that is 1 cm below and 1 cm medial to the tibial tuberosity. However, the distal femur, distal tibia, or iliac crest can also be used. Some areas are more likely for success depending on the age of the child. IO access can allow the infusion of any fluid, medication, or blood product, often at rates that exceed those of small-bore peripheral IVs.

- Be sure to address ongoing fluid needs, as well as volume deficits.
- The 4:2:1 rule is a convenient way to calculate pediatric maintenance IV rates:
  - ▶ 4 mL/kg/hr for the first 10 kg of body weight +
  - ▶ 2 mL/kg/hr for the next 10 kg of body weight +
  - ▶ 1 mL/kg/hr for the remaining kg of body weight

Example: a 25-kg child will require a maintenance rate of
$(4 \times 10) + (2 \times 10) + (1 \times 5) = 65$ mL/hr.

Judging Hydration Status in Children

The gold standard for assessing hydration status in children is the change in body weight relative to their baseline (hydrated state), as in:

% Dehydration = 100 × (Baseline weight – Illness weight) / Baseline weight

However, a child's baseline weight is not always known. In this case, studies involving rehydration usually consider the child's stable, post-resuscitation weight as a substitute for the baseline weight. While this is useful in a research study, it allows the severity of dehydration to only be assessed retrospectively if the child's baseline weight is not known.

In addition to weight, multiple assessment tools have been developed to determine the level of dehydration, all of which focus primarily on clinical signs. The World Health Organization scale is perhaps the most well-known:

Clinical Dehydration Scale

	A	B	C
Look at condition	Well, alert	Restless, irritable	Lethargic or unconscious
Eyes	Normal	Sunken	Sunken
Thirst	Drinks normally, not thirsty	Thirsty, drinks eagerly	Drinks poorly or not able to drink
Feel: skin pinch	Goes back quickly	Goes back slowly	Goes back very slowly

Scoring: Fewer than two signs from column B and C: no signs of dehydration <5%, >2 signs in column B: moderate dehydration 5-10%, >2 signs in column C: >10% severe dehydration.

Oral Rehydration Therapy

Oral rehydration therapy (ORT) is recommended as first-line therapy for children with mild to moderate dehydration. Researchers evaluated the use of ORT compared with IV fluid therapy in moderately dehydrated children and demonstrated that ORT was as effective as IVF, and that ORT was initiated more quickly for these patients. While only one-third of the ORT group required hospitalization, almost half of the IVF group was hospitalized, though this difference did not reach statistical significance.

Multiple oral rehydration fluids have been described, including the standard WHO oral rehydration solution: 1/2 teaspoon salt plus 6 teaspoons sugar dissolved in 1 liter of water. An alternative hypotonic solution containing 75 mmol/L each of glucose and sodium may reduce stool output and decrease the need for IV fluid therapy in children with diarrhea.

IV Fluid Choices for Initial Resuscitation

There are an enormous number of IV fluid formulations — some standard, some proprietary. Common prepared IV fluids vary in the amount of electrolytes, glucose, free water, and other additives they contain. Patients with normal cardiopulmonary and renal function allow more flexibility in the IV fluids they receive, as they can more effectively filter what they do not need and excrete it. Patients who are oliguric, anuric, or who have compromised cardiorespiratory function will require more precise fluid selection and management (much of which is beyond the scope of this chapter).

In adult patients, most reviews of the literature have found that there is no advantage of colloid over crystalloid solutions, however, crystalloid may be associated with lower mortality in trauma patients, and some argue that the expense of colloids is not justified.

Current literature supports a similar approach to the pediatric population. The Dutch Pediatric Society issued an evidence-based clinical practice guideline recommending isotonic saline as the first-line fluid for resuscitation of children with hypovolemia. Researchers also have found that hypotensive pre-term infants did equally well with saline compared to 5% albumin, and the saline caused less fluid retention in the first 48 hours.

For initial resuscitation, crystalloid fluids are the mainstay in modern practice, best exemplified by normal saline and lactated Ringer's. These fluids are isotonic, providing about the same osmolality as intra- and extra-cellular fluid under normal conditions. They contain only electrolytes (no proteins or glucose). In theory, they should provide minimal shifting of water across fluid compartments. Normal saline is a 0.9% solution of sodium chloride in water. The amount of sodium is in excess to that in blood – 154 mEq/L. In contast, lactated Ringer's solution contains sodium, chloride, potassium, calcium, and lactate in amounts closer to that of serum levels of these electrolytes.

While technically still crystalloid solutions, the dextrose-containing solutions such as D5, D10, etc., are not used in initial resuscitation. These solutions provide "free water." (After the dextrose is metabolized, solute-free water remains.)

Colloid solutions get their tonicity from albumin or synthetic polymers. It has been demonstrated that crystalloid solutions rapidly redistribute themselves in the body's various fluid compartments. For example, within several hours, approximately two-thirds of infused normal saline is extra-vascular. Colloid solutions were supposed to solve this problem. However, even the larger colloid particles can —and do — migrate out of the vasculature and, having done so, can occasionally worsen conditions such as peripheral edema. Colloid solutions also are more expensive and have allergenic potential. For all these reasons, crystalloid solutions have become the preferred solutions for initial resuscitation.

IV Fluid Choices for Fluid Maintenance

While isotonic crystalloids are ideal for initial resuscitation, they are poorly suited for maintenance. This is because they contain relatively large amounts of electrolytes; many crystalloids contain no glucose and no free water. Infusing normal saline for many days, for example, can lead to sodium overload (and consequent fluid retention).

The most common maintenance IV fluids are D5 ½ NS, and D10 ¼ NS for infants up to 6 months. These fluids contain ½ (or ¼, respectively) as much saline as NS, avoiding the problem of over-administration of saline. The solutions are hypotonic (providing some free water), and they contain dextrose (to help meet the body's glucose needs and reduce catabolism). The lower-sodium content of D10 ¼ NS is used with infants in the first 6 months of life because their renal concentrating ability is reduced compared to older children and adults.

Frequently, 10-20 mEq of potassium is added to each liter of maintenance fluid for patients with normal renal function.

Blood and Blood Products in Resuscitation

Blood transfusions may be required for any of a number of reasons in critically ill children, from blood loss through hemorrhage to acquired coagulopathy. While a detailed discussion of transfusion medicine is beyond the scope of this chapter, there are a few key concepts that can help guide you in selecting blood products.

While transfusion of blood products can provide lifesaving benefits to patients, there is a substantial risk of infusing blood products compared to other IV fluids. While the HIV epidemic has caused people to be concerned with the safety of transfusions from a blood-borne disease perspective, these are not the only dangers faced by transfusion recipients. Allergic reactions are not uncommon and can range from mild itching to full-blown anaphylaxis. Transfusion reactions from mistyped or non-cross-matched blood can result in hemolysis, renal failure, and death. Always take care when writing orders for blood transfusions and remember the simple maxim: *the most common cause of transfusion-related death is simple human error.*

There are three main blood products commonly used in transfusion:

Packed red blood cells are cells separated from plasma by centrifugation. They can be filtered further to remove white cells (leukoreduction), which helps reduce both disease transmission and immune-mediated transfusion reactions. Use packed red blood cells to replace blood lost in trauma if a patient fails to respond to initial crystalloid resuscitation, or for profound and symptomatic anemia.

As with adults, a conservative transfusion strategy appears to be well-tolerated. A threshold of 7g/dL before transfusing red blood cells is well-tolerated and is not associated with any significant adverse effects.[17] Transfusions to increase hemoglobin in nonanemic patients in septic shock do not further improve oxygen consumption.

Plasma (most commonly supplied as fresh frozen plasma [FFP]) contains plasma proteins, clotting factors, albumin, and other substances — all but the cellular components of blood. It is the honey-colored supernatant solution left behind when whole blood is centrifuged and the cells are separated from the plasma. While FFP can be used as a volume expander, it carries risks of disease transmission and allergic reaction not associated with crystalloid solutions. Use FFP to treat coagulopathy related to deficiencies in clotting factors when factor-specific therapy is not available. FFP is most commonly used by emergency physicians when treating dilutional coagulopathy from severe blood loss (typically after one to two blood volumes' worth of fluid has been infused into a patient) or DIC (disseminated intravascular coagulation).

Platelet preparations are used specifically for treating coagulopathy related to disorders of platelet number (thrombocytopenia) or platelet function. Like FFP, they are not typically replaced during acute blood loss, unless greater than 1-2 blood volumes has already been lost. Patients may need platelets if their counts are lower than 10,000-20,000 or if they are showing signs of active bleeding.

General Principles of Treatment

The first and most important intervention in fluid resuscitation is the prompt administration of one or more crystalloid boluses of 20 mL/kg. During and after the administration of initial fluid boluses, assess the patient for improvement in clinical parameters, such as decrease in heart rate, improvement in distal pulses, decreased capillary refill time, or improvements in mental status. Once hemodynamically stable, consider transitioning to fluid replacement that targets maintenance, deficits, and ongoing losses for correction over time.

While initial boluses are being administered, aggressively search for (and begin to treat) secondary causes of hypovolemia. For trauma patients, look for and control sources of bleeding. For patients with fever, administer acetaminophen or ibuprofen to reduce body temperature. Order laboratory studies to confirm or refute suspected diagnoses and to facilitate ongoing management.

Don't forget to monitor the volume and electrolyte status of your patients on IV therapy. A daily weight and BMP will allow you to check for volume status and assess the adequacy of resuscitation. For patients with bleeding concerns or those receiving blood products, a CBC is mandatory, as are coagulation studies (PT/PTT) for patients receiving plasma products or at risk for coagulopathy.

Special Considerations
Trauma

- One or more fluid boluses (20 mL/kg isotonic crystalloid).
- If still hypotensive after two fluid boluses, consider PRBCs at 10-20 mL/kg.
- Extensive resuscitation (>2 blood volumes) can lead to iatrogenic coagulopathy.
  - ▶ Watch for oozing from previously coagulated wounds and around IV sites!
  - ▶ Give FFP (10 mL/kg) and/or platelets.
- Stop ongoing hemorrhage. Direct pressure, in the absence of severe coagulopathy, will stop almost all bleeding. Bandage or suture as necessary to stop the rest.

Burns

- Calculate body surface area involvement (2nd- and 3rd-degree burns only)
  - ▶ Rough estimate: Surface area of patient's palm = 1% BSA
- **Parkland formula**
  - ▶ 24-hour requirement (mL) of lactated Ringer's = 4 mL × wt (kg) × % BSA burned
  - ▶ Add maintenance fluids if <20 kg.
  - ▶ Infuse first half of resuscitation fluids over 8 hours, second half over remaining 16 hours.
  - ▶ Re-check electrolytes within 2 hours and adjust fluids as needed.
  - ▶ Dressing burns is important not only to prevent infection, but to minimize ongoing fluid losses.

DKA

- Hyponatremia in the context of DKA is often pseudohyponatremia. As the glucose corrects, so will the sodium.
  - ▶ For every 100 mg/dL glucose over 200, **ADD** 1.6 to the measured Na$^+$
- Check electrolytes and replace as necessary (e.g., potassium).
- Patients tend to be K$^+$ depleted; as acidosis corrects, serum K$^+$ will drop.
- When blood glucose reaches 250 mg/dL, **ADD** glucose-containing fluids to prevent hypoglycemia.

Fever

- Normal insensible losses are 10-30 mL/kg/day.
- Insensible losses can increase 10% for each 1°C temperature increase.

Sepsis

- Initial management of hypotension is still IV crystalloid.
- Provide adequate fluids before using pressors.
- Prompt antibiotic therapy is crucial to the management of sepsis from any source.

Oral Rehydration

- May not be suitable for patients with continued vomiting.
- Encourage small sips of a balanced electrolyte solution (such as Pedialyte).
- If patient vomits, stop fluids for 1 hour and then resume with small sips.
- **SMALL AND FREQUENT** sips are the key. A 20-kg child requires 60 mL/hr for maintenance fluid. This is only about 4 tablespoons of fluid an hour (or 1 tbsp every 15 minutes)!

Hyponatremia

- Hyponatremia is common in vomiting children or infants whose lost fluids are replaced by hypotonic solutions (e.g., plain water).
- Replacement rate and fluid depend on clinical symptoms!
- For asymptomatic or mildly symptomatic patients, correct slowly.
- For seizures due to hyponatremia, more rapid correction with hypertonic saline is appropriate.
- Hypertonic saline should not be used to bring sodium level back to "normal" – merely to reduce clinical symptoms (risk of pontine myelinolysis).

- Calculate the sodium deficit (in mEq):
  $(0.6 \times \text{weight in kg}) \times (140 - [\text{serum Na}])$
- Correct the sodium at an appropriate rate based on duration of hyponatremia:
  - ▶ <24 hours – rapid correction OK
  - ▶ <2 days – max correction rate 2.5 mEq/hr
  - ▶ >2 days – max correction rate 0.6 mEq/hr (25 mEq/48 hours)

Cardiopulmonary Disease
- Use smaller boluses – 10 mL/kg.
- In these children, consider pump and rate problems as well as volume issues. Shock may not necessarily be due to (true) hypovolemia.
- Ensure adequate oxygenation.

Reassessment and Ongoing Management
- Reassess patients frequently for response to treatment.
- For patients requiring ongoing resuscitation, consider Foley catheter placement for strict monitoring of urinary output.
- If patients do not appear to be improving, re-double your search for hemorrhage, fever, GI, or other ongoing fluid losses.
- Remember to assess weights, electrolytes, and appropriate hematologic parameters on at least a daily basis.

Review Questions

1. **Which is the most important first intervention in hypovolemic shock?**
   - A. Stress-dose corticosteroids
   - B. Dopamine at 2-10 mcg/kg/min
   - C. One or more crystalloid IV fluid boluses at 20 mL/kg/min
   - D. Fluid restriction

2. **Which secondary causes of hypovolemia can be identified and treated?**
   - A. Sepsis
   - B. Diarrhea
   - C. Acute blood loss
   - D. All of the above

3. **Why is a balanced electrolyte solution important for oral volume replacement?**

   A. Rehydration with plain water alone can lead to hyponatremia and other electrolyte disturbances.

   B. Water alone causes more vomiting than balanced electrolyte solutions.

   C. Balanced electrolyte solutions contain large amounts of potassium to counteract the effects of contraction alkalosis.

   D. There is no benefit to balanced electrolyte solutions; their use should be discouraged.

4. **Which statement is true?**

   A. Crystalloid solutions may be cheaper, but they are inferior fluids for resuscitation.

   B. Crystalloid fluids lead to greater third-space accumulation of fluid compared to colloids.

   C. Colloid fluids have not been demonstrated to be superior to crystalloid fluids.

   D. Colloid fluids should be used for patients with congestive heart failure.

5. **An appropriate transfusion trigger for pediatric patients is:**

   A. 9 g/dL

   B. 7 g/dL

   C. 5 g/dL

   D. The optimal transfusion trigger for pediatric patients is unknown, so individual physician judgment is crucial in optimizing transfusion therapy.

Cardiopulmonary Arrest

22

Steve Groke, MD
Albert Fiorello, MD

Based on the most recent 2010 AHA Guidelines for Pediatric CPR and Emergency Cardiovascular Care[1,2,3]

Background/Epidemiology

- Pediatric cardiopulmonary arrest is uncommon (approximately 2.6-19.7 annual cases per 100,000 children).[4]
- Most pediatric cardiopulmonary arrests are due to primary respiratory arrest or decompensated shock.
  - ▶ SIDS 23%, trauma 20%, respiratory 16%, submersion 12%, cardiac 8%, CNS 6%.[5]
- Primary arrhythmia causing cardiac arrest in children is rare.
- Presenting rhythm asystole 67%, PEA 24%, ventricular fibrillation 9%.[5]
- Overall survival of pediatric out-of-hospital cardiac arrest is poor (about 4%).[4]
- Factors associated with greater overall survival include submersion injury-associated arrests, witnessed arrests, and bystander CPR.[4]
- Long-term survival is much greater for victims of respiratory arrest than of cardiac arrest (70% vs 21%).[6]
- The length-based Broselow tape simplifies resuscitations by providing size-appropriate doses and equipment sizes.

2010 Key Changes

- Initiate CPR with compressions, rather than ventilation. C-A-B, rather than A-B-C.
- Lay providers should start CPR immediately in a child who is unresponsive and not breathing normally.
- De-emphasis of the pulse check for health care providers.
- Chest compression depth should be at least 1/3 of the AP chest diameter.
- Elimination of "Look, Listen, and Feel" for breathing.

- Once circulation is restored, titrate FIO_2 to keep O_2 saturation 94%-99% (to avoid hyperoxia).
- Exhaled CO_2 detection (capnography or colorimetry) is recommended to confirm tracheal tube position, as well as during CPR to guide therapy (i.e., effectiveness of chest compressions, evidence of possible ROSC).
- **AED use in infants:** For defibrillation, a manual defibrillator is preferred over an AED. If an AED is used, a device with a pediatric dose attenuator is preferred.
- **Defibrillation:** Initial energy dose 2-4 J/kg (monophasic or biphasic); for second and subsequent doses, give at least 4 J/kg (not to exceed 10 J/kg or the adult dose).
- Routine calcium administration is not recommended in the absence of documented hypocalcemia, calcium channel-blocker overdose, hyperkalemia, or hypermagnesemia.
- Etomidate is not recommended for routine use in pediatric patients with evidence of septic shock.
- **Post-cardiac arrest care:** Therapeutic hypothermia (32°C to 34°C) may be considered for adolescents who remain comatose after resuscitation. It also may be considered for infants and children.

Circulation and Vascular Access (C of the C-A-Bs)
Chest Compressions

- If the child is unresponsive and not breathing, providers may take up to 10 seconds to check for a pulse prior to initiating CPR. If the provider doesn't feel a pulse or is unsure, begin CPR.
- If, despite oxygenation and ventilation, the pulse is <60 and there are signs of poor perfusion, begin chest compressions.
- "Push hard and push fast." Depress the chest at least 1/3 of the AP diameter of the chest at a rate of at least 100 compressions per minute. This is approximately 1½ inches in most infants and 2 inches in most children.
- Release completely after each compression to allow the chest to fully recoil.
- Limit interruptions of chest compressions to <10 seconds.
- For two-rescuer CPR without an advanced airway in place, provide 15 compressions followed by 2 ventilations. Rotate compressors every 2 minutes.

- When an advanced airway is in place, provide compressions at least 100 per minute and 8-10 ventilations per minute (do not pause compressions for ventilations).

Airway Obstruction and Management (AB of ABCs)

- "Look, Listen, and Feel" is no longer recommended
- In the absence of neck trauma, use a head tilt-chin lift method to open the airway.
- In the presence of possible neck trauma, use a jaw-thrust method without head tilt.
- If a jaw-thrust method fails, attempt to use an oral or nasopharyngeal airway. If this fails and advanced airway devices are not immediately available, use the head tilt-chin lift method; maintaining an airway and providing ventilation are crucial.
- Ventilate using bag-mask ventilation, which can usually be as effective as ventilating through an endotracheal tube for short periods and actually may be safer, especially in the pre-hospital setting.[7]
- Use an E-C clamp method to provide a tight seal when using bag-mask ventilation. A two-person technique is usually more effective than ventilation by a single rescuer.
- Provide high-flow supplemental oxygen.
- If prolonged ventilation is necessary, consider using advanced airway techniques and waveform capnography.
- A pediatric laryngeal mask airway may be useful for patients who are difficult to ventilate with a bag-mask, or as a rescue device for failed endotracheal intubation.
- Beyond the neonatal period, both cuffed and uncuffed endotracheal tubes may be used.
- Avoid excessive ventilation. This may be detrimental because it impedes venous return, cerebral blood flow, and coronary perfusion by increasing intrathoracic pressures; causes air trapping and barotrauma; and increases the risk of regurgitation and aspiration.
- Rapid-sequence intubation is not needed in a full cardiopulmonary arrest but may be useful in a patient with impending respiratory arrest requiring airway management. When using RSI, you must always have a backup plan for airway management in case initial attempts fail.

- After intubation with appropriate ETT size (see *Table 1*), confirm ETT placement with auscultation of bilateral breath sounds and lack of gastric insufflation sounds, observation of bilateral chest wall movement, exhaled CO_2 detection, and chest x-ray.

- Exhaled CO_2 detection is now recommended for tube placement, as well as during CPR to help guide therapy (i.e., effectiveness of compressions). Continuous capnography may be beneficial during CPR. If <10-15 mmHg, focus efforts on improving chest compressions and ensuring that the child is not receiving excessive ventilations. An abrupt increase in end tidal CO_2 can indicate ROSC; monitoring for this may allow for limited interruptions of chest compressions for pulse checks.

- **Initial ventilator settings:** TV 6-8 mL/kg, RR age-appropriate, FiO_2 100%, PEEP 3-5; adjust settings as needed.

- **RR rate by age:** Infants – 20-30 breaths/min; children – 16-20 breaths/min; adolescents – 8-12 breaths/min.

- Titrate FiO_2 as soon as possible to keep O2 saturation between 94%-99%.

- After intubation, consider placement of a NG tube to decompress the stomach.

- If an intubated patient's condition suddenly deteriorates, reassess the airway (**DOPE**).
  - ▶ **D**isplacement of the tube from the trachea
  - ▶ **O**bstruction of the tube
  - ▶ **P**neumothorax
  - ▶ **E**quipment failure (If the patient was on a ventilator, take him off the ventilator and provide ventilation via bag.)

Table 1. Helpful Formulas

Uncuffed ETT size $= \dfrac{\text{age in years}}{4} + 4$

Cuffed ETT size $= \dfrac{\text{age in years}}{4} + 3.5$

ETT placement at lip $= 3 \times$ tube size

Weight (kg) $= 8 + (2 \times \text{age in years})$

Length-based tapes such as the Broselow tape are the most accurate at estimating weight.

Vascular Access

- Attempt placement of a peripheral IV, but limit the time of this attempt. If immediate peripheral IV access is not obtained, move on.
- Intraosseous access can be achieved rapidly and is safe and effective for administering fluids, drugs, and blood products. Approved sites include proximal tibia, distal tibia, distal femur, and anterior-superior iliac spine. The humerus may be used in older children and adolescents.
- Central venous access may also be obtained, but usually takes more time than placement of an IO line.
- If attempts at vascular access fail, **n**aloxone, **a**tropine, **d**iazepam, epinephrine, and **l**idocaine ("NAVEL") may be administered via the endotracheal tube. Optimal doses are not known (see *Table 2*).
- To treat shock, give an initial bolus of 20 cc/kg of an isotonic crystalloid fluid (normal saline or lactated Ringer's), even if blood pressure is normal. Repeat as needed if systemic perfusion fails to improve.

Table 2. Medications for Pediatric Resuscitation and Arrythmias[2]

Medication	Dose
Adenosine	0.1 mg/kg (max 6 mg) given as a rapid IV bolus Repeat: 0.2 mg/kg (max 12 mg)
Amiodarone	5 mg/kg IV/IO, repeat up to 15 mg/kg (max 300 mg)
Atropine	0.02 mg/kg IV/IO 0.03 mg/kg ET*
Calcium chloride (10%)	20 mg/kg IV/IO (2 mL/kg). *Note: Routine calcium administration for cardiopulmonary arrest is not recommended in the absence of documented hypocalcemia, calcium channel-blocker overdose, hyperkalemia, or hypermagnesemia. It has no documented benefit and may be harmful.*
Epinephrine	0.01 mg/kg (0.1 mL/kg 1:10,000) IV/IO 0.1 mg/kg (0.1 mL/kg 1:1000) ET* (max dose 1 mg IV/IO, 10mg ET) *Note: No survival benefit has been demonstrated by use of high-dose epinephrine, and it actually may be harmful.[8]*
Glucose	0.5-1 g/kg IV/IO (D_{10}W: 5-10 mL/kg, D_{25}W: 2-4 mL/kg, D_{50}W: 1-2 mL/kg)

Lidocaine	Bolus: 1 mg/kg IV/IO (max dose 100 mg) Infusion: 20-50 mcg/kg/min ET*: 2-3 mg/kg
Magnesium sulfate	25-50 mg/kg IV/IO over 10-20 min, faster in torsades (max dose 2 g)
Naloxone	<5 years or ≤20 kg: 0.1 mg/kg IV/IO/ET* >5 years or >20 kg: 2 mg IV/IO/ET*
Procainamide	15 mg/kg IV/IO over 30-60 min
Sodium bicarbonate	1 mEq/kg per dose IV/IO slowly

*(Flush with 5 mL NS, follow with 5 ventilations.)

Pulseless Arrest

- Presenting rhythm may be asystole, PEA, ventricular fibrillation, or ventricular tachycardia.
- Asystole and wide-complex bradycardia are most common in asphyxia arrests.

Shockable Rhythms: Ventricular Fibrillation/Pulseless Ventricular Tachycardia

- Defibrillation is the definitive treatment.
- Survival declines with increased time to defibrillation, therefore attempt defibrillation immediately.
- Perform chest compressions while preparing defibrillator or AED.
- AED use in infants: For defibrillation, a manual defibrillator is preferred over an AED.
- Use largest paddles or pads that will fit on the chest wall, leaving about 3 cm between paddles (usually use adult paddles for children >10 kg or 1 year; infant paddles for children <10 kg).
- If using paddles, apply electrode cream or paste. Self-adhering defibrillation pads do not require additional gel.
- Place one paddle over the right side of the upper chest and the other at the apex of the heart (left of the left nipple). Apply firm pressure.
- Initial defibrillation (monophasic or biphasic) is at 2-4 J/kg. Subsequent attempts should be at least 4 J/kg (not to exceed 10 J/kg or the adult dose).
- Resume chest compressions immediately after delivering the shock, and continue for about 5 cycles or 2 minutes.

- Check the rhythm. If a shockable rhythm persists, give another shock at least 4 J/kg and give epinephrine (0.01 mg/kg IV/IO = 0.1 mL/kg 1:10,000). Repeat the dose of epinephrine every 3-5 minutes during cardiac arrest.
- After 5 cycles of CPR, check the rhythm. If the rhythm continues to be shockable, deliver another shock of at least 4 J/kg, resume chest compressions, and consider administration of amiodarone (5 mg/kg IV) **OR** lidocaine (1 mg/kg IV/IO, 2-3 mg/kg ET). **Amiodarone is preferred**.
- Continue CPR for 5 cycles, check rhythm, and defibrillate if necessary.
- If at any point an organized rhythm emerges, check for a pulse and proceed accordingly.
- Throughout the resuscitation, consider treatable, reversible causes (*Table 3*).
- Rotate rescuers performing compressions every 2 minutes to ensure continued adequate compressions.

Nonshockable Rhythms: Asystole/PEA

- Resume chest compressions.
- Administer epinephrine (0.01 mg/kg IV/IO = 0.1 mL/kg 1:10,000). Repeat every 3-5 minutes during cardiac arrest.
- Throughout the resuscitation, consider treatable, reversible causes (*Table 3*).

Table 3. Possible Treatable Causes of Cardiopulmonary Arrest

Hypovolemia
Hypoxia
Hydrogen ion (acidosis)
Hypo- or hyperkalemia
Hypoglycemia
Hypothermia
Toxins
Tamponade (cardiac)
Tension pneumothorax
Thrombosis (coronary or pulmonary)
Trauma

Bradycardia with Hemodynamic Compromise

- Treat patients with bradycardia that is causing cardiorespiratory compromise.

- If the patient develops pulseless arrest, treat as described above in the *Pulseless Arrest* section.

- Support airway, breathing, and circulation.

- Administer supplemental oxygen.

- Attach a monitor or defibrillator.

- Reassess patient to determine if cardiorespiratory compromise persists despite adequate oxygenation and ventilation. If perfusion, pulses, and respirations are normal, no emergency treatment is necessary. Proceed with further evaluation.

- If heart rate <60 beats per minute and there is evidence of poor perfusion despite adequate ventilation with oxygen, start chest compressions.

- If symptomatic bradycardia persists, administer epinephrine (0.01 mg/kg IV/IO = 0.1 mL/kg 1:10,000). Repeat every 3-5 minutes if needed. If bradycardia persists or if it only transiently responds to the dose of epinephrine, consider continuous infusion of epinephrine.

- If bradycardia is due to increased vagal tone, administer atropine (0.02 mg/kg IV/IO or 0.04-0.06 mg/kg ET; min dose 0.1 mg; max cumulative dose 1 mg).

- Consider transcutaneous pacing if bradycardia is due to heart block or sinus node dysfunction not responsive to prior treatment above, especially if it is associated with congenital or acquired heart disease.

- Throughout the resuscitation, consider treatable, reversible causes (*Table 3*).

Tachycardia with Hemodynamic Compromise

- If the patient develops pulseless arrest, treat as described above in the *Pulseless Arrest* section.

- If pulses are palpable and the patient has signs of hemodynamic compromise, ensure airway is patent, assist ventilations if needed, administer supplemental oxygen, and attach the patient to the monitor or defibrillator.

- **Assess the QRS duration:** ≤0.09 seconds = narrow complex tachycardia. >0.09 seconds = wide complex tachycardia

Narrow Complex Tachycardia (≤0.09 s)

- If the rhythm is sinus tachycardia, search for and treat reversible causes.
- If the rhythm is probable supraventricular tachycardia (SVT), infants usually >220, children usually >180:
  - ► Attempt vagal stimulation unless the patient is very unstable (*infants and young children:* apply ice to the face; *older children:* carotid sinus massage or Valsalva maneuver).
  - ► If IV access is readily available, administer adenosine (0.1 mg/kg *rapid* IV bolus). If conversion does not occur, may repeat a double dose (0.2 mg/kg *rapid* IV bolus).
  - ► *OR* synchronized cardioversion may be performed at 0.5-1 J/kg. If conversion does not occur, this may be repeated at 2 J/kg. Sedate the patient if possible, but do not delay cardioversion in an unstable patient.
  - ► If conversion fails after 2 doses of adenosine or 2 attempts at synchronized electrical cardioversion, or SVT quickly recurs after conversion, consider the use of an antiarrhythmic prior to additional attempts at conversion. Amiodarone (5 mg/kg over 20-60 minutes) *OR* procainamide (15 mg/kg over 30-60 min) may be used. (Use extreme caution when using multiple drugs that can cause QT prolongation.)

Wide-Complex Tachycardia (>0.09 s)

- In the setting of hemodynamic compromise, wide-complex tachycardia is usually ventricular in origin, but may be supraventricular with aberrancy.
- If patient is hemodynamically stable, consider adenosine (0.1 mg/kg *rapid* IV bolus).
- Treat with synchronized electrical cardioversion at 0.5-1 J/kg. If conversion does not occur, this may be repeated at 2 J/kg.
- If conversion fails after a second shock, consider the use of an antiarrhythmic (amiodarone or procainamide) prior to a third shock.

Tachycardia with Hemodynamic Stability

- Consider consultation with an expert in pediatric arrhythmias prior to treating children who are hemodynamically stable.
- For supraventricular tachycardia (SVT), follow the algorithm above.
- For ventricular tachycardia, administer an amiodarone infusion slowly. If amiodarone is not available, procainamide may also be used.

Post-Cardiac Arrest Care

- Although pediatric data is needed, therapeutic hypothermia (32°C to 34°C) may be beneficial for adolescents who remain comatose after resuscitation.
- Therapeutic hypothermia (32°C to 34°C) may also be considered for infants and children who remain comatose after resuscitation.

Special Resuscitation Situations
Trauma

- If spinal injury is suspected, restrict motion of the neck. If possible, use a jaw-thrust method to open the airway.
- Do not over-ventilate. Over-ventilation can decrease cerebral perfusion. Intentional brief hyperventilation may be used as a temporizing measure if signs of impending brain herniation develop.
- Suspect thoracic trauma in all thoracoabdominal trauma, even in the absence of obvious external injuries. Tension pneumothorax, hemothorax, and pulmonary contusions may impair breathing and cause deterioration.
- If the patient has facial trauma or has a suspected basilar skull fracture, insert an orogastric tube instead of a nasogastric tube.
- Blood pressure drops late in children. Even if the blood pressure is normal, treat signs of shock with a bolus of 20 mL/kg of normal saline or lactated Ringer's solution. Give additional 20 mL/kg boluses if signs of shock persist. After 40-60 mL/kg of crystalloid fluid, give 10-15 mL/kg of packed red blood cells. Use type-specific blood if possible. If type-specific blood is not available, use emergency release O-negative in females, and O-negative or O-positive in males.
- Always consider intra-abdominal hemorrhage, tension pneumothorax, pericardial tamponade, and spinal cord shock in children with signs of shock. Additionally, intracranial hemorrhage can cause shock in a small infant.

Toxicologic Emergencies

- Cocaine may cause cardiac arrhythmias. For coronary vasospasm, consider nitroglycerin, benzodiazepines, and phentolamine. Avoid the use of β-blockers, as they may potentiate marked hypertension from an unopposed α effect. For ventricular arrhythmias, consider sodium bicarbonate in addition to standard treatment.

- Tricyclic antidepressants may cause intraventricular conduction delays, heart block, bradycardia, prolongation of the QT interval, ventricular arrhythmias, hypotension, and seizures. Treat with sodium bicarbonate 1-2 mEq/kg boluses until arterial pH is >7.45 and then infuse 150 mEq $NaHCO_3$ per liter of D5W to maintain alkalosis. Do not administer quinidine, procainamide, flecainide, propafenone, amiodarone, or sotalol, as they may exacerbate cardiac toxicity. For hypotension, use normal saline boluses. Epinephrine and norepinephrine have been shown to be more effective at raising blood pressure than dopamine in TCA overdose.

- Calcium channel-blockers may cause hypotension, conduction delays, and arrhythmias. Mild hypotension may be treated with small boluses of normal saline. For more significant hypotension, calcium chloride (10%) may be administered at 20 mg/kg over 5-10 minutes, followed by an infusion of 20-50 mg/kg per hour if the initial dose was beneficial. For bradycardia and hypotension, consider a high-dose vasopressor such as norepinephrine or epinephrine.

- Beta blockers may cause bradycardia, heart block, decreased cardiac contractility, hypotension, and prolonged QRS and QT intervals. High-dose epinephrine may be effective. Consider the use of glucagon. Consider an infusion of glucose and insulin.

- Opioids may cause hypoventilation, apnea, bradycardia, and hypotension. Treat respiratory depression initially with assisted ventilation. Naloxone reverses the effects of opioids. For children less than 5 years old or less than or equal to 20 kg, administer 0.1 mg/kg IV/IO/ET. For children greater than 5 years old or over 20 kg, administer 2 mg IV/IO/ET.

Review Questions

1. For a 20-kg child, the appropriate dose of epinephrine used during a cardiac arrest is:

   A. 1 mg IV

   B. 0.2 mg IV

   C. 10 mg IO

   D. 0.01 mg IV

2. The most common presenting rhythm in pediatric cardiac arrest is ventricular fibrillation.

   A. True

   B. False

3. For two-rescuer CPR in a patient who is not intubated, the recommended compression to ventilation ratio is:

   A. 100:1

   B. 30:3

   C. 15:2

   D. 50:5

4. Endotracheal intubation has been shown to be far superior to bag-mask ventilation in children for short-term ventilation, especially in the pre-hospital setting.

   A. True

   B. False

5. Which of the following should NOT be administered down the ET tube?

   A. Lidocaine

   B. Epinephrine

   C. Sodium bicarbonate

   D. Atropine

6. In a pediatric cardiopulmonary arrest situation, if immediate peripheral IV access cannot be obtained, a _____ line should immediately be established.

   A. Internal jugular central venous

   B. Intraosseous

   C. Femoral central venous

   D. Ultrasound guided deep brachial venous

7. **For treatment of ventricular fibrillation, the initial defibrillation dose is:**

   A. 0.5 J/kg

   B. 20 J/kg

   C. 5 J

   D. 2 J/kg

8. **For wide-complex tachycardia with pulses, but with evidence of hemo-dynamic compromise, the initial synchronized cardioversion dose is:**

   A. 0.5-1 J/kg

   B. 10-20 J/kg

   C. 5-10 J

   D. 2-4 J/kg

9. **If bradycardia is suspected to be due to increased vagal tone, the following should be administered:**

   A. Amiodarone

   B. Lidocaine

   C. Naloxone

   D. Atropine

10. **A 2-year-old male ingested some his grandmother's amitriptyline. He presents with a heart rate of 120, blood pressure of 59/42, and has a wide QRS complex on the monitor. He should be treated with:**

    A. Naloxone

    B. Atropine

    C. Sodium bicarbonate

    D. Calcium chloride

11. **Following a return of spontaneous circulation after drowning, a 4-year-old male (20 kg) child should be placed on what ventilator settings?**

    A. Tidal volume 250 mL, RR 12, FiO2 at 100%

    B. Tidal volume 140 mL, RR 20, titrate FiO2 to keep sats at 94%-99%

    C. Tidal volume 200 mL, RR 35, titrate FiO2 to keep sats at 94%-99%

    D. Tidal volume 150 mL, RR 28, FiO2 at 80%

12. **A 3-year-old comes into the ED with a HR of 210. An EKG shows a QRS duration of 0.08 seconds with a regular interval. The child looks nontoxic and has an age-appropriate blood pressure. You should:**

A. Prepare for immediate cardioversion of 2 J/kg.

B. Administer 0.01 mg/kg of IV/IO epinephrine.

C. Attempt a Valsalva maneuver.

D. Administer a 20-cc/kg crystalloid bolus.

13. **An adolescent presents in ventricular fibrillation. He is immediately defibrillated unsuccessfully three times with appropriate CPR and administration of epinephrine IV between attempts. You should then:**

A. Administer atropine 0.5 mg IV.

b. Administer 5 mg/kg of amiodarone IV and consider reversible causes.

C. Administer 20 mg/kg of calcium chloride.

D. Increase the Joules used for defibrillation to 15 J/kg (max 400 J)

Key		
1. B	7. D	
2. B	8. A	
3. C	9. D	
4. B	10. C	
5. C	11. B	
6. B	12. C	
	13. B	

Rapid Sequence Induction (RSI)

Garrett S. Pacheco, MD
Chad Viscusi, MD

Critical Knowledge

- Most pediatric cardiac arrests are a consequence of a preceding respiratory arrest. Survival after cardiac arrest in children averages 7% to 11%, and most survivors are neurologically impaired. For this reason, early recognition and prompt management of airway compromise, respiratory distress, or respiratory failure in a critically ill child is essential to save a child's life and prevent permanent neurologic disability. As such, expert and efficient airway management and ventilatory support is a requisite skill for every provider of emergency care to children. Airway compromise is the most common cause of cardiac arrest, death and severe morbidity in acutely ill and injured children.

- **Indications for intubation**
  - ▶ Respiratory failure or anticipated respiratory failure
  - ▶ Inadequate ventilation or inadequate oxygenation
  - ▶ Airway protection
  - ▶ Anticipated airway obstruction

Anticipate respiratory failure if you see any of the following:

- Increased respiratory rate, particularly with signs of distress (e.g., increased effort/ accessory respiratory muscle use, nasal flaring, retractions, or grunting)
- Inadequate respiratory rate, effort, or chest excursion (e.g., diminished breath sounds, gasping, and cyanosis)
- Depressed mental status or inability to adequately protect the airway

Pediatric Airway Anatomy

- Proportionally larger head and occiput can cause neck flexion and airway obstruction when the infant and small child are supine.
- Infants are obligate nose-breathers, thus congestion causes respiratory distress.

- Larger, more intra-oral tongue results in less oral space.
- Decreased muscle tone causes passive airway obstruction by the tongue.
- The epiglottis is relatively larger and floppier, often requiring direct elevation.
- The larynx is higher and more anterior, making visualization more difficult.
- The trachea is shorter, increasing the risk of right main-stem intubation.
- The airway is narrower, increasing airway resistance.
- The subglottic cricoid ring is the narrowest portion of the airway.

Difficult Airway Indicators

- Inability to extend neck beyond 35 degrees
- Thyromental distance less than 2 adult finger widths (3 cm) – mandibular ramus to thyroid cartilage in adolescent or child, or less than one finger width in infants
- Limited mandible motion, (i.e., JRA, scoliosis, trismus, facial fractures)
- Congenital anomalies: cleft palate, micro/retrognathia, macroglossia, gloss-optosis, maxillary or mandibular anomalies, protruding maxillary incisors
- Airway obstruction due to bleeding, infection, burns, cervical fractures, inhalation injury, foreign body, etc.

Airway Adjuncts: Maintaining an Open Airway

- Proper airway positioning with small towel roll under the shoulders of children less than 2 years, or under the occiput of a teen or young adult.
- **Oropharyngeal Airways**
  - ▶ Used in unconscious patients (i.e., with no gag reflex). Select the correct size. An oropharyngeal airway that is too small will not keep the tongue from obstructing the pharynx; one that is too large may obstruct the airway. Correctly sized airway will extend from the corner of the patient's mouth to the angle of the mandible. Not tolerated in patients with a gag response.
- **Nasopharyngeal Airways**
  - ▶ Better tolerated than oral airways by patients who are not deeply unconscious. Small nasopharyngeal tubes (for infants) may be easily obstructed by secretions. Correctly sized airway will extend from the nare to the tragus, and should be inserted perpendicularly to the face.

- **Laryngeal Mask Airway**
  - ▶ There is insufficient evidence to recommend for or against the routine use of a laryngeal mask airway (LMA) during cardiac arrest. When endotracheal intubation is not possible, the LMA is an acceptable adjunct for experienced providers, but it is associated with a higher incidence of complications in young children.[1]

Rapid-Sequence Intubation

- Used by trained and experienced emergency care providers to facilitate safe, emergent endotracheal intubation and reduce the incidence of complications.
- Sedatives, neuromuscular blocking agents, and other medications are administered rapidly and sequentially to sedate and paralyze the patient for this procedure.
- Use of RSI requires thoughtful, meticulous preparation, individualized medication selection, and a reliable backup plan in the event that failure of intubation or ventilation is encountered.

Adverse Effects of Intubation

- Increased Intracranial pressure (ICP) (theoretical)
- Airway trauma
- Pain
- Bradycardia or tachycardia
- Dysrhythmia
- Gastric regurgitation
- Aspiration
- Hypoxemia or hypercarbia
- Death

Cuffed Versus Uncuffed Endotracheal Tubes

- In the hospital setting, a cuffed endotracheal tube is as safe as an uncuffed tube for infants beyond the newborn period and in children.[2]
- In certain circumstances (e.g., poor lung compliance, high airway-resistance, or a large glottic air leak) a cuffed tube may be preferable, provided that attention is paid to endotracheal tube size, position, and cuff inflation pressure.[2]
- Keep cuff inflation pressure <20 cm H_2O.

Helpful Pediatric Formulas and Mnemonics

- Weight estimation (kg) = (2 × age in years) + 8 (for ages 1 to 8 years)
- **Uncuffed** ETT size (mm) = (age in years/4) + 4
- **Cuffed** ETT size (mm) = (age in years/4) + 3.5 (i.e., ½ size less than uncuffed)
- ETT placement depth at lip = 3 × normal estimated tube size.
- Drugs that can be given through ETT: **NAVEL** (**N**arcan, **a**tropine/**A**tivan, **V**alium/**V**ersed, **e**pinephrine, **l**idocaine)

RSI Procedure

The Many Ps of Airway Management Success

- Patient history: **AMPLE**
- Properly positioning your patient: Place a towel between the shoulder blades to help align the oral, pharyngeal, and tracheal axis.
- Pre-oxygenation
  ▶ Preparation: **MAIDS** (**M**onitor, **a**irway equipment, **I**V, **d**rugs, **s**uction). Laryngoscopy blade choice: A Miller blade is typically used for children 2 years and younger. A mnemonic to remember is that you switch to a 2 blade size at age 2, and a 3 in the third grade (typically at 9 years old).
- **Premedication: LOAD**
  ▶ **L**idocaine (1.5 mg/kg) mixed evidence on transient decrease in ICP and intraocular pressure, therefore not commonly used.
  ▶ **O**piate (fentanyl 2-3 mcg/kg IV) sympatholytic theoretically lessens ICP.
  ▶ **A**tropine use has come under scrutiny. It is no longer routinely recommended for pretreatment, but it is best to have available at the bedside. Atropine (0.02 mg/kg IV minimum dose 0.1 mg, maximum 1 mg) is indicated if age <2 when using succinylcholine, or when bradycardic prior to intubation.
  ▶ **D**efasciculating dose (1/10 the paralytic dose); not commonly used.
  ▶ Try to pretreat with a 20-mL/kg bolus of IVF, as most children are fluid-down prior to intubation. This will help avoid preintubation hypotension.
- **Cricoid pressure**: Has become controversial in infants and small children with very pliable/collapsible airways. Cricoid pressure can impede the glottis view, the passage of the tube, or ability to ventilate. Use with caution, if at all.

- **Paralysis and sedation**
  - ► **RSI sedation**
    - Etomidate (0.3 mg/kg IV) is not FDA-approved for <10 years old but is commonly used without complications. Avoid in patients with septic shock.
    - Ketamine (0.5-2 mg/kg IV) is preferred in presence of broncho-spasm; avoid if signs or symptoms of elevated intracranial pressure.
    - Thiopental (3-5 mg/kg IV) is sometimes suggested in patients with suspected elevated ICP, as it may be neuro-protective, but is a strong cardiac depressant.
    - Midazolam (0.1-0.2 mg/kg) lowers BP, HR, and RR.
    - Apply gentle cricoid pressure immediately after giving induction agent.
  - ► **RSI paralysis**
    - Succinylcholine (1-2 mg/kg IV): Pretreat with Atropine if <2 years old for first and all subsequent doses. Avoid in suspected hyperkalemia, neuromuscular disorder, muscular dystrophy, or family history of malignant hyperthermia.
    - Rocuronium (0.6-1.2 mg/kg IV): Onset is one minute; effect lasts 30 minutes.
- **Passage of the ETT**
  - ► Gentle cricoid pressure may be placed after induction of sedation and paralysis.
  - ► The BURP maneuver can be used to obtain that best visual of the glottis (i.e., backward, upward (cephalad), and rightward pressure).
  - ► Bimanual laryngoscopy can be achieved by using an assistant's hand or the operator's right hand to improve the laryngeal view.
  - ► Avoid BVM ventilation to prevent gastric insufflation, helping to prevent emesis.
  - ► Passive oxygenation by high-flow nasal cannula is not well-studied in children, but can be used as an adjunct to RSI.
- **Proof of proper position (tube confirmation)**
  - ► In infants and small children, there is a high risk that an endotracheal tube will be misplaced (i.e., placed in the esophagus or in the pharynx above the vocal chords), right mainstemed, displaced, or become obstructed, especially when the patient is moved.

- No single confirmation technique is completely reliable, so providers must use both clinical assessment and confirmatory devices to verify proper tube placement.
- Confirmation of correct tube position must be completed immediately after intubation, again after securing the tube, and any time the child is moved.
- The operator should visualize the tube passing through the vocal cords.
- Bilateral chest movement and equal breath sounds over both lung fields, especially over the axillae.
- Listen for gastric insufflation sounds over the stomach (they should not be present if the tube is in the trachea).
- CO_2 detector (colorimeter or waveform) if there is a perfusing rhythm
- If the child has a perfusing rhythm and is >20 kg, you may use an esophageal detector device to check for evidence of esophageal placement.
- Check oxygen saturation with a pulse oximeter. Following hyperoxygenation, the oxyhemoglobin saturation detected by pulse oximetry may not demonstrate a fall indicative of incorrect endotracheal tube position (i.e., tube misplacement or displacement) for as long as 3 minutes.
- If you are still uncertain, perform direct laryngoscopy and look to see if the tube goes between the cords.
- In the hospital setting, perform a chest x-ray to verify that the tube is not in the right main bronchus and to identify a high tube position at risk of easy displacement.

- **Protect/secure the tube**
  - There is insufficient evidence to recommend any one method.
  - Maintain the patient's head in a neutral position.
  - Neck flexion pushes the tube farther into the airway
  - Neck extension pulls the tube out of the airway.

- **Failed airway**
  - LMA insertion
  - Video laryngoscopy
  - Cricothyroidotomy of value in severe facial trauma
  - Contraindicated in patients less than 8 years

- ▶ Needle cricothyroidotomy with transtracheal jet ventilation
- ▶ Digital tracheal intubation
- ▶ Retrograde endotracheal intubation

Troubleshooting an Intubated/Ventilated Patient

- DOPE
  - ▶ **D**isplacement of the tube from the trachea
  - ▶ **O**bstruction of the tube
  - ▶ **P**neumothorax
  - ▶ **E**quipment failure or malfunction
- Abdominal distension may impede ventilation. Children often have gastric insufflation from crying or preintubation ventilation. Place a nasogastric tube early to allow for gastric decompression and easier ventilation.

Review Questions

1. A 5-year-old boy is the victim of a near-drowning accident. Paramedics started CPR in the field, and the child's ventilation was assisted with BVM. On arrival, the child has cardiac activity and pulses. What size endotracheal tube should you use?

   A. 4
   B. 4.5
   C. 5
   D. 5.5

2. An 18-month-old child is suffering from respiratory failure in the ED from RSV. Upon evaluation for securing an airway, you notice that the patient's vitals are HR 95, BP 80/40, RR 70, temp 38.4°C. What pretreatment should you give this child?

   A. Lidocaine 1.5 mg/kg
   B. Atropine 0.02 mg/kg
   C. Lidocaine 0.02 mg/kg
   D. Atropine 1.5 mg/kg

3. **Which of the following alternative airway techniques would NOT be indicated for a 4-year-old after failing at RSI endotracheal intubation?**

   A. LMA

   B. Cricothyroidotomy

   C. BVM

   D. Transtracheal jet ventilation

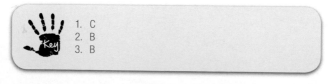

1. C
2. B
3. B

Electrocardiography

Kevin Reilly, MD
Lisa Chan, MD

Background

- Like many things in medicine, understanding the pediatric electrocardiogram (ECG) is daunting at first.
- **The key concept to understand in pediatric ECG interpretation is that the changing anatomy of the heart with growth is reflected in the ECG.** This is why there are large ECG variations with age; therefore, having readily available tables for normal age-related measurements is important.
- Many of the rules for reading pediatric ECGs are the same as they are in adults; having a good working knowledge of the basics of ECG interpretation will help a great deal.

Critical Knowledge

- The neonatal right ventricle is the predominate structure in the newborn heart; it is responsible for circulating most of the blood to the fetal body.
- This changes at birth as the ductus arteriosis closes, and then again over the next 3-5 years as the left heart enlarges in size to dominate the childhood heart.
- It is impossible for the average emergency physician to memorize the normal ranges for the developing heart. Fortunately, there are excellent tables of normal values and even mobile applications for smart phones that define age-related "normal." The rate, axis, QRS complex, and T waves undergo significant changes as the heart transitions from fetal to adult size.

Approach

- Use a stepwise approach to interpret the pediatric ECG, following the traditional approach of evaluating rate, rhythm, axis, intervals, QRS morphology, and ST/T waves.
- Addition of the V4R lead to the standard 12-lead EKG aids in identification of ventricular hypertrophy; some pediatric cardiologists advocate for replacing the standard V4 with V4R.

- Modern ECG machines are excellent at measuring intervals and voltages, but you should verify any abnormal results and recheck any measurements that do not pass the eyeball test.
- ECGs should be obtained with standard 10 mm/mv and 25 mm/sec, so measurements will be accurate. **It is important to check the tables to determine normal values.**
  - ► Rate
    - ECG rate is determined in children in the same fashion as it is in adults. The normal rates decrease with increasing age. Upper limits of normal (ULN) and lower limits of normal (LLN) reflect two standard deviations from the mean.

Normal Range of Heart Rate by Age (beats per minute)

Age	1 wk	1-3 wks	1-2 mos	3-5 mos	6-11 mos
HR LLN	90	100	120	105	110
HR ULN	160	180	180	185	170

Age	1-2 yrs	3-4 yrs	5-7 yrs	8-11 yrs	12-15 yrs	>16 yrs
HR LLN	90	70	65	65	60	50
HR ULN	165	140	140	130	130	120

Adapted from Sharieff GQ, Rao SO. The pediatric ECG. *Emerg Med Clin North Am.* 2006;24:195-208

  - ► Rhythm
    - As in adults, supraventricular tachycardia (SVT) is the most common abnormal rhythm in children.
    - Younger children are more likely to have atrioventricular re-entrant tachycardia (AVRT); older children are more likely to have atrio-ventricular nodal re-entrant tachycardia (AVNRT).
    - The rules for rhythm analysis are similar enough that no additional training is needed for the pediatric ECG.
  - ► P Waves
    - The P wave should be upright in II and aVF. In aVR, the P wave will be inverted. Inversion in II or aVF typically indicates a low atrial rhythm (usually around the coronary sinus) or limb lead reversal.

- Polysplenia may be associated with absence of the sinus node and a low ectopic atrial focus. Asplenia may have two right atria with duplication of the SA node resulting in two different P-wave axes.

- The P waves give information about atrial hypertrophy; the following patterns should be sought.
  Findings suggestive of right atrial enlargement (RAE) or P pulmonale are:
  - Peaked P waves in II and V1 >3 mm (age <6 months) or >2.5 mm (age >6 months)

  Findings suggestive of left atrial enlargement (LAE) or P mitrale are:
  - P waves >0.08 sec in duration (age <12 months) or >0.10 sec (age >12 months)
  - Notched contour in II
  - Terminal P in V1 inverted

► **Axis**

- The dominant right ventricle of the newborn shifts the axis to the right (>90°); however, at 3-5 years of age, the left ventricle catches up then exceeds the mass of the right ventricle, resulting in a more leftward axis (<90°).

- An abnormal axis is one of the first clues of congenital heart disease, as hypertrophy of one or both ventricles is common in this setting.

- Right-ventricular hypertrophy (RVH) often results in right-axis deviation (RAD) greater than would be expected for age.

- Left-ventricular hypertrophy (LVH) usually does not result in marked left-axis deviation (LAD) but is common with conduction defects.

Normal Range of Axis by Age *(Degrees)*

Age	1 wks	1-3 wks	1-2 mos	3-5 mos	6-11 mos
Axis low	60	45	30	0	0
Axis high	180	160	135	135	135

Age	1-2 yrs	3-4 yrs	5-7 yrs	8-11 yrs	12-15 yrs	>16 yrs
Axis low	0	0	0	-15	-15	-15
Axis high	110	110	110	110	110	110

Adapted from Sharieff GQ, Rao SO. The pediatric ECG. *Emerg Med Clin North Am.* 2006;24:195-208

- ► Intervals
  - ▪ The PR interval is much shorter in the neonate and may fool the eye that is accustomed to looking at normal adult PR intervals.
  - ▪ Remember that the PR interval measurement starts at the beginning of the P wave and extends to the first deflection of the QRS complex.
  - ▪ Accessory pathways, like WPW, are common sources of SVT in infants. Recognizing the short PR with a delta wave is more difficult in the younger child, in whom the PR interval is already quite short.

Normal Range of PR Interval (seconds)

Age	1 wk	1-3 wks	1-2 mos	3-5 mos	6-11 mos
PR low	0.08	0.08	0.08	0.08	0.07
PR high	0.15	0.15	0.15	0.15	0.16

Age	1-2 yrs	3-4 yrs	5-7 yrs	8-11 yrs	12-15 yrs	>16 yrs
PR low	0.08	0.09	0.09	0.09	0.09	0.12
PR high	0.16	0.17	0.17	0.17	0.18	0.20

Adapted from Sharieff GQ, Rao SO. The Pediatric ECG. *Emerg Med Clin North Am.* 2006;24:195-208

- ▪ Discovery of long QT is incredibly important, especially in the setting of seizure, syncope, or an apparent life-threatening event (ALTE). **It is critical to obtain an ECG in these settings.**
- ▪ QT is slightly longer in neonatal and early infancy ages, with an upper limit of normal (ULN) at 0.47 seconds in the first week of life, and 0.45 seconds during infancy. The ULN for QT in children is 0.44 seconds.
- ▪ As in the adult, it is important to correct the QT interval for heart rate with the Bazett formula (QT interval/square root of the RR interval).

- ► QRS Complex
  - ▪ The QRS duration lengthens with increasing age.

Normal Range of QRS Duration *(Seconds)*

Age	1 wk	1-3 wks	1-2 mos	3-5 mos	6-11 mos
QRS low	0.03	0.03	0.03	0.03	0.03
QRS high	0.08	0.08	0.08	0.08	0.08

Age	1-2 yrs	3-4 yrs	5-7 yrs	8-11 yrs	12-15 yrs	>16 yrs
QRS low	0.03	0.04	0.04	0.04	0.04	0.05
QRS high	0.08	0.08	0.08	0.09	0.09	0.10

Adapted from Sharieff GQ, Rao SO. The pediatric ECG. *Emerg Med Clin North Am.* 2006;24:195-208

- Evaluation of the QRS morphology is critically important in the pediatric population to detect ventricular hypertrophy reflecting congenital heart disease.
- The emergency physician should be familiar with the common patterns of right, left, and bilateral ventricular hypertrophy in the EKG.
- Right- and left-bundle branch patterns will assume the same QRS manifestations in children as they do in adults; however, determining an abnormal QRS duration will require consultation with the table of age-related "normal."
- In the presence of bundle-branch block, it is difficult to determine the presence of hypertrophy; an echocardiogram usually is needed.
- Successful recognition of ventricular hypertrophy starts by examining V1 and V6, as V1 overlies the right ventricle and V6, the left ventricle. Looking for a tall R wave in these leads will help the reader detect hypertrophy.

▶ **Findings suggestive of RVH are:**

- Tall R in V1/V2
- Tall R in V4R
- Deep S in V5/V6
- R/S ratio >ULN in V1
- R/S ration <LLN in V6
- Tall R in III and aVR
- Deep S in I and aVL

- Q in V1 is seen in L transposition and single ventricle
- Upright T in V1 after 3 days of age is suggestive of RVH.
- A pure R in V1 of more than 10 mm strongly suggests RVH.
- An rSR complex in V1 may be normal, but if the R is >10 mm in size in a child <1 year or >15 mm in a neonate, RVH should be suspected.

► **Findings suggestive of LVH are:**
- Tall R in V5/V6
- Deep S in V1/V2
- Deep S in V4R
- Large R/S ratio in V6
- Small R/S ratio in V1
- Tall R in I, II, aVL, aVR
- Deep Q >4 mm in V5/V6
- Deep Q in II, III, aVF
- Inverted T in V6

Normal Range of QRS Voltage by Age *(Millimeters)*

Age	1 wk	1-3 wks	1-2 mos	3-5 mos	6-11 mos
R in V1	5-26	3-21	3-18	3-20	2-20
S in V1	0-23	0-16	0-15	0-15	0.5-20
R in V6	0-12	2-16	5-21	6-22	6-23
S in V6	0-10	0-10	0-10	0-10	0-7

Age	1-2 yrs	3-4 yrs	5-7 yrs	8-11 yrs	12-15 yrs	>16 yrs
R in V1	2-18	1-18	0.5-14	0-14	0-14	0-14
S in V1	0.5-21	0.5-21	0.5-24	0.5-25	0.5-21	0.5-23
R in V6	6-23	4-24	4-26	4-25	4-25	4-21
S in V6	0-7	0-5	0-4	0-4	0-4	0-4

Adapted from Sharieff GQ, Rao SO. The pediatric ECG. *Emerg Med Clin North Am.* 2006;24:195-208

- To obtain proper measurements, be sure that the tracing is performed at 10 mV/cm. This can be determined by the calibration marking that precedes the ECG tracing.
- **Findings suggestive of biventricular hypertrophy are:**
  - Findings above of both RVH and LVH
  - Findings of RVH with waves falling short of LVH may indicate cancellation of opposing forces.
- **ST segment and T waves**
  - ST-segment and T-wave changes signify similar pathology to changes in the adult ECG.
  - Pericarditis, myocarditis, digitalis effect, ischemia, infarction, hypertrophy with strain, hypothyroidism, and electrolyte abnormalities can produce changes.
  - J-point elevation and ST depression (1 mm in limb leads and 2 mm in precordial leads) may be normal findings.

Summary

- The large variations of "normal" in pediatric ECG make ECG interpretation in the pediatric population more challenging than in the adult population for the average emergency physician.
- However, understanding how the developing heart is reflected in the ECG and having a readily accessible table of age-related normals will greatly aid in pediatric ECG interpretation.
- A strong knowledge base and experience of reading many adult ECGs will aid, as well.

Review Questions

1. **Which is the predominate structure in the newborn heart?**
   A. Right atria
   B. Right ventricle
   C. Left atria
   D. Left ventricle

2. **Which of the following aids in pediatric ECG interpretation?**
   A. Understanding how the developing heart is reflected in the ECG
   B. Having good tables for normal age-related measurements readily available
   C. Having a good knowledge base of the basics of ECG interpretation
   D. All the above

3. **When evaluating for RVH in children, which wave is most important to consider?**
   A. R in V1
   B. R in V4
   C. R in V6
   D. S in V1

4. **What diagnosis can be made in a 3-month-old with right-axis deviation and an R wave that is 12 mm in V1?**
   A. LVH
   B. RVH
   C. Biventricular hypertrophy
   D. Ventricular septal defect

1. B
2. D
3. A
4. B

Congenital Heart Defects

Dale P. Woolridge, MD, PhD

Critical Concepts

- It is not critical to determine the exact cardiac defect at hand in the emergency setting. It **IS** critical, however, to determine the hemodynamics at hand to be able to administer appropriate care.

- Left→right shunt lesions manifest in infancy with CHF (large cardiac lesions), or in adolescents or later with symptoms of pulmonary hypertension (small cardiac lesions).

- The hemodynamic effects of left→right shunt lesions are blunted by the high pulmonary vascular-resistance in the newborn. Symptoms become more evident after one month of life when this resistance drops.

- Transient cyanosis associated with crying may suggest pulmonary disease or a cardiac defect allowing right→left shunting. Very often, one will see the patient with a cyanotic heart defect to be "comfortably blue" at rest, only to worsen with agitation. On the other hand, patients with primary pulmonary processes will show cyanosis that improves with crying since the underlying defect is ventilatory in nature.

- Prostaglandin therapy can have complicating side effects, but should *not* be avoided. This therapy is lifesaving for the newborn in shock from a ductal-dependent lesion.

Background

Cardiac malformation accounts for approximately 10% of infant mortality and almost all deaths. The presentation of congenital heart disease (CHD) can be quite deceiving for two very important reasons. First, the diagnosis is relatively uncommon with an approximate incidence of 4 to 6 cases in 1,000 live births. Second, neonates with congenital heart disease are not always overtly symptomatic at birth and the diagnosis may be overlooked in the nursery.

The age when symptoms develop can serve as a valuable tool in discerning the underlying cardiac defect at hand. Patients who develop symptoms in the first week of life tend to have ductal-dependent lesions. The next crucial time at which these patients present is marked by the fall in pulmonary vascular-resistance

(PVR) and progressive left→right shunting (2-6 weeks of life). Patients who present at this time are those who have lesions that allow shunting in the face of unrestricted pulmonary blood flow. Examples that are typical of this scenario include transposition of the great arteries, total anomalous pulmonary venous return, and truncus arteriosus. In each of these, PVR *decreases* and left-to-right shunting *increases*, which results in progressively increased pulmonary perfusion. This results in pulmonary congestion and signs of congestive heart failure. To confound matters, the patient with a left→right shunt lesion is more susceptible to respiratory infections. Often it is an underlying infection that tips the patient into the decompensated state that requires medical care in the emergency setting.

It is not critical to determine the exact cardiac defect at hand in the emergency setting. This will be determined later, after echocardiographic imaging and cardiac catheterization is performed. It is, however, critical to determine the hemodynamics at hand to be able to administer appropriate care. One of the better categorization schemes for congenital cardiac lesion is to organize by the hemodynamic manifestation of these lesions. This physiologic categorization scheme is based on the presence or absence of hypoxia and the presence or absence of pulmonary over-perfusion (*Table 1*).

Table 1. Physiologic Classification of Congenital Heart Disease

Acyanotic
• **Left→right shunt lesions**
► Atrial septal defect
► Ventricular septal defect
► Patent ductus arteriosus
► Endocardial cushion defects
• **Left outflow tract obstruction**
► Coarctation of the aorta
► Aortic stenosis
► Hypoplastic left heart
► Interrupted aortic arch
Cyanotic
• **Decreased pulmonary blood flow (right→left shunt lesions)**
► Tetralogy of Fallot
► Pulmonary stenosis
► Pulmonary atresia *with* VSD
► Pulmonary atresia *without* VSD (hypoplastic right heart)
► Tricuspid atresia

> - **Increased pulmonary blood flow (abnormal intracardiac mixing)**
>   - ► Transposition of the great arteries (TGA)
>   - ► Truncus arteriosus (TA)
>   - ► Total anomalous pulmonary venous return (TAPVR)

Assessment

- History
  - ► Note genetic syndromes associated with congenital heart disease (*Table 2*).
  - ► Fussiness
  - ► Inadequate weight gain
  - ► Low-grade fever (due to patient's hypermetabolic state)
  - ► Feeding intolerance (Feeding for the infant is equivalent to exercise in adults.)
    - ▪ Length of feedings, sweating during feeds, taking frequent breaks

Physical Findings

- General appearance
  - ► Varies from consolable, irritable to lethargic
  - ► Dehydration and/or muscle-wasting may be present.
  - ► Cyanosis: Distinguish between cyanosis of *central* (always pathologic) and *peripheral* (may be a normal finding) (*Table 3*).
- Vital signs
  - ► Respiratory rate (An increased work of breathing, although sometimes subtle, is almost always present.)
  - ► Increased heart rate
  - ► Hypotension (late and ominous finding)
- Precordial exam
  - ► Presence and location of a precordial thrill or impulse
  - ► Nature of S1 and S2 heart sounds
  - ► Characteristic and timing of audible murmurs
    - — Concerning findings include harshness, louder than a Grade 3, thrill, and hyperdynamic precordium.
    - — Diastolic murmurs are *always* abnormal.

- Abdominal exam
  - In CHD, hepatomegaly is much more likely to be seen in an infant than jugular venous distention and isolated lower extremity edema.
- Extremities
  - Varying extremity pulses (i.e., decreased lower-extremity pulses in coarctation of the aorta).
  - Blood pressures should be measured in the right arm (pre-aortic arch) and lower extremity (post-aortic arch).

Table 2. Genetic Syndromes with Known Association to Congenital Heart Disease

Trisomy 21	Endocardial cushion defects
Turner (XO)	Coarctation of the aorta
Noonan	Pulmonary stenosis
DiGeorge	Conotruncal abnormalities (truncus arteriosus, Tetralogy of Fallot, interrupted aortic arch)
Williams	Supravalvular insufficiency, mitral valve prolapse
Holt-Oram	Atrial septal defects

Table 3. Central vs. Peripheral Cyanosis

• **Peripheral cyanosis: Manifestation of inadequate peripheral perfusion**
▶ Blue discoloration of the hands, feet, and circumoral region
▶ Common in the neonate and generally not indicative of a serious illness
• **Central cyanosis is *always* abnormal.**
▶ May be secondary to a cardiac, pulmonary, or central nervous system etiology
▶ Blue discoloration of the trunk, extremities, lips, and mucosal membranes

Evaluation/Tests

- **Pulse oximetry:** Pre- (right arm) and post- (either leg) ductal oxygen saturation
- Blood gas
  - Acidosis suggests inadequate oxygenation in cyanotic lesions or inadequate perfusion in acyanotic lesions.

- ► pCO2
  - ■ Patients with CHD in the absence of respiratory failure are unlikely to be hypercarbic (pCO2>40 mmHg).
  - ■ Most often, these patients will have increased ventilation at baseline, demonstrated by a pCO2 of 25-40 mmHg.
- • **100% oxygen test:** Administering 100% oxygen and assessing the rise in arterial oxygenation
  - ► **Theory:** Hypoxia secondary to pulmonary disease or hypoventilation is more likely to be overcome with 100% oxygen; while cyanotic cardiac defects that have a mixing of saturated and desaturated blood are less likely to be overcome with 100% oxygen.
    - ■ pO2 value <100 mmHg on 100% inhaled oxygen is highly suggestive that the cause of cyanosis is cardiac in nature.
    - ■ pO2 value >150 mmHg on 100% inhaled oxygen is highly suggestive that the cause of cyanosis is not cardiac.
    - ■ pO2 value >100 mmHg, but <160 mmHg despite 100% oxygen is equivocal.
- • Chest radiograph, evaluate for:
  - ► Size and shape of the cardiac silhouette
  - ► Almost all congenital heart defects, excluding total anomalous pulmonary venous return, will result in cardiomegaly.
  - ► "Boot-shaped" in Tetralogy of Fallot
  - ► "Egg on a string" in transposition of the great arteries
  - ► "Figure 8" in total anomalous pulmonary venous return
  - ► Right sided aortic arch is seen in Tetralogy of Fallot and transposition of the great arteries.
    - ■ In a normal radiograph, the airway will deviate slightly to the right above the carina. In a right-sided aortic arch, the airway will be either straight or deviate to the left.
  - ► Increased pulmonary vascular markings suggest pulmonary over-perfusion; decreased pulmonary vascular markings suggest right-heart obstructive lesions.
- • Electrocardiogram
  - ► Infants are born with a rightward axis (~90-180°) that converts by approximately 3-4 weeks of life to the axis more often seen in adults (~0-90°).

- ▶ Upright T wave in V1 is normal at birth, but should not persist beyond 3 days of age.
- ▶ Chamber hypertrophy (Refer to reference tables. Criteria for hypertrophy varies by age.)
- ▶ See *Table 4* for a summary of concerning EKG changes.
- Echocardiogram and cardiac catheterization are required for diagnosis and characterization of the altered hemodynamics.

Table 4. Concerning EKG Changes

Right Atrial Enlargement
- Peaked P waves >3 mm in any lead

Left Atrial Enlargement
- P-wave duration >0.10 sec **OR**
- P wave with notching or plateau contour **OR**
- Terminal or deeply inverted P wave in V3R or V1

Right Ventricular Hypertrophy
- R-wave amplitude in V1 >98%** **OR**
- S-wave amplitude in V6 >98%** **OR**
- Upright T wave in V1 after 3 days of age

Right Ventricular Hypertrophy in the Newborn
- Pure R wave in V1>10 mm **OR**
- R in V1 >25 mm or R In aVR >8 mm **OR**
- Right-axis deviation >180° **OR**
- Any Q wave in V1

Left Ventricular Hypertrophy
- R-wave amplitude in V5 or V6 >98%** **OR**
- S-wave amplitude in VI >98%** **OR**
- R-wave in V1 or V2 <5% **OR**
- Inverted T wave in V6 **OR**
- Q wave >4 mm in V5 or V6

Due to physiologic axis changes that naturally occur in utero, the above criteria are not as reliable in the premature infant.

Criteria may not be applicable in the event of incorrect lead placement, abnormal conduction, abnormal cardiac positions. or complex cardiac detects.

**Amplitudes vary with the age of the patient and are derived from population-based studies and can be obtained from published tables.

Management

- Consult with pediatric cardiology immediately when congenital heart disease is expected.
- "ABCs"
- Consider antibiotics; sepsis is a much more common cause of shock!
- Infants who present in the first week of life have almost exclusively ductal-dependent lesions.
- Treatment strategy is to maintain ductal patency.
- Intravenous PGE1 (ductal-dependent lesions)
  - ► Continuous infusion at 0.05 to 0.2 mcg/kg/min initiated at 0.1 mcg/kg/min
  - ► Consultation with a pediatric cardiologist is advisable.
  - ► Intravenous prostaglandins are lifesaving in the presence of a ductal-dependent lesion.
  - ► The physician who strongly suspects the presence of an underlying ductal-dependent defect in this age group should not hesitate to start prostaglandins.
  - ► Side effects: hyperpyrexia (14%), apnea (9 %-12%), and flushing (10%), tachycardia, bradycardia, hypotension.
    - ■ Close monitoring is essential.
    - ■ Strong consideration should be given to intubation prior to transfer.
- Hypotension
  - ► Crystalloid volume bolus (10-20 mL/kg)
  - ► Positive inotropic agents such as dobutamine and/or dopamine (not as effective in an acidosis)
    - ■ Correcting hypoglycemia (10 cc/kg of 10% glucose solution)
    - ■ Correct acidosis: ventilation, fluid resuscitation, sodium bicarbonate (0.5-1 mEq/kg)

Positive-pressure ventilation will help with pulmonary edema, but may antagonize issues of hypotension.

Consult with a pediatric cardiologist and intensivist.

Definitive diagnosis will require echocardiography and/or cardiac catheterization.

Specific Treatment
Congestive Heart Failure
- Treatment is directed at decreasing afterload and increasing cardiac output.
- Furosemide (0.5-1 mg/kg IV)
- Ace inhibitor (consider enalapril 0.005-0.01 mg/kg IV)
- Inotropic agents (consider dobutamine ggt)

Hypoplastic Left Heart Syndrome
- Prostaglandins IV
- Therapy is directed at increasing pulmonary vascular-resistance to promote left→right shunting across the PDA in order to promote systemic perfusion.
  - ▶ An increased PVR is promoted through hypercarbia and hypoxia.
  - ▶ Ventilate to target respiratory acidosis: $pCO_2 \sim 35$.
  - ▶ Oxygen restriction (target SaO_2 <90%) may require N_2 gas mixing into ventilator circuit.

Hypercyanotic "Tet" Spell
- Theory
  - ▶ Muscular component of pulmonary stenosis is dynamic, resulting in acute increases in obstruction to flow.
  - ▶ Decreases in SVR (dehydration, vagal tone, etc.)
- Treatment is directed at increasing SVR and promoting flow to the lungs.
  - ▶ Squatting/babies knees to chest
  - ▶ IVF boluses
  - ▶ Morphine (thought to decrease pulmonary obstruction)
  - ▶ Phenylephrine 0.1 mg/kg/dose IV/IM
  - ▶ Propranolol (relaxes the infundibular muscle spasm that causes the right ventricular outflow tract obstruction)

Postoperative Patients
- The key to therapy is to understand the hemodynamic physiology at hand.
  - ▶ This requires a general understanding of the patient's anatomy and surgical repair process. (Common surgical repair procedures are listed in *Table 5*.)
  - ▶ Rely heavily on the patient's guardian, who oftentimes is very knowledgeable about the child.

- All postoperative patients are at risk for dysrhythmia. This is especially true for Tetralogy of Fallot, where surgical repair requires instrumentation of the ventricle.
- Dysrhythmia is highest in the early postoperative period, but can occur *years* later.
- Determine when medications were last adjusted. Growing children will outgrow their doses (i.e., patients with left→right shunt lesions taking diuretics).

Table 5. Common Surgical Repair Procedures

Procedure	Description
Blalock-Taussig	Shunt anastomosis of subclavian to pulmonary artery
Fontan	Total cavo-pulmonary shunt; results in redirecting systemic venous return directly to the pulmonary artery. Final stage in surgery for single ventricles.
Mustard	Atrial switch using prosthetic material for intra-atrial baffle
Senning	Atrial switch using native material for intra-atrial baffle
Norwood	Palliative procedure in HLHS; involves reconstruction of hypoplastic aorta
Ross	Transplantation of pulmonary valve to correct defective aortic HLHS valve followed by conduit from right ventricle to pulmonary artery
Atrial septostomy	Catheter-mediated balloon dilation of foramen ovale with resultant disruption of atrial septum
Bidirectional Glenn	Anastomosis of superior vena cava to right pulmonary artery or hemi-Fontan
Arterial switch	Correction of TGA where aortic trunk is reconnected to the LV and the pulmonic trunk is reconnected to the RV
Rastelli	Patch closure of VSD with conduit connecting right ventricle to pulmonary artery

Review Questions

1. A hypercyanotic "Tet" spell is treated with all the following EXCEPT:
   A. Morphine
   B. Phenylephrine
   C. Ace inhibitors
   D. Squatting

2. All the following are true for ventricular septal defects EXCEPT:
   A. Left→right shunt lesions
   B. Present acutely in the newborn period with cyanosis
   C. May cause recurrent lower respiratory infections
   D. Can present in adolescents with pulmonary hypertension

3. All of the following are true for hypoplastic left heart syndrome EXCEPT:
   A. It's a ductal-dependent lesion.
   B. Hemodynamics result in over-perfusion of the lungs.
   C. Intravenous prostaglandins are helpful preoperatively.
   D. Hyperventilation and hyperoxygenation can improve hemodynamics.

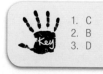

1. C
2. B
3. D

Endocrine Emergencies

Giselle Zagari, MD

26

Diabetic Ketoacidosis

Critical Knowledge

- ABCs, supplemental O2
- 2 large-bore IVs
- NPO
- Arterial line (shock, AMS, severe acidosis)
- Labs: immediate FSBS, ABG/VBG, UA with osmolarity, serum electrolytes, serum magnesium, serum calcium, CBC with differential, serum osmolarity
- Assess dehydration
- Begin with isotonic fluids, 20-ml/kg bolus over 30-60 min.
- Transition early to maintenance fluids for correction over 24-48 hours.
- Administer insulin.
- Empiric antibiotics (if infectious etiology thought to be present)
- Monitor (ICU admission, pediatric endocrine consult)

Background

- **Definition:** hyperglycemia, ketonemia, and acidosis due to untreated absolute (type I) or relative (type II) deficiency of insulin.
- **Hyperglycemia**: Results from impaired uptake from lack of insulin or insulin-insensitivity. Hyperosmotic serum pulls water out from cells, leading to osmotic diuresis and hypovolemia. Hypovolemia leads to hypoperfusion, resulting in lactic acidosis.
- **Ketonemia**: Glucagon is released to mobilize glycogen from liver for fuel for cells and also leads to lipolysis. Incomplete fatty acid oxidation leads to ketoacid formation: acetone, acetoacetate, and beta-hydroxybutyrate; only the former two are detected on UA. These (acetone and acetoacetate) increase as acidosis resolves, while beta-hydroxybutyrate decreases. As acidosis worsens, the opposite is true; **therefore, a UA may *not* reflect ketosis.**

- **Acidosis**: Combination of ketosis and lactic acidosis
  - ▶ Anion gap (AG) will be elevated (AG = $Na^+ - [Cl + HCO3]$)
- Hyperkalemia initially may be seen, even if a potassium deficit exists.
- As acidosis corrects, serum potassium levels will decrease.
  - ▶ **Must correct severe potassium deficits before insulin administration**.
  - ▶ Caused by an extracellular shift of K^+ as H^+ moves intracellularly due to excess (acidosis).
  - ▶ Also caused by decreased renal tubular excretion.
  - ▶ EKG may show tall, peaked T waves.
- Hypokalemia
  - ▶ May develop after insulin administration due to the correction of acidosis and the K^+ returning intracellularly.
  - ▶ Replace accordingly with IVF as described in *Treatment* section.
  - ▶ EKG may show low T waves or U waves.
- Hyponatremia
  - ▶ Often observed as a dilutional effect of free water moving extracellularly due to the increased serum osmolarity from hyperglycemia.
  - ▶ Measurement of true serum Na^+ during hyperglycemia: serum Na^+ + 1.6 mEq per 100 mg/dL glucose over a baseline glucose of 100.
- Hypophosphatemia
  - ▶ Results from acidosis, catabolism, insulin insufficiency, and osmotic diuresis.
  - ▶ Often occurs during treatment of DKA.

Complications

- Hypoglycemia
- Persistent acidosis
- Hypokalemia
- Cardiac dysrhythmias
  - ▶ Hyperkalemia, hypokalemia, and/or hypocalcemia
- Pulmonary edema/ARDS
  - ▶ May be due to low plasma oncotic pressure and increased pulmonary capillary perfusion in combination with excessive crystalloid infusion

- Cerebral edema/herniation
  - ▶ Cause is multifactorial
  - ▶ May occur from rapid correction of hyperglycemia and serum osmolarity.
  - ▶ Brain cells absorb glucose readily during hyperglycemia. If extracellular osmolarity drops rapidly due to correction of hyperglycemia, free water shifts intracellularly to the area of high-glucose concentration within brain cells, resulting in edema.
  - ▶ Occurs in 0.3-1% of all episodes of DKA.
    - ■ One-third of cases lead to death.
    - ■ One-third of cases lead to some type of neurological impairment.
  - ▶ High-risk indicators
    - ■ New-onset DM
    - ■ Age <2 yrs
    - ■ pH <7.1 or pCO_2 <20
    - ■ Severe dehydration
    - ■ Neurological changes
    - ■ Cardiovascular instability
    - ■ Rapid decline in blood glucose
    - ■ Rehydration with hypotonic solutions
    - ■ Use of bicarbonate
    - ■ Rate of hydration >50 cc/kg/hr
  - ▶ Usually occurs 4-24 hrs after therapy initiated
    - ■ Patient appears to be improving chemically/clinically
    - ■ 50% cases demonstrate neurological changes before collapse: HA, incontinence, behavior, papillary, BP, bradycardia, S7, temperature dysregulation.
    - ■ Treat by reducing ICP.
    - ■ ABCs
    - ■ Mannitol (0.2-1 g/kg IV over 30 min)
    - ■ Reduce fluids.
    - ■ Hyperventilation 5-10 breaths/min over regular rate for age
    - ■ Glucocorticoids

Differential Diagnosis

- **NOTE: Classic symptoms are often absent in toddlers!**
- **New onset diabetes:** presenting symptoms
  - ► Insidious
  - ► 3Ps: polyuria, polydipsia, polyphagia
  - ► Nausea/vomiting
  - ► Abdominal pain
  - ► Weight loss
  - ► Fever
- **Known diabetic:** precipitating factors
  - ► Missed insulin doses
  - ► Infection/current illness (**most frequent cause of DKA; evaluate aggressively**)
  - ► Drugs/alcohol
  - ► Psychosocial stressors
  - ► Poor compliance
  - ► Trauma
  - ► Pump failure
  - ► DKA in nondiabetics
  - ► Salicylate intoxication
  - ► Pneumonia/asthma
  - ► Head injury/CNS infection
  - ► Dehydration
  - ► Renal glucosuria
  - ► Alcoholic ketoacidosis
  - ► Large or small bowel obstruction
  - ► Pancreatitis
  - ► Gastroenteritis
  - ► Pyloric stenosis
- What not to miss on initial presentation
  - ► AMS without evidence of head trauma
  - ► Kussmaul respirations

- ► Acetone/fruity odor on patient's breath; **not everyone can detect this odor!**
- ► Don't forget the importance of a quick finger-stick!
- ► NOTE: Sedation is contraindicated due to neurological and respiratory impairment. **Do not give promethazine!**

Treatment

- ABCs
- Assess level of dehydration:
  - ► **Minimal**: 1%-2% (10-20 cc/kg)
    - Polydipsia
    - Mild oliguria
    - Mild: 3%-5% (child-infant; 30-50 cc/kg)
    - Dry lips
    - Thick saliva
    - Decreased tears
    - Anterior fontanelle flat
    - Decreased urine output
  - ► **Moderate**: 6%-9% (child-infant; 60-90 cc/kg)
    - Sunken eyes
    - Absent tears
    - Dry mucosa
    - Sunken fontanelle
    - Weak/rapid pulse
    - Decreased skin turgor
    - Cap refill >2 sec
    - Listless/irritable
    - Urine: dark, <1-2 cc/kg/hr, specific gravity = 1.030, increased BUN
    - pH <7.3
  - ► **Severe**: 10%-15% (child-infant; 100-150 cc/kg)
    - Limp and cold
    - Lethargy or coma
    - Acrocyanosis

- Thready pulse
- Grunting
- Deep and rapid RR
- Hypotension
- Skin retracts >2 sec
- Oliguria/anuria: specific gravity >1.035
- Cap refill >4 sec
- Markedly increased BUN
- pH <7.0

Fluid Replacement

- Determine volume of fluid replacement.
  - ▶ Deficit (% dehydration × body weight in kg) + maintenance given over 48 hours
  - ▶ Approximately 1½ times maintenance fluids
- Determine type of fluids to use:
  - ▶ Begin with 0.45 NS w/ 20 mEq KCl
- Order 2 bags of fluid and hang:
  - ▶ ½ NS +/- K⁺ and D10 ½ NS +/- K⁺
  - ▶ ½ NS +/- K⁺ will run at calculated rate.
  - ▶ D10 ½ NS +/- K⁺ may be titrated in while maintaining a constant rate once glucose drops to 250 mg/dL.
- Potassium (**Must be replaced prior to insulin administration**.)
  - ▶ Check EKG and urine output.
  - ▶ K⁺ must be >2.5 for insulin administration.
  - ▶ Recheck K⁺ levels hourly.
  - ▶ Replacement:
    - 2.5-3.5: *ADD* 40-60 mEq/L
    - 3.5-5.0: *ADD* 30-40 mEq/L
    - 5-5.5: *ADD* 20 mEq/L
    - >5.5: *OMIT* K from IVF
- Phosphorous
  - ▶ May drop with insulin therapy.

- ▶ Treat if there are cardiopulmonary effects (<0.5-1).
- ▶ Avoid excessive replacement; may lead to hypocalcemic tetany.
- ▶ Use 50:50 mix of Kphos and KCl for K^+ replacement in the first 8 hours.
- Bicarbonate (**Note: controversial**)
  - ▶ May worsen cerebral acidosis and edema.
  - ▶ Resultant alkalosis decreases O2 delivery to tissue due to a left-shifted O2 dissociation curve and hypokalemia due to intracellular shift of potassium.
  - ▶ May be indicated in severe, refractory acidosis (pH <7.1 after 1 hour resuscitation) with evidence of decreased heart contractility or hypoventilation.
  - ▶ Consult PICU attending/endocrinologist.
- Insulin
  - ▶ Begin drip at 0.1 units/kg/hr of regular insulin.
    - 50 units in 500 cc = 0.1 unit/cc
    - Note: Flush IV tubing with insulin prior to administration as it binds to plastic tubing.
  - ▶ Continue until acidosis is resolved.
  - ▶ Begin SC insulin and D/C drip 30 min after SC dose.
    - 0.1-0.25 units/kg q 6-8 hrs for new diabetic
    - Patient must be able to tolerate PO.
    - Resume prior regimen in known diabetic.
- Glucose
  - ▶ Decrease 50-100 mg/dL/hr during insulin gtt.
  - ▶ Maintain target blood sugar between 150-250.
    - Remember: Hyperglycemia is not killing your patient! Treatment goal is to resolve acidosis that is the result of ketogenesis, not hyperglycemia.
    - Acidosis reflects insulin deficiency; hyperglycemia reflects hydration status.
  - ▶ Begin glucose infusion when blood glucose is about 300 mg/dL or if blood glucose drops more than 100 mg/dL/hr.
    - Titrate the contents of the D10 ½ NS bag with the currently running fluids while maintaining the overall rate at a constant.
    - Insulin dose should not be adjusted!

- ICU Admission Criteria
    - ► Arterial pH <7.3 or venous pH <7.25
    - ► AMS
    - ► Severe vomiting/dehydration
    - ► Glucose >600
- Monitoring
    - ► Finger-sticks every hour
    - ► Neuro checks every hour
    - ► **Note: This includes watching for bradycardia and hypertension, which are part of Cushing's triad!**
    - ► VBG every 2-4 hours
    - ► Electrolytes every hour if unstable, or every four hours if stable
    - ► Urinalysis with each void to assess for ketones and glucose

Figure 3. Flow Sheet for Monitoring Diabetic Ketoacidosis

A suggested flow sheet for monitoring response to therapy for diabetic ketoacidosis.
(Pao_2 = partial pressure of oxygen; $Paco_2$ = partial pressure of arterial carbon dioxide)

Patient's name _____

Weight (Initial) _____ After 24 hours _____

Date _____ Hour _____	0	1	2	3	4	5	6
General information							
Mental status							
Temperature							
Pulse							
Respiration/depth†							
Blood pressure							
Serum glucose (mg/dL)							
Serum ketones							
Urinary ketones							
Electrolytes							
Serum sodium (mEq/L)							
Serum potassium (mEq/L)							
Serum chloride (mEq/L)							
Serum bicarbonate (mEq/L)							
Serum blood urea nitrogen (mg/dL)							

Effective osmolality:
   2 (measured serum sodium [mEq/L])
   + glucose (mg/dL)/18							

Anion gap (mEq/L)							
Arterial blood gases							
pH: venous (V); arterial (A)							
Pao$_2$							
Paco$_2$							
O$_2$ saturation							
Insulin							
Units in past hour							
Route							
Intake of fluids/metabolites							
0.45% saline (mL) in past hour							
0.9% saline (mL) in past hour							
5% dextrose (mL) in past hour							
Potassium chloride (mEq) in past hour							
Phosphate (mmol) in past hour							
Other							
Output							
Urine (mL)							
Other							

Adapted with permission from Kitabchi AE, Fisher JN, Murphy MB, Rumbak MJ. Diabetic ketoacidosis and the hyperglycemic hyperosmolar nonketotic state. In: Kahn CR, Weir GC, eds. *Joslin's Diabetes Mellitus*. 13th ed. Baltimore: Williams & Wilkins, 1994:738-70.

Hypoglycemia

Critical Knowledge

- ABCs, supplemental O2
- 2 large-bore IVs
- NPO
- Arterial line (shock, AMS, severe acidosis)
- Labs: Immediate FSBS, ABG/VBG, UA w/ osmolality, serum electrolytes, serum magnesium, serum calcium, CBC with differential, serum osmolarity
- **Important: Draw an extra heparinized tube and place on ice to be used for later testing by endocrinology, if necessary, for lactate, pyruvate, beta-hydroxybutyrate, amino acid profile, acylcarnitine profile, toxicologic, and hormonal studies.**

- Conscious patient *without* IV access taking POs: 5-10 grams glucose
  - ▶ 5-g glucose tablet
  - ▶ 240 cc milk
  - ▶ 1 teaspoon granulated sugar (5 g/tsp)
- *Unconscious* patient *with* IV access:
  - ▶ Peds: 1-2 mL/kg of 25% dextrose solution
  - ▶ Infants/neonates: 2.5-5 mL/kg of 10% solution
- *Unconscious* patient *without* IV access *OR* failure to respond to glucose:
  - ▶ Glucagon SC or IM:
    - Children: 30 mcg/kg
    - Neonates: 50 mcg/kg
- Refractory hypoglycemia
  - ▶ Empiric steroids: hydrocortisone 1-2 mg/kg IV q 6 hrs
- Suspected sulfonylurea overdose:
  - ▶ Octreotide 50-125 mcg SC
- Suspected hyperinsulinemic (endogenous insulin):
  - ▶ Diazoxide
    - Children/infants: 1-3 mg/kg q 8 hrs
    - Neonates: 3-5 mg/kg q 8 hrs.
- Correct electrolytes.
- Control seizures if patient is refractory to glucose therapy.
- Identify underlying cause and correct.
- Consult surgery if endogenous cause is suspected.
- Severely affected neonates of <3 months not responsive to above therapy may require surgical exploration and subsequent sub-total pancreatectomy.
- Monitor: PICU, endocrinology

Background

- Definition: blood glucose value <40 mg/dL; in neonates, <30 mg/dL for the first 24 hours of life, and <45 mg/dL thereafter.
- Whipple's triad (clinical definition): symptoms consistent with hypoglycemia; measured hypoglycemia; symptoms resolve as hypoglycemia resolves.
- Normal regulation of blood glucose: usually around 80-90 mg/dL.

- Glucose Increases transiently after meals to 120-140 mg/dL; should return to normal within 2 hrs post-prandial.
- Insulin: Secreted when glucose is present and stimulates liver to store glycogen and muscles to uptake glucose. Excess is stored as fat. Inhibits lipolysis and glycogenolysis.
- Glucagon: Increases blood glucose levels by stimulating liver to release glucose back into blood.
- Starvation: Liver maintains glucose by gluconeogenesis (amino acid and glycerol break down) and ketosis. Hypothalamus causes epinephrine release by adrenals to stimulate further glucolysis from liver.
  - ▶ Prolonged hypoglycemia over hours to days will result in growth hormone and cortisol release to preserve and decrease glucose utilization by most cells of the body.
- Newborn hypoglycemia: Serum glucose declines after birth until 1-3 hrs, rapidly depleting liver glycogen stores. Gluconeogenesis via alanine results in rapid, spontaneous glucose return.
- Older infants/children glucose homeostasis: Glycogenolysis in immediate post-feeding period and gluconeogenesis several hours after meals
- In diabetic patients (long-standing type 1):
  - ▶ Patients develop loss of glucagon secretion in response to hypoglycemia.
  - ▶ Epinephrine is released at a lower glucose threshold.
  - ▶ Hypoglycemic unawareness = loss of warning symptoms of hypoglycemia that previously prompted the patient to eat.
- Septic, liver/renal failure patients
  - ▶ Cause is multifactorial due to deficient cortisol or thyroid hormone.
- Recurrent, spontaneous hypoglycemia
  - ▶ Hyperinsulinism due to insulinoma, iatrogenic insulin or sulfonylurea drug use, insulin autoantibodies, or tumors
- Hyperinsulinism
  - ▶ Onset = birth-18 months
  - ▶ Inappropriately elevated insulin at time of hypoglycemia
  - ▶ Transient neonatal hyperinsulinism in macrosomic infants of diabetic mothers

- ▶ Due to diminished glucagon secretion and inhibited endogenous glucose production.
- ▶ Manifests as increasing demands for feeding, intermittent lethargy, jitteriness, and frank seizures.
- Ketotic hypoglycemia
  - ▶ Observed in children younger than 5 years who usually become symptomatic after an overnight or prolonged fast, especially with illness and poor oral intake.
  - ▶ Children often present inexplicably lethargic or frankly comatose, having only marked hypoglycemia with ketonuria.

Differential Diagnosis

Decreased Availability of Glucose	Increased Use of Glucose	Diminished Availability of Alternative Fuels	Unknown or Complex Mechanisms
Decreased intake: fasting, malnutrition, illness	Hyperinsulinism: islet cell adenoma or hyperplasia, ingestion of oral hypoglycemic agents, insulin therapy, infants of diabetic mothers, Beckwith-Wiedmann syndrome	Decreased or absent fat stores	Sepsis, shock, burns, cardiogenic shock, ARDS
Decreased absorption: acute diarrhea	Large tumors: Wilms' tumor, neuroblastoma	Inability to oxidize fats: enzymatic defects in fatty acid oxidation	Reye's syndrome, hepatitis, cirrhosis, hepatoma
Inadequate glycogen reserves: defects in glycogenolytic pathway enzymes	Hyperthermia		Ingestions: Salicylate, ethanol, isoniazid, propanolol, pentamidine, quinine, disopyramide, rat poison
Inability to mobilize glycogen: glucagon deficiency.	Polycythemia		Adrenal insufficiency
Ineffective gluconeogenesis: defects in enzymes of gluconeogenic pathway	Growth hormone deficiency		Hypothyroidism, hypopituitarism

What Not to Miss

- **Signs and symptoms of hypoglycemia are nonspecific and are often overlooked.**
  - ▶ Adrenergic symptoms
    - Palpitations
    - Anxiety
    - Tremulousness
    - Hunger
    - Sweating
  - ▶ Neurologic symptoms
    - Irritability
    - Headache
    - Fatigue
    - Confusion
    - Seizure
    - Unconsciousness

Treatment

- Treat initial hypoglycemia as presented above.
- Maintain blood glucose via infusion with D10W at 1½ times maintenance (6-8 mg/kg/min).
- Goal is to maintain blood sugar higher than 70 mg/dL.
- Admission criteria
  - ▶ **Any** child with documented hypoglycemia **not** secondary to insulin therapy
  - ▶ Continued or recurrent altered mental status
  - ▶ Decreasing serial glucose levels despite glucose therapy
  - ▶ Large doses of glucose required during replacement therapy
  - ▶ Known/suspected history of massive insulin or sulfonylurea overdose
  - ▶ Severe underlying disease, including sepsis, renal/hepatic failure, endocrine deficiency
  - ▶ No responsible caregiver to monitor blood glucose every 3 hours at home and give repeated feedings

Hypocalcemia/Hypocalcemic Crisis

Critical Knowledge

- ABCs
- IV
- O2
- Monitor and 12-lead EKG (long QT)
- Labs
  - ▶ Stat: calcium, phosphorus, magnesium, albumin, ionized calcium
  - ▶ Total protein, BUN/creatinine, parathyroid hormone, pH, urine calcium/phosphorous/mag
- Recognize and treat frank tetany, laryngospasm, seizures.

Background

- Total calcium level reflects bound and unbound (ionized) calcium.
- Ionized component is physiologically active.
  - ▶ Affected by albumin level, blood pH, serum phosphate, and serum magnesium.
  - ▶ Reduced by anything that may bind calcium, including citrate from blood transfusions or free fatty acids from TPN.
- Corrected serum calcium level in hypoalbuminemia
- $(0.8 \times$ [normal albumin-patient albumin]$) + Ca$
- CNS effects:
  - ▶ Hypocalcemia decreases the threshold of neuronal excitability, allowing repetitive responses from a single stimulus.
  - ▶ Affects both motor and sensory nerves.
- Tetany
  - ▶ Hypocalcemia should depress muscular excitability by impeding acetylcholine release at neuromuscular junction.
  - ▶ Results from an override of inhibitory muscle contraction and sensitive neuronal excitability.
- Calcium homeostasis
- Vitamin D (1,25[OH]2D3)
  - ▶ Raises serum calcium by absorbing calcium and phosphorous from the gut.

- ▶ Enhances PTH-dependent calcium mobilization from bone.
- ▶ Promotes renal conservation of calcium.
- Parathyroid hormone
  - ▶ Increases calcium resorption from bone.
  - ▶ Increases renal phosphorous excretion and decreases renal calcium excretion.
  - ▶ Enhances conversion of Vitamin D to active form.
- **Ergo, hypocalcemia results from a defect/deficiency in the above mentioned regulatory pathways**.
  - ▶ Vitamin D or PTH deficiency
  - ▶ End-organ resistance to these hormones due to lack of receptors or abnormal receptor binding

Differential Diagnosis
- **Do not miss life-threatening manifestations!**
- Tetany
- Seizure
- Laryngospasm/stridor
- Prolonged QT, conduction abnormalities with bradycardia

Treatment
- Acute treatment of symptomatic hypocalcemia
  - ▶ 0.5-1 mL/kg 10% calcium gluconate IV over 3-5 minutes
  - ▶ Up to 2 mL/kg IV over 20 minutes
  - ▶ Can repeat every 6-8 hours
  - ▶ **Note: Patient must remain on cardiac monitor and therapy stopped if HR <60.**
  - ▶ Therapy may be added to IV solution once symptoms are relieved or if administered orally.
    - ■ Maintenance infusion:
      <2 yrs= 8 mL/kg/day 10% calcium gluconate
      >2 yrs= 5 mL/kg/day 10% calcium gluconate
- **Note: Precautions for IV calcium**
  - ▶ Ensure diluted solution to minimize risk of burn.
  - ▶ Ensure proper IV flow to avoid SC tissue burn.

- ► Never mix with fluids containing phosphate or bicarb.
- ► Frequently monitor serum calcium.

Differential Diagnosis

Early/Neonatal (days 1-3)	Late Neonatal (3d-6 wks)	Infancy/Childhood
Prematurity: poor intake, decreased vitamin D responsiveness, increased calcitonin, hypoalbuminemia	Idiopathic hypoparathyroidism: transient vs. permanent	Hypoparathyroidism: autoimmune, post-surgical/post-irradiation, hypomagnesemia, pseudohypoparathyroidism (PTH receptor defect), infiltration (iron overload-Wilson's disease, hemosiderosis, thalassemia)
Hypoxic encephalopathy/birth asphyxia: delayed feeds, incr. calcitonin, increased phosphate, alkali therapy	Maternal hypercalcemia	Hyperphosphatemia: improper formula, inappropriate use of phos-containing enemas, loading in TPN, renal failure
IUGR	Congenital Aplasia: DiGeorge syndrome, velo-cardio-facial syndrome	Chelation, blood transfusions
Exchange transfusion (citrate load)	Cow's milk tetany: due to high phosphate load with cow's milk	Acute severe illness; malabsorption syndromes
Infant of diabetic mother	Chronic diarrhea: calcium/magnesium malabsorption, alkaline treatment for acidosis, renal losses of calcium/mag	Pancreatitis
Magnesium deficiency	Hypomagnesemia	Rickets; "hungry bone syndrome" after treatment of rickets
	Severe infantile osteopetrosis	Alkalosis: respiratory or metabolic

Acute correction of hypomagnesemia (mg <1.5 mg/dL)

- If thought to be the cause of hypocalcemia, administer magnesium first (IM route).
- Treat if hypocalcemia if refractory to calcium supplementation.
- 0.2 mL/kg IM of 50% mg sulfate
  - ► May repeat q 8-12 hours.

- Maintenance
  - ► Begin 250-500 mg PO qID when possible.
  - ► IV magnesium excreted rapidly
- **Significant hyperphosphatemia**
  - ► Correct before calcium replacement to prevent soft-tissue calcification.
  - ► Give phosphate binders such as calcium carbonate and aluminum hydroxide.
  - ► For cell lysis: NS boluses and IV mannitol
  - ► Dialysis in renal failure

Admission Criteria

Any newborn infant with hypocalcemia should be monitored in the NICU.

Any child with symptomatic hypocalcemia should be admitted to the hospital unless the diagnosis is hyperventilation.

Adrenal Crisis
Critical Knowledge
- ABCDs (D = dextrose level), O_2
- IV
- Monitor
- Labs: Electrolytes, fasting blood sugar, serum ACTH, plasma renin activity, serum cortisol, serum aldosterone
- Recognize diagnosis by hypoglycemia, hyponatremia, hyperkalemia, metabolic acidosis, shock, and ambiguous genitalia
- Immediate volume-expansion with 20 mL/kg IV NS boluses
- Maintain blood sugar with 10% dextrose.
- 50-100 mg IV hydrocortisone
- Order sepsis workup for precipitating cause and empiric antibiotics if suspected.

Background
- Definition: Adrenal cortex fails to produce enough glucocorticoid and mineralocorticoid in response to stress.
- May be primary: Adrenal disorder
- Secondary: Hypothalamic-pituitary disorder

- Mineralocorticoids/aldosterone
  - ▶ Maintain salt and water homeostasis.
  - ▶ Promotes salt resorption in distal renal tubules and collecting ducts.
  - ▶ Regulated by rennin-angiotensin system; therefore, not deficient in secondary adrenal insufficiency.
- Glucocorticoids/cortisol
  - ▶ Important hormone in mounting a response to stress, such as infection, surgery, or trauma; and promotes gluconeogenesis, and protein and fat breakdown.
  - ▶ Release is stimulated by corticotropin releasing hormone (CRH) from the hypothalamus to pituitary, and from ACTH from the pituitary to the adrenals.
  - ▶ Low levels of cortisol stimulate ACTH release; ergo, ACTH levels will be high in primary adrenal insufficiency.
- Congenital adrenal hyperplasia
  - ▶ 90% of all cases are due to 21-hydroxylase deficiency.
  - ▶ Enzyme necessary for cortisol and aldosterone production.
  - ▶ ACTH increases, precursors of cortisol/aldosterone accumulate.
  - ▶ Androgen production is increased due to shunting of the cortisol/aldosterone production pathway.
    - Females virilized in utero, born with ambiguous genitalia, and often identified at birth
    - Enlarged clitoris and fusion of labial folds
    - Males often have normal genitalia development, so are more likely to present with salt-wasting crisis in infancy or demonstrate precocious puberty.
    - Undervirilized males: small phallus, hypospadias, gonads in inguinal canals
    - Hyperpigmentation of labioscrotal folds and nipples
- Adrenal crisis often presents at 2-5 weeks of age.
  - ▶ Symptoms are often insidious and include poor feeding, lack of weight gain, lethargy, irritability, and vomiting.
  - ▶ Hyponatremia
    - Due to lack of aldosterone and inability to spare sodium ("salt-wasting")

- ▶ Hypoglycemia
  - ■ May be due to lack of cortisol and/or reduced caloric intake during acute illness.
- ▶ Hyperkalemia
  - ■ Serum levels are often between 6-12 mEq /L without EKG changes.
  - ■ May appear to be within normal limits if vomiting and diarrhea have occurred.
- ▶ Metabolic acidosis
  - ■ Reflected by low bicarb
  - ■ Due to retention of hydrogen ions in exchange for sodium loss

Differential Diagnosis

Primary Adrenal Insufficiency	Secondary Adrenal Insufficiency
Hereditary: Congenital adrenal hyperplasia, adrenoleukodystrophy, mineralocorticoid deficiency, Refsum disease, Wolman disease	Iatrogenic: inadequte glucocorticoid administration, withdrawal from glucocorticoid therapy
Autoimmune: Addison's, IDDM, thyroiditis	Tumors: pituitary or hypothalamic
Infection: tuberculosis, meningococcal septicemia, systemic fungal infections, HIV	CNS surgery or irradiation
Adrenal hemorrhage	Structural abnormalities: septo-optic dysplasia
Meds that increase steroid metabolism: rifampin, phenytoin, phenobarbitol	Congenital hypopituitarism
Meds that decrease steroid synthesis: etomidate, ketoconazole	Isolated ACTH deficiency

Treatment
- Immediate volume expansion with 20 mL/kg IV NS
- Immediate hydrocortisone IV
  - ▶ <3 yrs = 25 mg
  - ▶ 3-12 yrs = 50 mg
  - ▶ >12 yrs = 100 mg
  - ▶ Subsequent = 50 mg/m2/24 hours IV or q 6 hours

- Hyperkalemia
- Correct if cardiac arrhythmias present:
  - ▶ 10% calcium gluconate: 1 mL/kg IV over 3-5 min.
  - ▶ Kayexalate: 1-2 mg/kg PO (if taking POs)
  - ▶ Insulin: 0.1 units/kg IV with 2 mL/kg of 25% glucose 1-2 mEq/kg IV
  - ▶ Bicarb: 1-2 mEq/kg IV over 5-10 min
  - ▶ **NOTE:** Flush line after giving calcium gluconate, as bicarb not compatible.
- Identify and treat any precipitating cause, including infection and/or trauma.
- Long-term mineralocorticoid replacement:
  - ▶ 0.05-0.2 mg/day fludrocortisone acetate PO
  - ▶ **NOTE:** initial hydrocortisone at 50 mg/m2/day will supply initial maintenance amount of necessary mineralocorticoid.
- Admit to PICU
- Closely monitor hydration and blood sugar.
- Check electrolytes q 2-4 hours.
- Replace 50% fluid deficit in first 8 hours with NS and 10% dextrose and remainder over next 24 hours.

Review Questions

1. Which ketoacid is not detected by urinalysis?
2. Which electrolyte must be corrected prior to insulin administration?
3. What is the leading cause of mortality in DKA?
4. What is normal, fasting blood sugar?
5. What does glucagon do in blood sugar homeostasis?
6. At what age is surgical consultation considered in cases of hypoglycemia?
7. What two cardiac dysrhythmias are seen with hypocalcemia?
8. What electrolyte disturbance should be considered if hypocalcemia is refractory to therapy?
9. What liver function abnormality must be considered with low serum calcium levels?
10. What are the electrolyte disturbances encountered in acute adrenal crisis?
11. What immediate intervention will resolve most of these abnormalities?
12. What physical manifestations might be observed in the neonate that would suggest the diagnosis of congenital adrenal hyperplasia?

1. Beta-hydroxybutyrate (remember – the detectable ones may not be present in severe acidosis!)
2. Potassium
3. Cerebral edema
4. 80-90 mg/dL
5. Increases blood glucose levels by stimulating liver to release glucose back into blood
6. Infants <3 months not responsive to glucose therapy
7. Prolonged QT, bradycardia
8. Hypomagnesemia
9. Hypoalbuminemia.
10. Hyponatremia, hypoglycemia, hyperkalemia, metabolic acidosis
11. Immediate fluid resuscitation
12. Ambiguous genitalia in females, hypospadias, hyperpigmented nipples, and undescended testes in males

Sport-Specific Injury

Becky Doran, MD

27

Critical Concepts

- Individual sports are highly associated with specific injury patterns.
- Recognize and address acute issues of specific sports.
- Recognize the signs and symptoms of concussion and refer for long-term care.
- Re-injury syndrome following closed head injury can have devastating consequences.
- Be a true advocate for the child by exercising caution when giving guidelines for return-to-play.

Introduction

Sports injuries are one of the most common reasons pediatric patients will be brought to the ED. As an emergency physician it is important to be cognizant of the common injuries associated with a particular sport and with the high-risk injuries that can lead to poor outcomes (*Table 1*). Child athletes have different injury mechanisms, types, and distribution than their adult counterparts. An understanding of this can help the emergency medicine physician guide treatment and address the unique concerns of child athletes and their parents.

Table 1. Common Sports-Specific Injuries

Sport	Common Injuries
Baseball	"Little league elbow"/shoulder injuries
Basketball	Hand fractures/dislocations
	Knee injuries
Bicycling	Head injury
	Genitourinary injury
Boxing	Fifth metacarpal fracture
	Eye injury
Dancing	Base of fifth metatarsal fracture
Diving	Spinal cord injury
Football	Concussion/C-spine injury
	ACL tears

Golf	Elbow injury
Gymnastics	Back fractures
Hockey	Intracranial injury
Horseback Riding	C-spine/back fractures Shoulder injury
Ice Skating	Ankle injury
Running	Lower extremity stress fractures Heat injury
Soccer	ACL tear
Swimming	Rotator cuff injury
Tennis	Elbow injury
Wrestling	Rotator cuff injury Lower extremity ligamentous injury

Concussion Critical Knowledge

Concussion is a common injury in adolescent contact sports. Often the signs of a concussion are not obvious and can easily be mistaken for other processes by emergency physicians. Return to play is the ever-present question from parents, athletes, and coaches, and a firm and educated response is required. Second impact or re-injury syndrome is a real threat to athletes who have had a prior injury.

Background

- Definition: A concussion is an injury to the brain that results in temporary loss of normal brain function.[1]

- A concussion does not always include a loss of consciousness.

- Concussions can occur in any sport from contact or from falls.

- 15%-20% of high school football players will receive a concussion during a single season, according to the American College of Neurosurgeons.

- Emergency physicians will be approached for evaluation of the patient and for advice or permission regarding the athlete's ability to return to play *(Table 2)*.

Table 2. Concussion Symptoms

Prolonged headache	Balance impairment
Vision disturbance	Difficulty concentrating
Memory loss	Sensitivity to light
Irritability	Ringing in ears
Sleep disturbance	Loss of smell or taste
Nausea or vomiting	Dizziness

Diagnostics

- Complete neurologic exam
  - ► Cranial nerves
  - ► Cerebellar exam
  - ► Strength testing
- Visual acuity exam
- Head CT, if warranted
  - ► Loss of consciousness
  - ► Abnormal exam
  - ► Persistent symptoms

Treatment/Disposition

- Neurosurgery consultation for any abnormal head CT
- Symptomatic treatment for headache, nausea, etc.
- Close follow up with primary care provider for repeat exams and return to play advice
- Potential follow up with neurology or neuropsych testing if symptoms persist.

Second Impact Syndrome

Critical Knowledge

An uncommon, but devastating, injury is reported in those athletes who have sustained a prior concussion and suffer a "second hit." The lifetime accumulation of concussion and brain injury leads to long-term effects. Athletes who have had one concussion prior are much more likely to suffer a second than those who have never had a head injury.

Background

- Risk of concussion is **6 times** more likely in a player who has previously suffered a concussion.
- Second-impact syndrome is reported in the literature and is thought to have caused several instances of athlete sudden death on the playing field.
- After a brain injury, the brain needs recovery time; a second injury during that recovery period can lead to irreversible damage.

Treatment/Disposition

- Emergent airway management and immediate consultation with neuro-surgery for ICP monitoring
- Evaluation with head CT and MRI for injury assessment
- During recovery, complete restriction from contact sports

Return to Play Critical Concepts

Knowledge of return to play guidelines is critical for the emergency physician. Parents, coaches, and athletes want to return as soon as possible, often for compelling reasons (scholarships, etc.). A working understanding of guidelines and risks, and an educational approach for families, will best protect young athletes from re-injury.

Background

- The American Academy of Neurology and the International Conference on Concussion in Sport have recently posted a strong position statement on concussion and return to play guidelines.

Table 3. Graduated Return to Play Protocol

Rehabilitation Stage	Functional Exercise at Each Stage of Rehabilitation
1. No activity	Complete physical and cognitive rest
2. Light aerobic exercise	Walking, swimming or stationary cycling keeping intensity <70% MPHR; no resistance training
3. Sport-specific exercise	Skating drills in ice hockey, running drills in soccer; no head impact activities
4. Non-contact training drills	Progression to more complex training drills, e.g., passing drills in football and ice hockey; may start progressive resistance training
5. Full contact practice	Following medical clearance, participate in normal training activities
6. Return to play	Normal game play

Recommendations should require 7 days in Stage 1 with movement through the next stages in slow increments. If at any time symptoms return, go back to the prior stage and begin again. Moving through these stages should be done under the advisement of the PCP.

Treatment

- Follow up with primary care physician before return to play is always indicated for young athletes to ensure the subtle signs of continued brain recovery are not missed.

- Using the most conservative guidelines when setting up athlete and family expectations for return to play is recommended.

Ligamentous Injury and Dislocations

Critical Concepts

Although becoming more common in adolescents, ligamentous injury and dislocations in isolation (ACL tears) are, in general, relatively infrequent in the pediatric population. An astute emergency physician will search for the hidden fracture or other injury in a young child who at first glance appears to have only a ligamentous injury or dislocation.

Background

- Ligamentous injury – and in their most severe form, dislocations – are uncommon in very young children and generally are associated with fractures.

- Ligaments in children are much more elastic and stronger than boney structures.[1]

- Subluxation of the radial head in toddlers, or "nursemaid's elbow," is the one exception to this general principle.

  ▶ *Subluxation of radial head*

    - Exam: Arm held pronated and extended (limp by child's side); child is not distressed until limb is moved.

    - If signs and symptoms are typical of nursemaid's elbow, a radiograph is not mandatory. If the history is atypical, or there is focal swelling, a radiograph should be done to exclude supracondylar or radial head fracture.

    - Treat by holding child's hand; and with the other hand, encircle the elbow, thumb over radial head. Apply traction and supinate the hand while flexing the forearm at the elbow. You should feel a "pop" as the radial head is relocated. The child should move the arm normally within 30 minutes.

Treatment

- Pain control
- Stabilization of the injury with splinting in functional position
- Close follow up in consultation with orthopedic surgery
- Joint dislocations from injury are emergent because they can be associated with arterial injury, which places the entire distal limb at risk. Most are managed with immediate closed reduction. These patients should receive urgent follow up as some of these injuries in young athletes (shoulder dislocations, ACL tears) do very poorly with conservative treatment and usually require surgical intervention.

Fractures
Critical Concepts

A fracture should be suspected in any child presenting with deformity, swelling, or localized boney tenderness of a limb after an injury. In very young children, not moving the limb or weight-bearing refusal may be indicative of an injury. Fractures in children follow a different injury pattern due to the growth plate and the relative strength imbalance between the growth areas and ligaments.

Background

- Salter-Harris fractures are common.
- Watch for Greenstick and buckle fractures in young children.
- May be missed in acute injury period; if still suspicious, repeat x-rays in 5-7 days.

Diagnostics

- An x-ray should be obtained of any suspected fracture site and should often include the joints on either side.
- Comparison views of the contralateral side should NOT be done routinely, but on occasion may be helpful in interpretation (elbow).

Treatment

- Fractures are painful; early effective splinting, along with adequate pain medication, can greatly improve the patient's outlook.
- If fracture is not immediately apparent, but mechanism and suspicion are high, splinting and repeat films in 5-7 days are recommended to rule out an occult fracture.

- Fracture follow up should include referral to an orthopedist for further management, and repeat imaging after 1 week to ensure proper alignment of fracture area.

Salter–Harris classification of epiphyseal injuries[1]

Fracture Type	Description
Salter-Harris I	Slipped growth plate
Salter-Harris II	Fracture through metaphysis
Salter-Harris III	Fracture through epiphysis
Salter-Harris IV	Fracture through epiphysis and metaphysis
Salter-Harris V	Crush or compression of growth plate

Sprains and Strains

Critical Knowledge

Sprains and strains do occur in the young athlete and may indicate overuse of a particular muscle group. These injuries should be considered a diagnosis of *exclusion* in the younger age group because a disproportionate number of children complaining of painful areas after a sports injury will have a fracture.

Background

- **SPRAIN:** Overstretching and stress to a ligament
- Sprains are most common in sports that require a high frequency of twisting/cutting movements.
- Sprains are more common in adolescent athletes and do not tend to occur in younger children because the epiphyseal plates are the weak link in an injury event and are more likely to fracture.
- **STRAIN:** Damage to the muscle as a result of forceful contraction
- Children and adolescents who have recently gone through a growth spurt are at higher risk of suffering from strains.
- The most common sites for strains are the hamstrings, quadriceps, and calf muscles.[1]

Treatment

- Management of the mild to moderate sprain (fracture excluded) should follow the **RICE** pneumonic.

  REST: minimal weight bearing until acute pain subsides, then encourage mobilization and range of motion exercise.
  ICE: applied every 4 hours for 15 minutes over the first 48 hours
  COMPRESSION: firm bandaging for 48 hours only
  ELEVATION: elevate whenever possible to allow swelling to subside

- Follow up should be ensured for all of these children from the emergency department to a primary physician, who can assess progress and make rehabilitation decisions.

Heat Stress Injury

Critical Knowledge

Heat injuries include heat cramps; heat exhaustion; and heat stroke, which is a life-threatening emergency. These injuries must be recognized early and immediately treated to prevent complications. Education for the parents and coaches of child athletes is crucial in reducing heat-related injury.

Background

- Children acclimate to heat more slowly than adults because of their lower heat dissipation and sweat rates.
- Children can adjust to temperatures with proper clothing (breathable), hydration (frequent breaks), and proper monitoring.
- If any signs of heat emergency are present, the child should be brought to medical attention and cooling should begin immediately.

Treatment

- Protect airway, breathing circulation in critical patients, and respond appropriately.
- Assess core temperature.
- Begin immediate cooling measures, including the removal of all clothing, cooling blankets, cold water baths, etc.
- Rehydration
- Restrict activities following a heat emergency, educate patients and caregivers, and ensure close follow up with a primary care physician.

Review Questions

1. A 15-year-old male football player presents to the emergency department with a persistent headache after a tackle in his game 4 days prior. He also complains of trouble sleeping and concentrating in school over the past few days. His neurologic exam is normal. What is your recommendation on the big district game this weekend, which is 3 days away?

    A. Head CT; if negative, allow play.

    B. Head CT; if negative and headache is gone by game, allow play.

    C. Give acetaminophen and continue to monitor; have school trainer re-examine prior to game; if no focal neurologic findings, allow play

    D. No resumed activity until 7 consecutive symptom-free days, then gradual return to activity in a step-wise fashion.

    E. Suspend play for the season.

2. A 2-year-old child is brought in after her parents noted that she would not use her right arm at dinner. They were at the zoo during the day and had been swinging her through the parking lot on the way to the car. She complained about the arm at the time, but fell asleep in the carseat and "seemed okay." She is now in no distress, with her right arm hanging limply at her side; no external signs of injury/swelling are present. What should your plan be?

    A. X-ray then reduction of subluxed radial head

    B. Immediate reduction of subluxed radial head with a post-reduction observation period for function return

    C. X-ray of the entire arm and consultation with orthopedics

    D. Splinting of the arm after x-ray and follow up in one week as an outpatient

    E. IV pain medication, conscious sedation, and closed reduction

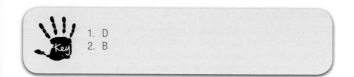

Key
1. D
2. B

Sports Dysrhythmias/ Sudden Cardiac Death 28

Anna L. Waterbrook, MD
Nathan Holman, MD

Critical Knowledge

- Pre-participation physical examination (PPE) has been the mainstay of screening for participation in athletics for many years.
  - ▶ The PPE includes taking a detailed, but targeted, personal and family history, as well as physical exam with a focus on the cardiovascular and musculoskeletal systems.[1]
- Patients with abnormal findings on history, physical examination, family history, or ECG (electrocardiogram) are referred for further testing.
  - ▶ This may include echocardiography, ambulatory monitoring, exercise treadmill testing, or cardiac magnetic resonance imaging.
- Standard ECG screening and/or other formal cardiac testing for all athletes prior to competition is controversial.
- It is very important to understand the differences between normal ECG adaptations to training and exercise versus pathological changes on the ECG that require further workup prior to participation in sports.
- Not all identified congenital heart disease requires disqualification from sports.
  - ▶ Many patients can be treated effectively and allowed safe participation in selective sports or activity.

Background/Epidemiology

- Sudden cardiac death (SCD) in young athletes (age <35 years) is a rare, but tragic, event.
- Most young athletes are otherwise healthy, and underlying heart disease is not known until SCD occurs.
- Oftentimes SCD is the initial presentation of underlying heart disease; however, it sometimes can be suspected early by prodromal symptoms such as chest pain, dyspnea, dizziness, palpitations, near syncope or syncope, or a family history of heart disease in young family members.[2,3]

- Malignant arrhythmias cause most cases of sudden cardiac death and are most often due to underlying structural heart disease or inherited arrhythmia syndromes.
- Occasionally, SCD can be a sporadic event in a normal heart due to such phenomena as commotio cordis or other idiopathic arrhythmias.
- Although still controversial, ECG screening recently has been implemented in many institutions.
- The American Heart Association (AHA) has proposed guidelines for pre-participation screening based on the athlete's age.[4]
  - ▶ Include a detailed personal history, family history of cardiac and pulmonary disease, and a detailed physical examination focusing on the cardiac and vascular systems.
  - ▶ Further testing is warranted in all patients for whom concern is identified.
  - ▶ Further testing can include 12-lead ECG, 24-hour ambulatory monitoring, exercise testing, echocardiography, cardiac catheterization, and electrophysiologic testing.
  - ▶ If the history and physical examination are normal, no further testing is warranted; only those over the age of 40 need routine ECG screening.
- The European Society of Cardiology (ESC) recommends routine 12-lead ECG screening for all athletes in addition to detailed history and physical exam, with further testing recommended for any abnormalities.[5]
- Much of the data in support of ECG screening of all athletes stems from several studies from the Veneto region of Italy, which showed a decrease in mortality by sudden cardiac death of 90% as a result of disqualification of those athletes identified to have cardiac abnormalities.[6]
- Many argue that this Italian study population is not generalized to other populations.
  - ▶ The most common cause of SCD was due to arrhythmogenic right ventricular cardiomyopathy (ARVC), a rare cause of SCD in the U.S. population.
  - ▶ Screening did not decrease the incidence of SCD due to other causes, such as hypertrophic cardiomyopathy (HCM) – the most common cause of SCD due to structural heart disease in the U.S.[7,8]

- Arguments against ECG screening in young athletes primarily involve concern about the number of false positives (the number of athletes who are unnecessarily disqualified may outweigh the number of lives saved), as well as cost of follow up regarding abnormal ECGs.
- ECG abnormalities that *require* further evaluation include:[9]
  - Q waves greater than 3 mm in depth and/or 40 ms duration in at least 2 leads, excluding aVR, III, and V1.
  - Conduction delay with a QRS duration greater than or equal to 120 ms
  - Isolated QRS axis deviation that is NOT between –30 and +115°
  - Atrial abnormalities including P-wave amplitude greater than 2.5 mm (right) atrial abnormality and/or a negative component of the P wave in V1 or V2 of 40 ms duration and 1 mm amplitude, and a total P-wave duration greater than 120 ms (left).
  - T wave inversions >**OR** = 1 mm in inferior or lateral leads, ST depression greater than 0.5 mm
  - QT abnormalities include QTc >470 ms in *men* and QTc >480 ms in *women*, as well as QTc <340 ms in *all*.
  - Brugada type I pattern (RBBB morphology with a 2 mm coved ST segment elevation that descends into inverted T wave)
  - Ventricular pre-excitation including a delta wave (slurring of the initial QRS and a short PR interval (<120 ms), documented atrial fibrillation/ flutter, supraventricular tachycardia, **OR** >/= 2 PVCs on an ECG.
- Benign ECG findings *not* requiring further evaluation include:[10]
  - Sinus bradycardia greater than or equal to 30 beats per minute
  - Benign early repolarization (ST elevation in leads V3 through V6 with an elevated J point and a peaked upright T wave)
  - Isolated increased QRS voltage criteria for left ventricular hypertrophy
  - Sinus arrhythmia
  - Junctional escape rhythm
  - Ectopic atrial rhythm
  - First-degree AV block
  - Mobitz type I (Wenckebach) second-degree AV block
  - Incomplete right bundle branch block

Note: These changes are largely due to increased vagal tone and enlarged cardiac chamber size seen in response to regular exercise.

Differential Diagnosis[11]

- Structural
  - ▶ Hypertrophic cardiomyopathy (HCM)[12,13]
    - ▪ Hypertrophy of heart muscle
    - ▪ HCM is the most common cause of SCD in young athletes in U.S. population.
    - ▪ May affect several areas of the left ventricle, but often affects the intraventricular septum.
    - ▪ Causes obstruction of the left ventricular outflow tract.
    - ▪ Inherited and has variable penetrance.
    - ▪ Usually asymptomatic; the first manifestation of the disease is often SCD as a result of vigorous physical activity.
    - ▪ Many associated arrhythmias, including atrial fibrillation, atrial flutter, ventricular ectopy, ventricular tachycardia, and ventricular fibrillation.
    - ▪ Some patients may benefit from placement of internal cardioverter-defibrillators.
    - ▪ Most recommend disqualification from participation in most competitive sports, except some low-intensity sports.[14,15]
  - ▶ Congenital coronary artery abnormalities
    - ▪ These include several aberrant coronary artery malformations, as well as premature atherosclerotic disease.
    - ▪ Often do not present until SCD, and can be difficult to detect.
    - ▪ Usually restricted from competitive athletic activity, unless patient has undergone surgical correction and normal cardiac workup 3 months after surgery.[16]
  - ▶ Myocarditis
    - ▪ Inflammatory condition of myocardium, usually due to viral infectious process such as Coxsackie.
    - ▪ May lead to fibrosis and/or cardiomyopathy and, ultimately, arrhythmias.
    - ▪ May be diagnosed with biopsy and histology.
    - ▪ Athletes need to be withdrawn from activity for a period of approximately 6 months to allow for healing and remodeling.

- Patients may return to sport if normal ECG, normalization of inflammatory markers, no arrhythmias, and normal echocardiogram.[14]
- ► Arrhythmogenic right ventricular cardiomyopathy (ARVC)[17]
  - Disease of heart muscle
  - Right ventricular myocardial atrophy and fibrofatty replacement
  - ECG changes associated with ARVC include inverted T waves in the precordial leads, a low-voltage QRS complex <1 mV in the peripheral leads, incomplete right bundle branch block, and inverted T waves in the inferior leads.
  - Associated ventricular arrhythmias include spontaneous sustained ventricular tachycardia, nonsustained ventricular tachycardia, and isolated or coupled premature ventricular beats.
  - Patients should be excluded from most competitive sports except for low-intensity activities.[14,15]
- ► Mitral valve prolapse
  - Myxomatous degeneration
  - High prevalence in population, but low rate of adverse cardiac events.
  - Usually diagnosed on cardiac auscultation with mid-systolic click and/or on echocardiography by displacement of mitral valve leaflets.
  - Most may participate in competitive sports if there is no personal or family history of cardiac events such as syncope, presyncope, arrhythmia or systolic dysfunction.[14]
- ► Marfan syndrome
  - Autosomal dominant connective tissue disorder
  - Involves primarily skeletal, ocular, and cardiovascular systems.
  - Cardiovascular abnormalities include dilatation of aortic root and descending aorta, which can lead to dissection and rupture.
  - Can also predispose patients to mitral valve prolapse and left ventricular systolic dysfunction.
  - Athletes may participate in low to moderate static/low dynamic sports[15] based upon the amount of aortic root dilatation, evidence of mitral valve regurgitation, and family history.
  - These patients need close echocardiographic surveillance.[14]

- Inherited arrhythmia syndromes
  - ▶ Congenital long QT syndrome (LQTS)[18]
    - LQTS is characterized by prolongation of the QT interval on ECG, leading to ventricular tachyarrhythmias.
    - Clinical manifestations include syncope, cardiac arrest, or sudden death.
    - A QT interval greater than 0.44 seconds is considered long.
    - It is caused by mutations in the genes for cardiac ion channels; there are several variants.
    - A variety of stimuli, including exercise, emotion, and noise may precipitate an arrhythmic response.
    - Some of the variants have been shown to respond more favorably to pharmacotherapy.
    - LQTS also may occur without stimuli.
    - Drug-induced QT prolongation can also predispose individuals to tachyarrhythmia.
    - The prognosis of those individuals with LQTS treated with pharmacologic agents is good, but athletes remain at risk for sudden cardiac death; participation should be restricted in most cases.[19]
    - Patients may also benefit from implanted cardioverter-defibrillator.
    - Most athletes should be restricted from competitive sports, except minimal contact activities (in some cases).[15,19]
  - ▶ Brugada syndrome
    - ECG changes, including incomplete right bundle branch block (RBBB) and ST elevations of the anterior precordial leads
    - Predisposes the patient to ventricular tachyarrhythmias and sudden death.
    - One of the most common causes of sudden death among young men with no history of structural heart disease.
    - Can be treated with internal cardiac defibrillation devices (ICD), but athletes should be restricted from all activities, except for minimal contact activities (in some cases).[15,19]

- ► Catecholaminergic Polymorphic Ventricular Tachycardia (CPVT)
  - CPVT is a rhythm disorder that affects the ventricles in predisposed individuals.
  - Affects approximately 1 in 10,000 people and is a significant cause of sudden cardiac death in young people.
  - Due to a mutation in a voltage-gated ion channel in cardiac cells.
  - Release of catecholamines can lead to ventricular tachycardia and death.
  - Most often, there is no evidence of underlying heart disease and the diagnosis is made based on ECG abnormalities during exercise or emotional stress.
  - Treatment includes beta blockers and calcium channel blockers
  - Most symptomatic patients should be treated with an implantable defibrillator.[19]
- ► Short QT syndrome[99]
  - Characterized by shortening of the QT interval (<300 ms) on ECG that can lead to ventricular tachyarrhythmia, especially ventricular fibrillation.
  - Short QT interval does not significantly change with heart rate.
  - Patients have tall, peaked T waves with a structurally normal heart.
  - Due to mutations in genes that affect the potassium channels of cardiac cells.
  - Clinical manifestations include syncope, cardiac arrest, or sudden death.
  - Treatments include antiarrhythmic agents and implantable cardioverter-defibrillator as a preventative measure from life-threatening arrhythmias.
  - Athletes should be restricted to low-intensity sports.[15,19]
- ► Wolf Parkinson White (WPW)[20]
  - Characterized by presence of an abnormal accessory electrical conduction pathway between the atria and the ventricles known as the "bundle of Kent."
  - May cause the ventricles to contract prematurely, causing a rapid heart rate, such as supraventricular tachycardia (SVT).

- Usually asymptomatic, patients may experience palpitations, dizziness, shortness of breath, syncope, or SCD.
- Classic ECG changes include a delta wave (an abnormal upward sloping of the QRS complex), but it also may be absent.
- Treatment of SVT includes electrical cardioversion and pharmacologic therapy.
- Definitive treatment includes electrical ablation of the accessory pathway.
- Athletes who are asymptomatic and have structurally normal hearts and/or who have had a successful ablation may be able to participate in sports without restrictions.[19]
- Younger athletes and those with history of arrhythmias need further workup with possible ablation prior to participation in sports.[19]

► Syncope
- Defined as transient loss of consciousness with loss of postural tone followed by rapid recovery.
- Not uncommon among athletes or the general population.
- Most cases are benign and self-limiting and can be classified as vasovagal syncope.
- Syncope also can be a symptom of cardiac disease or abnormalities of the cardiac system; unexplained syncope warrants further cardiac evaluation prior to sports participation.[19]

Critical Concepts

- It is important to be able to distinguish *normal* physiologic adaptations of exercise and competitive training from *pathologic* changes on ECG.
- Most structural and malignant arrhythmias associated with SCD ultimately lead to tachydysrhythmias, bradydysrythmias, or asystole as cause of death.
- Other causes include aortic dissection (Marfan's syndrome) and syncope.
- Any athlete suspected of underlying CHD should be referred to a cardiologist for further evaluation prior to any further participation in sports.

Treatment

- Please reference specific disease entities listed above for specific treatments.
- Treat cardiac arrhythmias per ACLS protocols (not covered in this chapter).
- It is very important to remember that any young athlete suspected of underlying cardiac disorder – either based upon symptoms, family history, or other clues such as ECG abnormalities seen in the ED – should be instructed to not participate in any athletic activity and/or exercise until they have followed up with a cardiologist for further evaluation.
- Not all athletes with underlying congenital heart disease need to be disqualified from sports.

Review Questions

1. **Which of the following ECG findings is considered NORMAL for an athlete?**

   A. Sinus bradycardia at 35 beats per minute

   B. QTc *less* than 340 ms

   C. QTc *greater* than 490 ms

   D. Presence of a delta wave

2. **What should an emergency physician do if there is a suspicion of underlying congenital heart disease in an athlete?**

   A. Clear for full participation in sporting events, but refer to a cardiologist for further management.

   B. Clear for limited participation in sporting events, but refer to a cardiologist for further management.

   C. Obtain a stat cardiology consult in the emergency department for all cases prior to discharge.

   D. Disqualify from participation in all athletic events until further evaluation by cardiologist.

3. **What is the most common cause of SCD in young athletes in the U.S. population?**

   A. Marfan's syndrome

   B. Myocarditis

   C. Arrhythmogenic right ventricular cardiomyopathy

   D. Hypertrophic cardiomyopathy

   E. Mitral valve prolapse

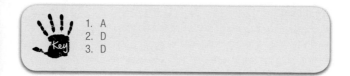

1. A
2. D
3. D

Hyperbilirubinemia

Sara Aberle, MD
Thomas Hellmich, MD
James Colletti, MD

Acknowledgement: Scott Thielen, MD, MS

Neonatal Jaundice

Background

Definition

Jaundice is a yellowish pigmentation of the sclera and/or skin caused by deposition of bilirubin.

Diagnosis

- Laboratory evaluation
  - ▶ Total serum bilirubin (TSB) >5 mg/dl
- Physical exam
  - ▶ Yellowish pigment in sclera
  - ▶ Blanch/press on skin to look at underlying pigment. (The extent of clinical jaundice does not correlate with clinician estimation of bilirubin levels or risk of developing neurologic dysfunction.)

Pathophysiology

- General causes of hyperbilirubinemia
  - ▶ Increased bilirubin production/load
  - ▶ Decreased bilirubin clearance
- Bilirubin forms
  - ▶ **Unconjugated bilirubin = indirect bilirubin**
    - Toxic breakdown product of hemoglobin
    - Difficult to excrete
    - Able to cross the blood-brain barrier (BBB) into the central nervous system, resulting in acute bilirubin encephalopathy (ABE) and kernicterus
    - Liver converts it into conjugated bilirubin with the enzyme, uridine diphosphate glucuronyltransferase (UDPGT)

- ▶ Conjugated bilirubin = direct bilirubin
  - Nontoxic and water-soluble
  - Easy to excrete
  - Unable to cross the blood-brain barrier
  - Eliminated in stool, but can be broken down to unconjugated bilirubin in the GI tract then re-absorbed back into the bloodstream (enterohepatic circulation)
- ▶ Total bilirubin = conjugated and unconjugated forms

Table 1. Conjugated and Unconjugated Bilirubin

	Unconjugated	Conjugated
Bilirubin	Indirect	Direct
Toxicity	Toxic breakdown product (hgb)	Nontoxic
Metabolism	Converted to conjugated form by UDPGT in liver	Enterohepatic circulation converts back to unconjugated bilirubin
Excretion	Difficult to excrete	Easy to excrete (water-soluble), eliminated in stool
Neurologic involvement	Crosses BBB	Does not cross BBB

Risk Factors

Major

- Jaundice present in the first 24 hours of life
- History of sibling needing phototherapy
- Prematurity (gestational age 35-36 weeks)
- Significant bruising, cephalohematoma, known hemolytic disease, or blood group incompatibility
- Exclusive breastfeeding
- East Asian race

Minor

- Jaundice present before hospital discharge
- History of sibling with jaundice
- Prematurity (gestational age ≤38 weeks)

- Maternal age ≥25 years old
- Macrosomia (secondary to maternal diabetes)
- Male sex

Signs of Pathologic Jaundice

- Onset in first 24 hours of life
- Rapidly rising total serum bilirubin (>5 mg/dL per day)
- Elevated direct bilirubin concentration (>2 mg/dL or >20% of total serum bilirubin)
- Presence of anemia or hepatosplenomegaly
- Prolonged jaundice (>/ to 10 days in a full-term infant)

Differential Diagnosis by Etiology

Unconjugated Hyperbilirubinemia

- Increased bilirubin load/production
  - ▶ Hemolysis
    - ▪ Intrinsic defects
      - — G6PD deficiency: oxidative stress leads to hemolysis. Occurs in about 12% of African Americans; common in Mediterranean, Middle East, Africa, and Southeast Asia
      - — Abnormality of the red blood cell membrane or hemoglobinopathies: hereditary spherocytosis, hereditary elliptocytosis, sickle cell
    - ▪ Extrinsic defects
      - — Autoimmune hemolytic anemia
      - — Fetal-maternal blood group incompatibility
  - ▶ Sepsis
  - ▶ Hematoma, occult hemorrhage, or polycythemia
  - ▶ Physiologic jaundice: breakdown of fetal RBCs and hepatocytes are unable to conjugate (and therefore handle) the indirect bilirubin.
  - ▶ Others: medications, DIC
- Decreased bilirubin excretion/uptake
  - ▶ Delay in intestinal transit time

- ▶ **Crigler-Najjar syndrome**
  - ▪ Type I: Extreme jaundice with bilirubin >25 mg/dL, high risk of bilirubin encephalopathy
  - ▪ Type II: Lower bilirubin levels, kernicterus rare, treatment is with phenobarbital (diagnostic and therapeutic)
- ▶ **Gilbert's syndrome:** mild jaundice, most common hereditary cause of hyperbilirubinemia (decrease in glucuronyltransferase activity)
- ▶ Neonatal hypothyroidism
- ▶ **Breastfeeding and breast milk jaundice**
  - ▪ Breastfeeding jaundice: develops 2-5 days postpartum (Inadequate breastfeeding can lead to decreased caloric intake and subsequently increased enterohepatic circulation.)
  - ▪ Breast milk jaundice: develops 4-7 days to 2-3 weeks postpartum (thought to be possibly due to deconjugating enzymes in breast milk, but this has not been proven). For healthy newborns, the danger is minimal and switching to formula is unnecessary. Breast milk jaundice may take up to 3 months to resolve.

Conjugated Hyperbilirubinemia

- Lacks toxicity, but is a marker for a serious underlying disease
- Generally presents with clinical jaundice in the first 4 weeks of life
- Causes:
  - ▶ Hepatitis
  - ▶ Cholestasis
  - ▶ Cystic fibrosis
  - ▶ Sepsis (CMV, TORCH infections, hep B) usually presents with other signs (i.e., vomiting, abdominal distention, respiratory distress, and poor feeding)
  - ▶ Inborn error of metabolism
  - ▶ Inflammation
  - ▶ Mass lesion

Complications

Bilirubin-induced neurologic dysfunction (BIND), acute bilirubin encephalopathy (ABE), and kernicterus are rare but potentially devastating consequences of neonatal hyperbilirubinemia.

Emergency Medicine Implications

There should be a sense of clinical urgency for the assessment and management of the jaundiced/hyperbirubinemic neonate. To better serve these patients, it is important to establish a systems-based approach to ensure timeliness of evaluation and treatment.

Emergency Department Evaluation

- Full history and physical exam
  - ▶ Look especially at the patient's vitals, extent of jaundice, and for neurologic abnormalities.
  - ▶ Note: Visual assessment is not consistent with the extent of bilirubin levels or risk of developing neurologic dysfunction.
- Lab testing (tailor to clinical scenario)
  - ▶ **Well-appearing afebrile infant:** total, direct and indirect bilirubin, CBC (consider urinalysis and urine culture)
    - ▪ Transcutaneous bilirubin (represents TSB; can use for immediate data if available at your facility)
  - ▶ **Sepsis:** above labs and blood, urine, and stool cxs, CSF studies, TORCH panel, hepatitis B serologies, urine for CMV
  - ▶ **Hemolysis:** Coombs test, haptoglobin, peripheral smear, maternal and fetal ABO types, G6PD
  - ▶ **Other etiologies/testing considerations:**
    - ▪ If mostly direct bilirubinemia, consider complete LFTs (AST, ALT, alk phos, ammonia, albumin, total protein, coagulation studies).
    - ▪ Basic metabolic panel
    - ▪ Urine for reducing substances
    - ▪ Alpha-1-antitrypsin, sweat chloride, red blood cell galactose-1-phosphate uridyltransferase
    - ▪ G6PD if poor response to phototherapy or clinical suspicion.
  - ▶ **Biliary atresia or obstruction:** abdominal ultrasonography
- Decision-making
  - ▶ Well-appearing, afebrile infant with unconjugated hyperbilirubinemia and normal hemoglobin = no further labs
  - ▶ Concern of sepsis, hemolysis, or inborn errors of metabolism = further workup

- ► Use www.bilitool.org for risk assessment and recommendations for follow up vs. admission/phototherapy.
- ► Plot infant on *Table 2* and *3*, or www.bilitool.org to determine need for phototherapy or exchange transfusion with possible admission for further workup and therapies.
- ► If questions or concerns exist, consult with pediatrician or neonatologist.

Emergency Department Treatment

- Goals: Identify and treat threats to life and risk-stratify.
  - ► Identify hyperbilirubinemia and most immediate potential threats to life (i.e., sepsis).
  - ► Treat underlying cause of hyperbilirubinemia.
  - ► Risk-stratify patients and develop evaluation, treatment, and follow-up plans accordingly.
    - ▪ Consider admission, phototherapy, further workup, and need for additional monitoring (sepsis, ABO incompatibility, etc.).
- Dehydration: Correct dehydration with *normal saline* boluses.
  - ► Frequent feeds and stools help excrete bilirubin.
  - ► Options for feeding with or without phototherapy
    - ▪ Continuation of breastfeeding with close monitoring
    - ▪ Supplementation with formula as needed
    - ▪ In breast milk jaundice, temporary cessation of breastfeeding is not generally recommended as long as infant is thriving, not losing weight, and breastfeeding well.
- Phototherapy *(Table 2)*
  - ► Blue light that causes photoconversion of the bilirubin molecule to a water-soluble product that is excreted in the urine and stool
  - ► Consider early goal-directed phototherapy in the ED during the evaluation and prior to return of a bilirubin level. Monitor temperature during phototherapy. Infants should wear eye-protection masks.
  - ► May lead to greater water loss (less so with LED lights)
    - ▪ Fluid intake must be increased (by up to 20%).
    - ▪ Breastfeeding may be continued.

- ▶ Rules for starting phototherapy: Use *Table 2*, www.bilitool.org, or existing American Academy of Pediatrics guidelines to determine if phototherapy is needed.
- Exchange transfusion *(Table 3)*
  - ▶ Emergent treatment is warranted for markedly elevated bilirubin with signs of bilirubin encephalopathy.
  - ▶ Exchange transfusion is recommended for term infants with hemolysis if phototherapy is unable to maintain the total bilirubin level below 17.5 – 23.4 mg/dL.
- Correction of anemia secondary to isoimmune hemolytic disease
  - ▶ Reduces the bilirubin concentration by approximately 50%
  - ▶ Should be used with concurrent phototherapy.
- Future directions in therapy
  - ▶ Medications to block bilirubin production from hemoglobin *(tin-mesoporphyrin* is currently in clinical trials).
  - ▶ High-dose intravenous immunoglobulin may decrease the need for exchange transfusion, as well as result in a shorter length of phototherapy and hospitalization in infants with isoimmune hemolytic jaundice.
- Disposition and discharge
  - ▶ Education to parents/caregivers should be both verbal and written.
  - ▶ Information to provide should include:
    - A basic explanation of hyperbilirubinemia and jaundice
    - Data regarding epidemiology and risks
      - — Two-thirds of neonates will have some physiologic, brief jaundice within the first weeks of life.
      - — One-third necessitate admission for evaluation and/or therapies.
    - Information regarding the general workup for the neonate's risk level
    - Potential therapies that may need to be initiated
    - Symptomatic management, including continuing with breastfeeding and supplementing with formula if needed
    - Worrisome signs/symptoms for which patients should return to the ED or see their primary care physician (PCP)

► Follow-up appointment/bilirubin testing should be absolutely clear and, if possible, arranged for close (e.g., next day) follow up for the patient prior to discharge from the ED. The ED provider should consider notifying the patient's PCP about the visit and evaluation, and should help facilitate follow up.

See flow chart below for a general approach to neonatal jaundice.

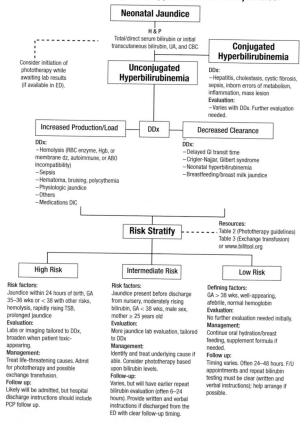

Neonatal Jaundice

H & P
Total/direct serum bilirubin or initial transcutaneous bilirubin, UA, and CBC

Consider initiation of phototherapy while awaiting lab results (if available in ED).

Unconjugated Hyperbilirubinemia

Conjugated Hyperbilirubinemia

DDx:
−Hepatitis, cholestasis, cystic fibrosis, sepsis, inborn errors of metabolism, inflammation, mass lesion
Evaluation:
−Varies with DDx. Further evaluation needed.

Increased Production/Load — DDx — **Decreased Clearance**

DDx:
−Hemolysis (RBC enzyme, Hgb, or membrane dz, autoimmune, or ABO incompatibility)
−Sepsis
−Hematoma, bruising, polycythemia
−Physiologic jaundice
−Others
−Medications DIC

DDx:
−Delayed GI transit time
−Crigler-Najjar, Gilbert syndrome
−Neonatal hyperbilirubinemia
−Breastfeeding/breast milk jaundice

Risk Stratify

Resources:
Table 2 (Phototherapy guidelines)
Table 3 (Exchange transfusion)
or www.bilitool.org

High Risk

Intermediate Risk

Low Risk

Risk factors:
Jaundice within 24 hours of birth, GA 35–36 wks or < 38 with other risks, hemolysis, rapidly rising TSB, prolonged jaundice
Evaluation:
Labs or imaging tailored to DDx, broaden when patient toxic-appearing.
Management:
Treat life-threatening causes. Admit for phototherapy and possible exchange transfusion.
Follow up:
Likely will be admitted, but hospital discharge instructions should include PCP follow up.

Risk factors:
Jaundice present before discharge from nursery, moderately rising bilirubin, GA < 38 wks, male sex, mother ≥ 25 years old
Evaluation:
More jaundice lab evaluation, tailored to DDx
Management:
Identify and treat underlying cause if able. Consider phototherapy based upon bilirubin levels.
Follow-up:
Varies, but will have earlier repeat bilirubin evaluation (often 6–24 hours). Provide written and verbal instructions if discharged from the ED with clear follow-up timing.

Defining factors:
GA > 38 wks, well-appearing, afebrile, normal hemoglobin
Evaluation:
No further evaluation needed initially.
Management:
Continue oral hydration/breast feeding, supplement formula if needed.
Follow up:
Timing varies. Often 24–48 hours. F/U appointments and repeat bilirubin testing must be clear (written and verbal instructions); help arrange if possible.

Kernicterus (Bilirubin Encephalopathy)

Definition

Bilirubin-Induced Neurologic Dysfunction

Spectrum of manifestations that occurs when unconjugated bilirubin crosses the BBR and binds to the basal ganglia and nuclei of the brain stem

Acute Bilirubin Encephalopathy (ABE)

Acute presentation of BIND with signs of toxic encephalopathy due to accumulation of bilirubin in the first days to weeks postpartum

Kernicterus

Chronic and permanent sequelae secondary to ABE

Diagnosis

Unconjugated hyperbilirubinemia and clinical signs of neurologic compromise

Clinical Picture

- Initial manifestations
  - ► Lethargy, decreased tone and poor suck
  - ► Differentiated from botulism by jaundice
- Intermediate manifestations
  - ► Irritability, moderate stupor, high-pitched cry, hypertonicity
  - ► Retrocollis (arching of neck backwards) or opisthotonus (backwards arching of trunk)
- Later manifestations
  - ► Irritability, fever, shrill or high-pitched cry, hypertonicity (retrocollis and/or opisthotonus), apnea, stupor, or coma
  - ► Differentiate hypertonicity from Infant *C. tetani* infection by jaundice.
- Chronic manifestations of kernicterus include extrapyramidal movement disorders, athetoid cerebral palsy, spasticity, gaze abnormalities, weakness, hearing difficulties, and mental retardation.

Pathophysiology

Unconjugated bilirubin is capable of crossing the BBB and is directly toxic to brain cells. Basal ganglia and brainstem nuclei appear to be more susceptible than other areas of the brain. This toxicity is manifested in the signs listed above.

Emergency Department Management

(Please see section on hyperbilirubinemia for a complete discussion.)

- Any infant with hyperbilirubinemia and signs of encephalopathy needs immediate exchange transfusion in a neonatal intensive care unit. Consider contacting the available neonatologist early to facilitate this.

- In isoimmune hemolytic disease, can use intravenous γ-globulin (0.5-1 g/kg over 2 hours) if the TSB continues to rise despite phototherapy, or the total bilirubin is within 2 to 3 mg/dL of the level requiring an exchange transfusion. The initial dose can be repeated once in 12 hours if needed.

- Please use www.bilitool.org or see *Table 2* for phototherapy and *Table 3* for exchange transfusion threshold levels.

- Workup to determine cause of hyperbilirubinemia (see previous section on hyperbilirubinemia).

- Contact a pediatrician or neonatologist for premature infants <35 weeks with suspected hyperbilirubinemia.

Table 2. Total Bilirubin Levels and Phototherapy Initiation

	Hours From Birth						
	Birth	12	24	48	72	96	>96
High Risk	>4	>6	>8	>11	>13.5	>14.5	>15
Medium Risk	>5	>7.5	>9.5	>13	>15	>17	>18
Low Risk	>7	>9	>11.5	>15	>17.5	>20	>21

Total serum bilirubin (mg/dL)

(NOTE: Low risk implies gestation >38 weeks and well; medium risk is >38 weeks with risk factors; and high risk is 35-38 weeks gestation with risk factors. The above table is not applicable to gestations <35 weeks.)

Table 3. Level to Initiate Exchange Transfusion

	Hours From Birth						
	Birth	12	24	48	72	96	>96
High Risk	>12	>13	>15	>17	>18.5	>19	>19
Medium Risk	>14	>15	>16.5	>19	>21	>22	>22
Low Risk	>16	>17.5	>19	>22	>24	>25	>25

Total serum bilirubin (mg/dL)

(NOTE: Low risk implies gestation >38 weeks and well; medium risk is >38 weeks with risk factors; and high risk is 35-38 weeks gestation with risk factors. The above table is not applicable to gestations <35 weeks.)

Review Questions

1. Which of the following is most consistent with physiologic jaundice?

   A. Jaundice within the first 24 hours of life

   B. Rapidly rising serum bilirubin

   C. Prolonged jaundice (>7-10 days in a full-term infant)

   D. Elevated direct bilirubin level (>2 mg/dl)

   E. Indirect bilirubin of 11 at 48 hours of life in a low-risk, otherwise healthy full-term infant

2. Which of the following is NOT in the differential diagnosis of unconjugated hyperbilirubinemia?

   A. Sepsis with hemolysis

   B. Physiologic jaundice

   C. Cystic fibrosis

   D. Crigler-Najjar syndrome

3. A 6-day-old infant is brought to your ED for poor feeding. She was born via an uncomplicated vaginal delivery. On physical exam, you note that the child is jaundiced. The child appears lethargic and has increased tone in her extremities. Appropriate management for this child should include all of the following, EXCEPT:

A. Admission to the neonatal intensive care unit

B. Sepsis workup

C. Immediate initiation of exchange transfusion

D. Phototherapy

E. Discharge to home

4. A 72-hour-old male infant, delivered vaginally at 38 weeks to a 32-year-old mother, was noted to be jaundiced. He has a total serum bilirubin of 16. For this patient you should:

A. Initiate exchange transfusion.

B. Discharge home, but recheck levels in 48-72 hours.

C. Initiate phototherapy.

D. Discharge home with no need for additional follow up.

5. Which of the factors below would classify a child as having "medium" level risk factors?

A. 37 weeks gestation and history of a jaundiced sibling

B. 37 weeks gestation and healthy/well-appearing

C. 38 weeks gestation and jaundice presentation within first 12 hours of birth

D. B and C

E. All of the above

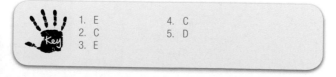

1. E   4. C
2. C   5. D
3. E

Neurologic Emergencies

Nathaniel Johnson, MD
Barrett Adams, MD

Seizure

Critical Knowledge

- ABCs, IV, monitor, oxygen, blood glucose
- Consider and evaluate for inciting event
- Status epilepticus
- First-line treatment = benzodiazepines, then consider phenytoin/fosphenytoin and/or phenobarbital
- Pyridoxine (in infants or suspected isoniazid exposure)

Definition

- Transient, involuntary alteration in consciousness, motor activity, behavior, sensation, or autonomic function.
- Caused by abnormal discharges from a group of cerebral neurons.

Background

- Seizure is a relatively common presenting complaint in the pediatric emergency department.
- Approximately 4%-6% of the population suffers a seizure by age 16.
- 1%-2% of all pediatric emergency department visits are seizure-related.
- 1%-2% of the general population has recurrent seizures/epilepsy.
- Status epilepticus (SE) is traditionally defined as a seizure or multiple seizures without return to baseline, and duration of longer than 30 minutes.
- 6%-12% of SE events in children are first-time seizures with no known precipitating cause.
- In a true emergency, timely efforts need to be made to control both *clinical* and *electrical* seizure activity.
- Morbidity/mortality from SE is related to seizure duration (increased neuronal death with duration >1 hour), age (mortality is higher in adults, particularly older adults, than it is in children), and cause of event.

Classification of Seizures

Partial (Focal Involvement of Brain)

Simple
— No impairment of consciousness.
— Symptoms may indicate location of cortex involved.

Complex
— Impairment in consciousness; symptoms can include prolonged staring/confusion (>30 seconds), automatisms.

Generalized (Involve Majority of Cerebral Cortex, Consciousness Usually Impaired)

Absence
— Brief loss of awareness (usually <5-10 seconds), multiple reoccurrences throughout the day are common.

Tonic
— Muscle contraction and rigidity

Clonic
— Alternating contraction and relaxation of involved muscles

Tonic-clonic
— Both tonic and clonic components

Myoclonic
— Brief muscle contractions

Atonic
— Loss of all muscle tone

Differential/Critical Concepts

- The most common etiology of seizures in children is fever, although this is a diagnosis of exclusion.
- One must consider other causes based on age and co-morbidities.
- For patients taking antiseizure medications, sub-therapeutic medication levels or simple withdrawal are common causes of seizures.
- Things that mimic seizure activity and should be considered in the differential when evaluating a patient include:
  ▶ Cardiac dysrhythmia
  ▶ Sleep disorders
  ▶ Migraines

- ► Breath-holding spells
- ► Nonepileptic convulsions (i.e., pseudo seizures)
- ► Toxic exposures (e.g., scorpion envenomation)
- ► Normal behavior/movements

Potential Seizure Etiologies Based on Age

Neonatal
Hypoxia, drugs, trauma, infection, hypo/hyperglycemia, pyridoxine deficiency, drug withdrawal, inborn errors of metabolism, hyper/hyponatremia
0-6 months
Infection, hypocalcemia, hyperphosphatemia, hyponatremia, developmental malformation, inborn errors of metabolism
6 months-3 years
Fever, infection, toxin, trauma, metabolic disorder
Over 3 years
Idiopathic, infection, trauma, sleep deprivation, mass

Treatment and Workup

General principles

- ABCs and D (D = dextrose)
- Maintain oxygenation and airway.
- Check glucose.
- Establish IV access (consider placing intraosseous access).
- Protect child from further harm (seizure pads, remove obstacles).

Status epilepticus

- Benzodiazepines are 80% effective in controlling SE (RAMPART study recently showed equivalency of IM midazolam to IV lorazepam for seizure treatment in the pre-hospital setting).
- Second-line antiepileptics:
  - ► Phenobarbital – 20 mg/kg IV, IM
  - ► Fosphenytoin – 20 phenytoin equivalents/kg IV; can administer as a bolus
  - ► Phenytoin – 20 mg/kg IV, **SLOW** IV infusion to avoid hypotension

- If refractory, consider intubation and sedation with propofol or barbiturates, and administer pyridoxine (particularly in infants or suspected isoniazid exposure).
- EEG monitoring
- Workup considerations
  - ► Head CT
  - ► Blood glucose
  - ► Chemistry panel
  - ► Therapeutic drug levels
  - ► CBC
  - ► Toxicology screen
  - ► Urinalysis
  - ► In the neonatal period, consider pyridoxine in the refractory seizure.

Febrile Seizure

Critical Knowledge

- Seizure is a self-limited, relatively common event in the febrile child.
- The source of the fever, however, must be considered and further evaluated when indicated.

Background

- Febrile seizures are the most common seizure event observed in the young pediatric population.
- Approximately 5% of children will experience a febrile seizure.
- In its most common form, a *simple* febrile seizure is self-limited and benign, requiring only supportive measures and no extensive diagnostic evaluation, aside from that normally performed for a fever in the respective age group and co-morbid state.
- A *complex* febrile seizure may be associated with a more severe pathology; however, risk of meningitis in patients presenting with an apparent complex febrile seizure is minimal.
- Consider lumbar puncture if:
  - ► Meningeal signs
  - ► <1 year old

- ▶ Hib/PCV immunizations not up-to-date
- ▶ On antibiotics, which can mask symptoms
- By definition, febrile seizures cannot be caused by intracranial infection or other neurologic disease.

Simple Febrile Seizure

- Fever present and age >6 months, <6 years
- Generalized convulsions (no focality)
- Last less than 15 minutes
- Do not reoccur within 24 hours

Table 1. 2011 AAP Guidelines for Neurodiagnostic Evaluation of Simple Febrile Seizures

Action Statements
• A lumbar puncture should be performed in any child who presents with a seizure and a fever and has meningeal signs and symptoms, or in any child whose history or examination suggests the presence of meningitis or intracranial infection.
• In any infant between 6-12 months who presents with a seizure and fever, a lumbar puncture **is an option** when the child is considered deficient in *Haemophilus influenzae* type b (Hib) or *Streptococcus pneumoniae* immunizations (i.e., has not received scheduled immunizations as recommended) or when immunization status cannot be determined because of an increased risk of bacterial meningitis.
• A lumbar puncture is an option in the child who presents with a seizure and fever and is pretreated with antibiotics because antibiotic treatment can mask the signs and symptoms of meningitis.
• An electroencephalogram (EEG) should not be performed in the evaluation of a neurologically healthy child with a simple febrile seizure.
• The following tests should not be performed routinely for the sole purpose of identifying the cause of a simple febrile seizure: measurement of serum electrolytes, calcium, phosphorus, magnesium, blood glucose, or complete blood cell count.
• Neuroimaging should not be performed in the routine evaluation of the child with a simple febrile seizure.

Complex Febrile Seizure

- Lasts more than 15 minutes and/or
- Reoccurs within 24 hours and/or
- Has a focal component

Differential/Critical Concepts

- Most febrile seizures occur between the ages of 9 months to 3 years, with range from 6 months to 5 years.
- Febrile seizures have a strong familial component and may be associated with a slightly higher lifetime risk of epilepsy, estimated to be 2% versus 1% in the general population.
- 30% of children will have a recurrent febrile seizure in a subsequent illness.
- The differential should include consideration of trauma, toxic ingestions, or meningitis.
- Risks of meningitis include a doctor visit within the previous 48 hours, seizure activity at presentation to the ED, focal or prolonged seizures, concerning physical exam findings, or an abnormal neurologic exam.

Treatment and Workup

- Febrile seizures are given a very narrow definition since, by making the diagnosis, the examining physician is essentially declaring that no underlying CNS pathology exists.
- The extent of workup for a child presenting to the ED with a febrile seizure will vary greatly based on the clinical picture and circumstances at hand.
- In 2011, the AAP published updated practice parameters for the management of simple febrile seizures.
- *Table 1* outlines the AAP's guidelines for the neurodiagnostic evaluation of a child with a simple febrile seizure between the ages of 6 months and 5 years.
- In the absence of suspicious history, such as vomiting or diarrhea, physical exam findings, CBC, electrolytes or blood glucose are of limited value in the examination of children older than 6 months with a simple febrile seizure.
- Lumbar puncture in the 6- to 12-month age group is no longer "strongly recommended," but is now considered an *option*, particularly in children deficient or suspected to be deficient in the *Haemophilus influenzae* type b (Hib) and *Streptococcus pneumonia* (Prevnar) vaccines.

- The pathophysiology of febrile seizures is still unknown.
- A child with a single simple febrile seizure has no increased risk of developing epilepsy when compared to the general population.
- Approximately 1/3 of children with their first febrile seizure will experience a recurrence, with 10% of these having three or more febrile seizures in a lifetime.
- The cognitive abilities of children are not affected by simple febrile seizures.
- *Table 2* outlines risk factors associated with recurrent febrile seizures and the risk of developing epilepsy.

Table 2. Risk Factors for Recurrent Febrile Seizures and Development of Epilepsy

	Recurrent Febrile Seizures	Epilepsy
Definite risk factor	Family history of febrile seizure	Neurodevelopmental abnormality
	Age <18 months	Complex febrile seizure
	Height of temperature	Family history of epilepsy
	Duration of fever	Duration of fever
Possible risk factor	Family history of epilepsy	More than one complex feature
Not a risk factor	Neurodevelopmental abnormality	Age at first febrile seizure
	Complex febrile seizure	Height of temperature
	More than one complex feature	Gender
	Gender	Ethnicity
	Ethnicity	

Migraine Headache

Critical Knowledge
- Common complaint in pediatric population
- May be associated with broad neurologic symptoms

Background
- Migraine headaches are relatively common in children and may mimic other disease entities, and often have broad associated symptomology.
- Generally, onset is around 7-10 years, with girls overtaking boys in prevalence after puberty.
- Migraine headaches are episodic, uni- or bilateral, moderate to severe in intensity, and often exacerbated by activity.
- Frequently, migraine headaches in children are associated with abdominal pain, nausea and vomiting, photo- and phonophobia.
- Migraine headaches can also be associated with dramatic neurologic findings, including stroke-like symptoms of hemiplegia, aphasia, ataxia, and visual changes.
- Classic migraines are preceded by neurosensory aura visual complaints.
- Common migraines are more prevalent and without auras.
- Multiple complex diagnostic criteria for migraine exist, but – in general – these include an episodic headache with three of the following:
  - ▶ Abdominal pain with nausea/vomiting
  - ▶ Unilateral headache
  - ▶ Throbbing quality
  - ▶ Preceding aura
  - ▶ Family history
  - ▶ Relieved by sleep

Differential/Critical Concepts
- The differential for headache is broad, and a careful history and exam is important to differentiate between benign and malignant causes.
- Generally, a diagnosis of migraine is longitudinal observation.
- Although less common, consider the dangerous causes of headache:
  - ▶ Carbon monoxide
  - ▶ Seizure

- ► Any intracranial pathology
  - ▪ Mass
  - ▪ Hydrocephalus
  - ▪ Traumatic injury and intracranial hemorrhage
  - ▪ Vascular pathology
  - ▪ Idiopathic intracranial hypertension (pseudotumor cerebri)

Treatment and Workup

- Children with recurrent headaches with normal neurologic findings do not routinely need neuro imaging.
- Consider CT or MRI and a neurology consult in the child with:
  - ► Dramatic change in the severity of headache
  - ► New neurologic dysfunction
  - ► New neurologic exam findings
- Migraine headache therapy in children can include:
  - ▪ NSAIDs
  - ► Anitemetics
  - ► IV fluids
  - ► Dark, quiet environment
  - ► Consider 5-DHT agonist such as sumitriptan
  - ► Narcotics (though be aware of rebound headache phenomena and addictive potential)

Shunt Malfunction

Critical Knowledge

- Shunt malfunction may progress rapidly to coma and death.
- Presenting complaint may mimic many childhood illnesses.

Background

- Cerebrospinal fluid shunts are frequently used in the pediatric population as a treatment for hydrocephalus.
- The majority are vetriculoperitioneal (VP), although shunt drainage may also be ventriculopleural or ventriculoatrial, draining into the pleural space or atria, respectively.

- 75% of shunts will malfunction within 10 years, with failure rates as high as 40% in the first year.
- Symptoms of malfunction are vague and nonspecific with headache, lethargy, vomiting, and irritability being most common.
- A low index of suspicion must be maintained in the shunt patient, particularly with any neurologic complaint.

Causes of shunt malfunction may include:
- Obstruction (most frequent)
- Infection
- Tubing disruption, disconnection, or migration
- Valve malfunction

Differential/Critical Concepts
- Evaluation of the shunt patient involves palpation of fluid reservoir and shunt tubing for signs of breaks, tenderness, swelling, or erythema.
- History should include underlying pathology and cause of hydrocephalus.
- A complete neurologic exam should be performed.
- The differential is broad and should include:
  - ▶ Meningitis
  - ▶ Worsening underlying disease
  - ▶ Sepsis
  - ▶ Otitis
  - ▶ Gastroenteritis

Treatment and Workup
- Concern for shunt malfunction mandates
  - ▶ Head CT/MRI, especially if signs of increased or changed hydrocephalus
  - ▶ Shunt series x-ray (skull, neck, chest, abdomen) to evaluate for kinks, interruptions
- Low threshold for antibiotics if fever or other signs of infection
- Neurosurgical consultation for any concern for shunt malfunction
- Shunt tap may be appropriate in consultation with neurosurgery.

Review Questions

1. An otherwise healthy 2-year-old toddler is brought to the emergency department by his mother after a witnessed 3-minute tonic-clonic seizure 30 minutes prior to arrival. Your exam reveals a nontoxic appearing child with a fever of 39.3°C, clear rhinorrhea, and an occasional cough. Your management should include:

   A. Appropriate fever workup, then discharge with instructions on symptom relief

   B. CT scan of the head, finger-stick glucose

   C. Admission to pediatrics to workup first-time seizure

   D. Load with phenytoin and pediatric neurology follow up

2. A 7-year-old boy with a known seizure disorder is brought to the emergency department by paramedics from school after a 15-minute seizure on the playground. Upon arrival, child begins with tonic-clonic activity and is unresponsive. Medics had been unsuccessful establishing IV access and no medication has been given. Initial appropriate management would include:

   A. Phenytoin 20 mg/kg IM

   B. Fosphenytoin 20 mg/kg IM

   C. Diazepam PO

   D. Midazolam IM

Key

1. A
2. D

Hematologic Emergencies

Nathaniel Johnson, MD
James Lehman, MD

31

Acute Anemia

Definition

- Low red blood cell (RBC) count, as assessed by hemoglobin and hematocrit
  - ► Must be determined using age-adjusted norms.

Critical Knowledge

- Age, sex, and racial predominance vary with the disease process.
- Not a true disorder, but the presenting sign of many disease processes.
- After ABCs are addressed, treatment and workup are directed toward the inciting cause.
  - ► Physical exam and history may be particularly instructive in identifying the underlying cause.

Background

- Incidence is 2-3 per 100 in the U.S.; there is higher incidence globally, particularly in regions such as Africa.
- Nutritional iron-deficiency anemia is by far the most common cause of anemia in children
  - ► It increases global morbidity and mortality.
- Age, sex, and racial predominance varies with the disease process.
  - ► Common anemias by age
    - ■ Newborns
      - — Blood loss at birth
      - — Prematurity (causes an earlier nadir in hemoglobin levels)
      - — Isoimmune hemolytic disease of the newborn
      - — Congenital red cell disorders
    - ■ Infants
      - — Iron deficiency anemia, usually found between 12 and 24 months of age
      - — May present earlier in premature infants.

- — Other nutritional anemia (e.g., vitamin B12 and folic acid deficiencies)
- — Transient erythroblastopenia of childhood (TEC)
- Young children
  - — Iron deficiency anemia
  - — Infectious anemias (e.g., parvovirus B19, Epstein-Barr virus)
  - — Autoimmune hemolytic anemias
  - — TEC; median age of onset is between 1½-2 years
- Adolescence
  - — Iron deficiency anemia
  - — Nutritional anemias
  - — Menstruation-related anemia
- Sex variations
  - — X-linked disorders such as hemophilia and glucose-6-phosphate dehydrogenase (G6PD) deficiency affect males.
  - — Von Willebrand disease may cause heavy menses in females.
- Racial variations
  - — Alpha-thalassemia affects Asian, Middle Eastern, and African-American populations.
  - — Beta-thalassemia affects Mediterranean and Middle Eastern populations.
  - — Sickle cell anemia affects African-American populations.
  - — G6PD deficiency affects African-American and Mediterranean populations.

Differential Diagnosis

- Inadequate RBC production
  - ▶ Bone marrow failure
    - Anemia of chronic disease (e.g., systemic lupus erythematosis [SLE])
    - Aplastic anemia (e.g., parvovirus B19 infection, idiopathic, etc.)
    - Chronic renal or liver disease
    - Drugs (e.g., chemotherapeutic agents, antiepileptics)
    - Transient erythroblastopenia of childhood (TEC)

- Congenital red cell aplasia (e.g., Diamond Blackfan anemia)
- Malignant bone marrow infiltration (e.g., leukemia, lymphoma)
- Hypothyroidism
- Fanconi anemia
- ► Defective hemoglobin synthesis
  - Iron-deficiency anemia
  - Lead poisoning
  - Nutrient deficiencies (e.g., pyridoxine, copper)
- ► Defective DNA synthesis
  - B12/folate deficiency
  - Drugs (e.g., phenytoin, trimethoprim, methotrexate)
- • Increased RBC destruction (hemolysis)
  - ► Hemolytic anemias
    - Isoimmune
      - — Isoimmune hemolytic disease of the newborn (i.e., Rh factor incompatibility, seen with sensitized Rh(-) mothers)
    - Autoimmune
      - — Idiopathic
      - — Autoimmune disease (e.g., SLE, rheumatoid arthritis)
      - — Infection (e.g., Epstein-Barr virus, mycoplasma)
      - — Drugs (e.g., penicillin, quinidine)
    - Membrane defects leading to early destruction
      - — Hereditary spherocytosis
      - — Hereditary elliptocytosis
      - — Paroxysmal nocturnal hemoglobinuria (PNH)
    - Hemoglobinopathies
      - — Sickle cell anemia
      - — Thalassemias
    - Enzymopathies
      - — G6PD deficiency
      - — Pyruvate kinase deficiency

- Other causes
  - — Microangiopathic anemia (DIC, HUS, TTP, HELLP syndrome)
  - — Mechanical destruction (e.g., artificial heart valve)
  - — Hypersplenism
  - — Toxins (e.g., snakebite)
  - — Thermal burns
  - — Infections (e.g., malaria)
- RBC loss from bleeding
  - Blood loss at birth (e.g., birth trauma, twin-twin transfusion, maternal-fetal transfusion)
  - GI bleeding
  - Menstrual bleeding
  - Traumatic blood loss
  - Coagulation defects (e.g., hemophilia, Von Willebrand disease)

Critical Concepts/Evaluation

- Age is an important factor when diagnosing anemia in children
  - ► Hemoglobin levels peak at birth and hit a nadir within 2-3 months.
    - Nadir occurs earlier in premature infants.
    - Diagnosis of anemia must be made using age-adjusted norms.
- Age determines the most likely causes of anemia (see above).
- History can be a key to diagnosis.
  - ► Birth history: prematurity, blood loss at birth, twinning, excessive bleeding at circumcision or from umbilical cord
  - ► Family history: anemias, splenectomy, inherited disorders, need for transfusions
  - ► Ethnicity and race (see above)
  - ► Diet/feeding history
    - Infants
      - — Iron-fortified vs. non-fortified formula
      - — Breastfeeding is normally adequate for 6 months.
      - — Whole milk is not a good source of iron, and may cause GI bleeding.

- Older children
  - Sources of iron:
    - Good sources of iron include meats, cereal, and green vegetables
    - Excessive soda and fatty snacks have been associated with anemia.
  - Assess for eating disorders.
- Growth history (poor growth may signal anemia of chronic disease)
- Medications (e.g., chemotherapeutic agents, antiepileptics, penicillin, trimethaprim, etc.)
- Pica (eating inedible substances such as dirt or paint chips, which may signify iron deficiency)
- Lead exposure

Clinical Signs/Symptoms

- Symptoms: pallor, weakness, malaise, lethargy, lightheadedness, anorexia
- Signs: tachycardia, tachypnea, systolic ejection murmur
- In severe anemia, CHF may occur with cardiomegaly, hepatomegaly, hypotension, and auscultative gallop
- Jaundice, dark urine→hemolysis
- Petechiae, purpura→hemophilia, microangiopathic diseases, autoimmune hemolysis
- Splenomegaly→malignant infiltration, hemolysis, Epstein-Barr virus
- Dysmorphic face and/or limbs→congenital diseases (e.g. Diamond Blackfan anemia, Fanconi anemia)
- Frontal bone prominence ("bossing")→chronic hemolysis with extramedullary hematopoiesis (e.g., thalassemia)
- Hypothermia, thin hair, dry skin, failure to thrive→hypothyroidism
- Glossitis→B12 deficiency and iron deficiency

Diagnostic Findings

- CBC findings
  - Anemia (based on age-adjusted norms)
  - Pancytopenia→aplastic anemia, microangiopathic anemia, chemotherapeutic agents

- ▶ Pancytopenia, except elevated/normal lymphocytes→leukemia
- Mean corpuscular volume (MCV)
  - ▶ Elevated MCV (macrocytic anemia)→B12/folate deficiency, hypothyroidism, reactive reticulocytosis (from RBC loss)
  - ▶ Decreased MCV (microcytic anemia)→iron deficiency, anemia of chronic disease, thalassemia
- Indexed/corrected reticulocyte count
  - ▶ Reticulocyte index = (patient Hgb/normal Hgb) × (retic.%)
  - ▶ Elevated count signifies increased RBC production by marrow in response to a loss of red cells→hemolysis, acute blood loss.
  - ▶ Decreased count signifies inadequate RBC production by the marrow→marrow failure anemias (see above).
- Peripheral smear
  - ▶ Schistocytes→microangiopathic anemia
  - ▶ Ghost/bite cells→G6PD deficiency
  - ▶ Target cells (leptocytes)→hemoglobinopathies, thalassemias
  - ▶ Elliptocytes→Hereditary elliptocytosis
  - ▶ Spherocytes→Hereditary spherocytosis, autoimmune hemolytic anemias
  - ▶ Basophilic stippling→lead poisoning, reticulocytosis
  - ▶ Sickled cells→sickle-cell anemia
  - ▶ Heinz bodies→hemolytic anemias, oxidant damage
  - ▶ Blast cells→malignant bone marrow infiltration
- Further testing is directed by age, clinic findings, and above tests.
  - ▶ LDH, bilirubin→hemolysis
  - ▶ Iron, ferritin, and total iron binding→iron deficiency anemia
  - ▶ Direct/indirect Coombs test→autoimmune hemolytic anemia
  - ▶ Hemoglobin electrophoresis→hemoglobinopathies, thalassemias
  - ▶ RBC enzyme studies→enzymopathies
  - ▶ B12 and folate levels→B12/folate deficiency
  - ▶ Osmotic fragility testing→spherocytosis
  - ▶ Blood typing with crossmatch→isoimmune hemolytic disease of the newborn

- ▶ Bone marrow biopsy→malignant bone marrow infiltration
- ▶ TSH/free T4→hypothyroidism
- ▶ Stool occult→GI bleeding
- Imaging is rarely useful in initial screening for anemia.

Treatment

- Should be directed at the cause of anemia.
- Supportive care
  - ▶ Packed red blood cell (PRBC) transfusions (10 15 mL/kg) as necessary (e.g., significant symptoms).
  - ▶ Stop medications that may cause anemia.
- Iron deficiency anemia
  - ▶ Diagnosis is often made presumptively in otherwise healthy children with microcytic anemia and otherwise normal CBC and peripheral smear findings.
  - ▶ Iron supplementation: 3 6 mg of elemental iron/kg/d
  - ▶ If RBC count and MCV are not improving, other diagnoses should be considered.
- Anemia from marrow failure (e.g., chronic disease, renal disease, chemotherapeutic agents)
  - ▶ Erythropoietin 50-250 units/kg SC/IV 1-3 times weekly
  - ▶ Not indicated for acute anemia as effects take 2-8 weeks.

Acute Leukemia

Definition

- A malignancy of white blood cells (WBCs) and their precursors resulting from clonal proliferation of a single cell line within the bone marrow/hematopoietic tissues

Critical Knowledge

- Most common childhood malignancy with variable presentations.
- Evaluate ABCs first.
- Be aware and address complications of acute, emergent presentations, including:
  - ▶ Tumor lysis syndrome (TLS), electrolyte abnormalities, renal failure, sepsis

Background

- The most common childhood malignancy (29% of all cancers in children 0-14 years).
- Incidence is 30-40 per 1 million in the U.S.
- Male predominance; more common in Caucasians
- Peak incidence between ages 3 and 7
- Causes remain largely unknown, but associations/risks include:
  ▶ Genetic disease (e.g., trisomy 21, ataxia telangiectasia, etc.)
  ▶ Environmental factors (e.g., ionizing radiation, benzene, chemotherapeutic agents)

Differential Diagnosis

- Aplastic anemia
- Idiopathic thrombocytopenia purpura
- Juvenile rheumatoid arthritis
- Infectious mononucleosis
- Infectious leukocytosis
- Disseminated intravascular coagulation
- Other malignancies
  ▶ Non-Hodgkin lymphoma
  ▶ Neuroblastoma
  ▶ Rhabdomyosarcoma

Critical Concepts

- Leukemia is a progressive cancer that proliferates at the expense of other bone marrow cell lines (i.e., neutrophils, thrombocytes, erythrocytes)
  ▶ Signs/symptoms of disease are a result of this lymphocytosis, with resulting neutropenia, thrombocytopenia, and anemia.
- Clinical signs/symptoms—often insidious
  ▶ General: fatigue, malaise, weight loss, low-grade fever, bone pain
  ▶ Pulmonary: dyspnea
  ▶ Hematologic: pallor, petechiae, easy bruising, mucosal bleeding, lymphadenopathy
  ▶ Renal: oliguria, occasional testicular pain/enlargement (from infiltration)
  ▶ Gastrointestinal: splenomegaly

- ► CNS: headache, vomiting, lethargy, nuchal rigidity, seizures, papilledema (found in CNS involvement, but not common at time of initial diagnosis)
- Diagnostic findings
  - ► Leukocytosis (present at diagnosis in only 50% of cases)
  - ► Neutropenia, thrombocytopenia, anemia
  - ► Peripheral smear (shows lymphoblasts and/or other immature forms)
    - ■ This is diagnostic (although bone marrow aspirate is used to confirm diagnosis).
    - ■ Should be examined by a trained hematologist.
  - ► Coagulation studies (generally normal)
  - ► Electrolyte abnormalities: hyperuricemia, hyperphosphatemia, hyperkalemia, hypokalemia/hyperkalemia
  - ► Elevated liver function tests with leukemic infiltration
  - ► Elevated lactate dehydrogenase (may indicate pending tumor lysis syndrome)
  - ► Cerebrospinal fluid for evidence of CNS infiltration.
  - ► CXR (may show a mediastinal mass in 5%-10% of patients)
  - ► Bone marrow aspirate: inpatient study for ultimate diagnosis, staging, and molecular analysis
- High-risk features that indicate a worse long-term prognosis:
  - ► Age <1 year or >10 years
  - ► WBC count >50,000 mm3 at diagnosis
  - ► Male sex
  - ► Black race
  - ► Large lymphadenopathy or splenomegaly at diagnosis
  - ► Certain chromosomal abnormalities and antigen expression patterns

Treatment

- Supportive care
  - ► Hydration therapy without (initial) potassium replacement
  - ► Blood transfusions as necessary

- Infection
  - ▶ Use broad-coverage antibiotics for identified infection.
    - Neutropenia requires trimethoprim/sulfamethoxazole prophylaxis for *Pneumocystis jiroveci* (PCP).
    - Neutropenia with fever requires antibiotics, admission, and isolation.
- Chemotherapy induction therapy (initiated by a pediatric oncologist)
  - ▶ Drug regimen is determined by phenotypical findings and risk stratification.
  - ▶ Intrathecal methotrexate should be added for CNS treatment or prophylaxis.
  - ▶ Can achieve remission rates >90%.
- Bone marrow transplant is a treatment option for relapse.
- Tumor lysis syndrome (TLS) is a triad of hyperuricemia, hyperkalemia, and hyperphosphatemia.
  - ▶ Caused by rapid cellular destruction with resulting release of large quantities of potassium, phosphate, and urea (may be seen before or after initiation of chemotherapy).
  - ▶ Secondary effects include:
    - Hypocalcemia
    - Acute renal failure (ARF)
  - ▶ Prophylaxis
    - Administer maintenance fluids at twice the normal rate (though judicious use in cases of severe anemia is advisable).
    - NO potassium supplementation, at least initially, in IV fluids.
    - Alkalization of urine with IV sodium bicarbonate.
      — Promotes the solubility of urea and increases its excretion.
      — Goal is a urine pH of 7.0-8.0.
    - Suppress uric acid formation.
      — Allopurinol 50-100 mg PO q8 hrs
      — Recombinant urate oxidase (e.g., rasburicase)
  - ▶ Monitor EKG, for hyperkalemic changes (e.g. peaked T-waves, widened QRS).

- ▶ Treatment for:
  - ■ Hyperkalemia
    - — Calcium gluconate 10% (0.5 mL/kg IV over 2-5 minutes) if EKG changes are seen
    - — Sodium bicarbonate (1-2 mEq/kg IV over 5-10 minutes)
    - — Insulin/glucose (0.1 unit/kg IV regular insulin with 2 mL/kg IV D25
    - — Sodium polystyrene resin (i.e., sodium polystyrene sulfonate) (1-2 g/kg with sorbitol PO)
    - — Furosemide (0.5 2 mg/kg IV bolus)
    - — Dialysis
  - ■ Hyperphosphatemia
    - — Aluminum hydroxide (50-150 mg/kg/day PO divided every 4-6 hours)
    - — Mannitol 0.25-1 g/kg IV bolus in normal saline
    - — Dialysis
  - ■ Hyperuricemia
    - — Allopurinol (10 mg/kg/d PO/IV in 3-4 divided doses) decreases urea production.
    - — Recombinant urate oxidase (rasburicase: 0.15-0.2mg/kg/day IV infusion over 30 minutes increases urea excretion by converting it to allantoin, a compound with 5x the solubility of urea).
    - — Alkalization of urine
- ● Survival rate with treatment is 80%.
  - ▶ Prognosis depends heavily on genetic factors.
  - ▶ Overall highest survival rates are seen in children ages 1-10.

Aplastic Anemia

Definition

- A condition with various causes characterized by pancytopenia (thrombocytopenia, anemia, and neutropenia) **AND** hypocellular bone marrow.

Critical Knowledge

- Consider histocompatibility testing of patient and siblings prior to non-emergent transfusions (transfusions may later impact the success of bone marrow transplant).

Background

- Incidence is 2-6 per 1 million in the U.S.
- No age, sex, or racial predominance
- 50% or more are idiopathic. Other causes include:
  - ▶ Genetic (e.g., Fanconi anemia, Diamond Blackfan anemia, etc.)
  - ▶ Acquired
    - ▪ Infection (e.g., Epstein-Barr virus, parvovirus B19, HIV, hepatitis)
    - ▪ Drugs (e.g., chloramphenicol, sulfonamides, carbamazepine, cimetadine, phenylbutazone, etc)
    - ▪ Toxins (e.g., radiation, benzene)
    - ▪ Graft-versus-host disease (GVHD)
    - ▪ Others
      - — Pregnancy
      - — Autoimmune disease (e.g., SLE)

Differential Diagnosis

- Bone marrow infiltration (e.g., leukemia, lymphoma, myelofibrosis)
- Myelodysplasia
- Megaloblastic anemia
- Chemotherapy effects
- Paroxysmal nocturnal hemoglobinuria (PND)
- Splenic sequestration

Critical Concepts

- Pathophysiology varies and is unknown much of the time; it often involves immune suppression.
- Insidious onset with signs of thrombocytopenia are often first noted.
- Historical points
  - ▶ Family history of anemia
    - Identifying an inherited aplastic anemia can have consequences for later treatment.
    - Penetrance varies, making family history unreliable.
  - ▶ Recent infection (e.g., parvovirus, etc.)
  - ▶ Recent radiation or medication usage
- Clinical signs/symptoms
  - ▶ General: fever, weakness, lethargy, pallor
  - ▶ Hematologic: bruising, petechiae, jaundice, mucous membrane bleeding
  - ▶ Gastrointestinal: GI bleeding, normal-sized liver and spleen
  - ▶ Eyes: retinal hemorrhages
  - ▶ CNS: symptomatic CNS bleeding (uncommon)
  - ▶ Cardiovascular: systolic flow murmur
  - ▶ Developmental: abnormal facies and/or extremities seen in some congenital diseases (e.g., Fanconi anemia, Diamond Blackfan anemia)
- Diagnostic findings
  - ▶ Anemia: macrocytic, reticulocyte count <0.1%
  - ▶ Thrombocytopenia (5,000-50,000 per mL)
  - ▶ Neutropenia with toxic granulation; no blast cells
  - ▶ Bone marrow aspirate/biopsy (hypocellular marrow)
  - ▶ Folate and B12 testing
  - ▶ Specialized testing
    - Ham test (tests stability of red cells, e.g., paroxysmal nocturnal hemoglobinuria)
    - Serologic viral testing (HIV, EBV, hepatitis, etc.)
    - Autoimmune panel (e.g., SLE)
    - Chromosomal studies to rule out genetic disease

Treatment

- Supportive therapy
  - ► Stop exposure to all possible causative agents!
  - ► Blood transfusions
    - Minimize when possible; better bone marrow transplant results occur with lower rates of transfusion.
    - Leuko-reduced blood products minimize alloimmunization.
  - ► Infection treatment
    - Use broad coverage antibiotics for identified infection.
    - Neutropenia requires trimethoprim/sulfamethoxazole prophylaxis for *Pneumocystis jiroveci* pneumonia (PCP)
    - Neutropenia with fever requires antibiotics, admission, and isolation.
- HLA-matched bone marrow transplant (BMT) is the therapy of choice for children with severe aplastic anemia.
  - ► Requires an HLA-compatible sibling
  - ► Survival rates better than with immunosuppression therapy alone.
  - ► Unrelated-donor BMT is less successful.
- Immunosuppression
  - ► Antithymocyte globulin (ATG), high-dose prednisone, and cyclosporine
  - ► Combination therapy has shown better results than monotherapy.
- Survival rate is between 85-95% with BMT.

Hemolytic Uremic Syndrome (HUS)

Definition

- A disease process with the common triad of microangiopathic hemolytic anemia, thrombocytopenia, and acute renal failure/kidney injury.

Critical Knowledge

- ABCs
- Transfuse platelets and PRBCs only when bleeding is ongoing and life-threatening, or if needed prior to invasive procedures.
- If cardiac arrest occurs, consider hyperkalemia as a cause.

Background

- Most common cause of pediatric acute renal failure.
- Rare disorder with less than 1,000 new cases per year.
- Peak age is under age 10, with a majority being under age 5.
- Can be epidemic, with clusters occurring during the summer.
- No sex predominance; rare in African Americans.
- Two diagnostic types with different natural histories:
  - 90% of all HUS is "typical" (D+) HUS and often occurs after a prodromal gastroenteritic illness with Shiga toxin-producing *Escherichia coli* (i.e., *E. coli* 0157:H7)
  - Atypical (D-) HUS encompasses all other forms of HUS; the pathogenesis of these is not well understood.

Differential Diagnosis

- Thrombotic thrombocytopenic purpura (TTP)
- Disseminated intravascular thrombosis (DIC)
- Hemolytic anemias with accompanying thrombocytopenia
- Vasculitis

Critical Concepts

- Clinical effects of D+ HUS are a direct result of damaged endothelial cells caused by bacterial toxins.
  - Endothelial cell wall damage leads to red blood cell hemolysis and the release of vasoactive substances.
  - Thrombocytopenia results from platelet destruction and consumption at the sites of endothelial damage.
  - Renal failure results from a decreased glomerular filtration rate secondary to microthrombi in the renal vasculature.
- Conflicting evidence suggests a risk that antibiotic treatment of gastroenteritis caused by *E. coli* 0157:H7 may trigger HUS.
  - 10%-15% of children with culture-documented 0157:H7 will develop HUS.
- HUS is a spectrum of disease that can range from subclinical to life-threatening, with a mortality rate of 3%-12%.
- Clinical signs/symptoms

- ► General: fever, elevated blood pressure, signs of dehydration
- ► Hematologic: pallor, petechiae, purpura,
- ► Gastrointestinal: prodromal diarrhea (often bloody), abdominal pain, pancreatitis (usually mild)
- ► Renal: decreased urine output
- ► CNS: lethargy, irritability, ataxia, seizures, coma (caused by microthrombi and cerebral edema)
- ► Cardiovascular: signs of heart failure, peripheral edema
- Diagnostic findings
  - ► Anemia with signs of hemolysis (elevated lactate dehydrogenase and bilirubin, schistocytes, decreased haptoglobin)
  - ► Coagulation defects (increased fibrin split products, increased or normal fibrinogen, normal INR/PT/PTT)
  - ► Leukocytosis is commonly found.
  - ► Renal failure (elevated BUN and creatinine, hyponatremia, hyperkalemia, hyperphosphatemia, microscopic hematuria and proteinuria, RBC casts)
  - ► Pancreatitis (elevated lipase and amylase)
  - ► Microbiology (positive stool culture for *E. coli* 0157:H7; this has a low sensitivity)

Treatment

- Renal care
  - ► Fluid-volume resuscitation with strict attention to input and output.
    - If *hypovolemic*, give normal saline or lactated ringers (patient is likely to be hyponatremic).
    - If *hypervolemic*, fluid restriction may be needed.
  - ► Hyperkalemia may require treatment with calcium gluconate, sodium bicarbonate, insulin/glucose, and/or kayexalate.
  - ► Antihypertensives may be required.
  - ► Dialysis in severe cases (peritoneal or hemodialysis)

- Transfusion
  - ► PRBC transfusion for hemoglobin below 6.0-7.0 or with signs of cardiac dysfunction.
  - ► Platelet transfusion only for children with life-threatening bleeding or prior to invasive procedures (transfusing platelets inappropriately can worsen intravascular coagulation).
- Immunoglobulin G (2 g/kg IV over 2-5 days) has shown conflicting results and should only be given in concert with pediatric consultation.
- Survival rate is 85%-95% with D+ HUS, but lower with D HUS, which can often be chronic.

Henoch-Schonlein Purpura (HSP)

Definition
- A small-vessel, IgA-mediated vasculitis causing purpura, arthralgias, and abdominal pain in children.

Critical Knowledge
- IgA-mediated vasculitis that clinically may cause purpuric-lesions (usually in gravity-dependent portions of the body), arthritis, and/or abdominal pain
- After tending to the ABCs, care is mainly supportive.

Background
- Incidence is 150 per 1 million in the U.S.
- Male predominance is 2:1
- Prevalence peaks between ages 4 and 15.
- Peak incidence is in the spring.
- Caucasians are affected more often than African Americans.

Differential Diagnosis
- Thrombocytopenia purpura (e.g., TTP, ITP)
- Meningococcemia
- Rocky Mountain spotted fever
- Other vasculitities (e.g., leukocytoclastic vasculitis, polyarteritis nodosa, SLE, etc.)
- Child abuse

Critical Concepts

- HSP is an immunoglobulin A (I_gA)-mediated vasculitis of small vessels.
  - ▶ Antigens may play a role, stimulating an autoimmune response.
  - ▶ Viral/bacterial antigens are suspected, as children often have preceding symptoms 1-3 weeks prior to onset of HSP.
- The hallmark of the disease is palpable purpura on dependent parts of the body, especially the legs and buttocks, but not all patients will have this rash early on in the illness.
- Though there is no treatment for HSP, a majority of children recover spontaneously over weeks or months.
- Clinical signs/symptoms
  - ▶ General: low-grade fever, preceding URI symptoms common
  - ▶ Hematologic: symmetrical erythematous rash in lower extremities, which spreads and later becomes palpable purpura
  - ▶ Gastrointestinal (30%-50% of patients)
    - GI bleeding (occasionally massive) with melena, hematochezia and/or hematemesis
    - Abdominal complaints, including nausea, vomiting, diarrhea and pain (Obstruction, infarction, and intussusception of the bowel can rarely occur.)
  - ▶ Renal: rare oliguria or gross hematuria, scrotal/testicular pain
  - ▶ Rheumatologic (60%-80% of patients): arthralgias and arthritis, especially in the knees and ankles
  - ▶ Skin: subcutaneous edema of scalp common in infants
- Diagnostic findings
  - ▶ Diagnosis is generally clinical, but in subtle or early cases, workup may be required; renal testing is mandatory if HSP is considered.
  - ▶ CBC is nonspecific, but may show leukocytosis, thrombocytosis, and eosinophilia.
  - ▶ Renal findings can vary and occur in approximately 50% of patients.
    - Glomerulonephritis: elevated creatinine, hematuria, proteinuria, RBC casts
    - Nephrotic syndrome (significant proteinuria with edema)
    - Oliguria and hypertension are rare.

- ▶ Stool guaiac-positive in patients with GI symptoms.
- ▶ Elevated IgA levels
- ▶ Joint examinations
  - ▪ Plain films may show joint effusion.
  - ▪ Effusion is serous, not bloody, if arthrocentesis is performed.
- ▶ Other imaging
  - ▪ Abdominal radiographs: bowel edema, thumb-printing
  - ▪ Ultrasound: bowel edema, free fluid, intussusception

Treatment

- Supportive care
  - ▶ Limitation of strenuous physical activity
  - ▶ Pain management
- Renal care
  - ▶ Fluid hydration
  - ▶ Low-salt diet
  - ▶ Antihypertensives
- Azithioprine has been used in cases of severe renal disease.
  - ▶ Limited data suggests improvement in long-term renal outcome.
  - ▶ Therapy is generally continued for several weeks.
- Corticosteroid therapy is not recommended unless severe renal disease occurs.
  - ▶ Improves arthritic and abdominal symptoms
  - ▶ Limited data suggests improvement in long-term renal outcome.
  - ▶ Increases the rate of relapse
- Survival rate is excellent at >98%.
  - ▶ Chronic renal disease develops in <5% (<1% with ESRD).
  - ▶ Relapse rate is up to 50%.
    - ▪ Usually occurring within 1-2 months
    - ▪ Increased rate in those who undergo steroid treatment

Idiopathic Thrombocytopenia Purpura (ITP)

Definition

- Thrombocytopenia without identifiable cause and with no abnormalities of the bone marrow or other blood cell lines.

Critical Knowledge

- Mental status changes or seizures in a child with ITP might signify intracranial hemorrhage. Respond with immediate platelet transfusion, imaging, and neurosurgical consultation.

Background

- Incidence is 50 per 1 million in the U.S.
- Two predominant forms with different natural histories:
  - ▶ Acute ITP
    - Peaks at ages: 2-4 years, no sex predominance.
    - Often severe anemia, full recovery is the norm.
    - Peaks in the winter and spring.
  - ▶ Chronic ITP
    - Defined as having symptoms for over 6 months.
    - More likely after age 10 and twice as common in females.
    - Generally insidious; worse long-term prognosis.

Differential Diagnosis

- TTP/HUS
- Congenital thrombocytopenia purpura (e.g., Fanconi syndrome, etc.)
- Infection (e.g., HIV and other viruses)
- Drugs (e.g., heparin, sulfonamides, alcohol, quinidine)
- Pseudothrombocytopenia secondary to EDTA use
- Liver disease
- Neonatal isoimmune thrombocytopenia
- Pregnancy
- Hypothyroidism
- Bone marrow infiltration (e.g., ALL, AML, myelofibrosis)

Critical Concepts

- Pathogenesis is thought to be immunologic.
    - ► Autoantibodies are thought to lead to platelet destruction.
    - ► Megakaryocytes are generally normal or increased, suggesting normal platelet formation.
- ITP is a diagnosis of exclusion.
- Physical exam may be normal.
- Clinical signs/symptoms:
    - ► General: children generally appear well
    - ► Hematologic: purpura and mucosal bleeding (often appear suddenly)
    - ► Gastrointestinal: no hepatosplenomegaly, occasional GI bleeding
    - ► Renal: hematuria
    - ► CNS: altered mental status from CNS hemorrhage (<1% of patients)
- Diagnostic findings
    - ► Thrombocytopenia: platelets normal in size and morphology
    - ► Normal INR/PT/PTT
    - ► No anemia or neutropenia (unless significant bleeding has occurred)
    - ► No evidence of hemolysis
    - ► Further studies
        - Imaging: CT head if intracranial bleeding suspected
        - When necessary: TSH, ANA, pregnancy testing, liver function panel, bone marrow aspirate

Treatment

- Supportive therapy
    - ► Stop exposure to medications that can cause thrombocytopenia.
    - ► Encourage limitation of strenuous activity and contact sports.
    - ► Blood transfusions
        - Platelets (1 unit/10 kg): Give only for ongoing life-threatening bleeding; do not treat based on the level of thrombocytopenia (serious bleeding is rare — 2%-4%).
            - — Packed-RBCs for anemia secondary to bleeding

- Observation alone is appropriate for patients with minimal mucosal bleeding and platelet counts >30,000/mm^3.
  - ▶ 80% of children will recover spontaneously in 4-8 weeks.
- Prednisone (2 mg/kg/day) does not alter time course of disease, but will transiently increase platelets and decrease bleeding.
- Intravenous immunoglobulin (IVIG)(1 g/kg/dose IV): Single- or multiple-dose therapy will increase platelets.
  - ▶ Appears more effective than corticosteroids.
  - ▶ Consider pre-dosing acetaminophen and diphenhydramine to counteract side effects of headache, nausea, and allergic reactions.
- Anti-D(Rh) immunoglobulin (0.025-0.1 mg/kg): similar effects as IVIG administration
  - ▶ Only effective in Rh(+) patients.
  - ▶ Side effect is hemolysis, limiting its usefulness in anemic patients.
- Splenectomy is an effective treatment, but used only for persistent and symptomatic thrombocytopenia.
- Survival rate is over 95%; most fatalities are from intracranial bleeding (incidence of less than 0.5%).

Hemophilia A and B

Definition

- Sex-linked, heritable bleeding disorders characterized by absence or dysfunction of factor VIII (hemophilia A) or factor IX (hemophilia B) of the clotting cascade.

Critical Knowledge

- Appropriate factor replacement is based on the severity of factor deficiency and bleeding.
- Do not delay factor replacement for imaging in children suspected of intracranial hemorrhage!
- Bleeding around the airway requires early airway stabilization; surgical airway is relatively contraindicated.

Background

- Incidence is 200 per 1 million in the U.S. (80% of which are hemophilia A).
- X-linked disorders predominantly affect males.
  - ► Females generally are asymptomatic carriers.
  - ► Show x-linked inheritance, although spontaneous mutations occur.
- Congenital diseases with diagnosis generally in infancy or before birth.
- No racial predominance.

Differential Diagnosis

- Von Willebrand disease (VWD)
- Other factor deficiencies (factor XI is the most common)
- Acquired factor VIII or IX deficiencies due to inhibitor (rare)
- Vitamin K deficiency
- Child abuse
- Isolated prolonged coagulation times without bleeding
  - ► Heparin therapy
  - ► Factor XII deficiency

Critical Concepts

- Factors VIII and IX are necessary for clot formation.
  - ► Both are involved in the intrinsic pathway of the clotting cascade.
  - ► The absence or abnormal function of either factor causes abnormal bleeding.
- Severity of disease is based on the severity of factor deficiency.
  - ► **Mild** (factor activity 5%-25% [of normal])
  - ► **Moderate** (factor activity 1%-5%)
  - ► **Severe** (factor activity <1%)
- Clinical signs/symptoms (vary with age)
  - ► Neonates
    - Bleeding from umbilical site or after circumcision is often the presenting sign.
    - Intracranial bleeding affects 1%-2% of neonates.

- ► Infants
    - Major bleeding is relatively uncommon.
    - Mucosal bleeding, especially the lips and tongue
- ► Toddlers and children
    - Hemarthrosis and soft-tissue bleeding become more common.
- Specific bleeding events
    - ► Hemarthrosis is common in weight-bearing joints (i.e., knees, ankles, elbows)
        - May start with only slight discomfort.
        - Warmth, swelling, pain, and ROM limitation follow.
        - Can lead to chronic arthropathy and joint destruction.
    - ► Soft-tissue bleeding occurs at sites of minor trauma.
        - Painful and may be swollen.
        - Ecchymosis is not always present; petechiae is uncommon.
        - Retroperitoneal bleeding may mimic an acute abdomen.
        - Compartment syndrome may occur.
    - ► Intracranial bleeding (even after relatively minor trauma)
    - ► Hematuria is common and generally benign; may be persistent.
    - ► GI bleeding is uncommon.
    - ► Post-surgical/dental bleeding can be life-threatening; requires prior treatment by surgeons familiar with care of hemophiliacs.
- Diagnostic studies
    - ► Prolonged partial thromboplastin time (PTT)
        - PTT may be normal in mild disease
        - It also may be prolonged in VWD.
    - ► Normal prothrombin time (PT), bleeding times, and platelet count
    - ► Special testing
        - Factor VIII C assay (low in hemophilia A)
        - Factor IX assay (low in hemophilia B)
        - Von Willebrand antigen assay (vWF:Ag) (normal in hemophilia, but may be low in VWD)

Treatment

- Treatment of acute bleeding events is intravenous replacement of the appropriate factor.
  - ▶ Factor VIII
    - 1 unit (U) of factor VIII raises circulating levels by 2%.
    - Serum half-life is 8-12 hours.
  - ▶ Factor IX
    - 1 unit (U) of factor IX raises circulating levels by 1%.
    - Serum half-life is 24 hours.
  - ▶ Dosing of factor replacement varies with the site and severity of injury.
- Factor replacement
  - ▶ Recombinant factors
    - Now standard treatment for newly diagnosed patients
    - Low or no risk of blood-borne pathogens (e.g., HIV, hepatitis)
  - ▶ Concentrated plasma-derived factors
    - Slightly higher risk of blood-borne pathogens.
    - Cheaper than newer recombinant treatments.
    - Not recommended for newly diagnosed patients or those who have been previously maintained on recombinant factors.
- Factor replacement therapy for specific injuries
  - ▶ Hemarthosis (level of activity required is 30%-50%)
    - Factor VIII 20-40 U/kg
    - Factor IX 30-40 U/kg
    - Other: consider immobilization, orthopedic consultation
  - ▶ Muscular bleeding (level of activity required is 40%-50%)
    - Factor VIII 20-40 U/kg
    - Factor IX 40-60 U/kg
    - Other: elevate area, observe for compartment syndrome
  - ▶ Epistaxis (level of activity required is 80%-100%)
    - Factor VIII 40-50 U/kg
    - Factor IX 80-100 U/kg
    - Other: treat bleeding appropriately

- ▶ Oral bleeding (level of activity required is 50%)
  - Factor VIII 25 U/kg
  - Factor IX 50 U/kg
  - Other: aminocaproic acid
- ▶ GI bleeding (level of activity required is 100%)
  - Factor VIII 40-50 U/kg
  - Factor IX 80-100 U/kg
  - Other: consult gastroenterology
- ▶ Intracranial bleeding (level of activity required is 100%)
  - Factor VIII 50 U/kg
  - Factor IX 100 U/kg
  - Other: consult neurosurgery
- Inhibitors (I$_g$G antibodies to factors VIII or IX, which shorten the half-life of replacement factor)
  - ▶ Inhibitors complicate the treatment of hemophilia by decreasing the effectiveness of common factor replacement therapies.
  - ▶ Frequency
    - Factor VIII inhibitor occurs in up to 35% of children with severe hemophilia A.
    - Factor IX inhibitor occurs only in 1%-3% of children with hemophilia B.
  - ▶ Inhibitors are described based on the intravenous titer levels.
    - Low-level titers can generally be treated with normal or high-dose factor replacement therapies.
    - High-level titers require alternative therapies.
      - — Immune tolerance induction
      - — Porcine factor VIII (e.g., antihemophilic factor injection)
      - — Anti-inhibitor coagulant complex (e.g., FEIBA)
      - — Recombinant factor VIIa (e.g., NovoSeven)
- Other medical therapies
  - ▶ Aminocaproic acid (100 mg/kg orally every 4-6 hours)
    - Inhibits activation of plasminogen, stabilizing clot formation
    - Useful in oral bleeding, counteracts fibrinolysin found in saliva

- ▶ Desmopressin (0.3 micrograms/kg IV every 12-24 hours)
  - Dose-dependent increase in factor VIII release.
  - Effective treatment for mild to moderate hemophilia A only.
    - — Can be used for minor bleeding or prior to surgery.
- Chronic (prophylactic) therapy
  - ▶ Now considered primary treatment for many patients; prophylactic factor replacement; often 3 times weekly is given to keep factor activity levels above 25%.
  - ▶ This treatment may be more cost beneficial than symptomatic treatment due to decreased episodes of acute bleeding.
  - ▶ This often requires IV port placement due to frequent IV administrations of factor.

Review Questions

1. **Which is NOT associated with autoimmune hemolytic anemia?**
   - A. Positive Coombs' test
   - B. Elevated corrected reticulocyte count
   - C. Blast cells on peripheral smear
   - D. Elevated LDH

2. **Which supports the diagnosis of iron deficiency anemia?**
   - A. 1-month-old child, formula-fed
   - B. Macrocytosis on peripheral smear
   - C. Jaundice and splenomegaly noted on exam
   - D. Anemia improved after one month of ferrous sulfate treatment

3. **Which is NOT a known cause of aplastic anemia?**
   - A. Chloramphenical
   - B. Hepatitis
   - C. Fanconi anemia
   - D. Folate deficiency

4. **Which lab finding might you expect to find with HUS?**
   A. Leukocytosis
   B. Elevated conjugated bilirubin
   C. Hypernatremia
   D. Hypophosphatemia

5. **Which renal finding is uncommon with HSP?**
   A. Red blood cell casts
   B. Peripheral edema
   C. Oliguria
   D. Proteinuria

6. **Which is an inappropriate treatment for an asymptomatic child with ITP and a platelet count of 15,000/mm³?**
   A. Anti-D immunoglobulin
   B. Intravenous immunoglobulin (I_gG)
   C. Prednisone
   D. Platelet transfusion

7. **Which would NOT be expected in a child with ITP and GI bleeding?**
   A. Thrombocytopenia
   B. Decreased haptoglobin
   C. Normal INR/PT/PTT
   D. Anemia

8. **Which is NOT generally seen in hemophilia?**
   A. Petechiae
   B. Easy bruising
   C. Oral bleeding
   D. Epistaxis

Key			
1. C		5. C	
2. D		6. D	
3. D		7. B	
4. A		8. A	

Special Health Care Needs

Melanie S. Heniff, MD

32

Developmental Disabilities/Cerebral Palsy/ Spina Bifida

Critical Knowledge

- A useful question for a patient's primary caregiver during the initial assessment is: "Can you tell me how (insert patient's name) is affected by (name of syndrome/developmental disability)?"

- Carefully check weight for medication dosing since standard age- or height-based dosing often is not reliable in this patient population.

- Do not use succinylcholine in patients with neuromuscular disorders such as muscular dystrophy. Succinylcholine can be used in patients with CP, however, the effects may be prolonged.

- VP shunt malfunction can be life-threatening; consider this diagnosis in VP shunt patients who have altered mental status, headache, or vomiting.

- Baclofen pump malfunction can be life-threatening. Consider the diagnosis of baclofen withdrawal in patients with a baclofen pump, altered mental status, hypotension, fever, increased spasticity, muscle rigidity, and pruritus. Treat baclofen withdrawal with IV benzodiazepines until pump can be refilled.

- Consider overdose of baclofen if patient has somnolence, respiratory depression, seizures, or coma; treat by supporting the ABCs and empty reservoir from the center of the pump.

Background

- "Special needs" = developmental disabilities (impairments in motor function, self-care, language, and cognition)

- Children with developmental disabilities (DD) often have multiple associated medical problems, medications, and implanted devices (VP shunts, tracheostomies, baclofen pumps, and gastrostomy tubes) that must be considered.

- Many medical complications are common in patients with all types of DD.
- A consistent, organized approach with review of problems by organ system is a useful way to evaluate this complex patient population.
- Identify the patient's baseline level of function to establish a basis for comparison at the time of evaluation.
- Cerebral palsy (CP) is the single most widespread permanent physical disability in the U.S.
- Neural tube defects/spina bifida/meningomyelocele (MMC) are the most common major birth defects in the U.S.

Cerebral Palsy

- A nonprogressive central motor deficit with multiple causes and manifestations.
- Spasticity leads to muscle contracture, which shortens muscle and limits use.
- Musculoskeletal problems; pain, spasticity
- Pain may be difficult to localize.
- Patient should be undressed for thorough exam of skin and joints.
- Increased risk of hip subluxation due to spasticity
- Osteopenia may result in fractures after seemingly insignificant trauma.
- Check for pressure sores.
- Increase in spasticity may come from medication withdrawal/toxicity, baclofen pump malfunction, pain, UTI, or constipation.

Seizures

- Occur in 50% of children with CP.
- Consider in altered mental status; it is hard to recognize seizures such as partial complex seizures, or psychomotor seizures.
- Standard approach to status epilepticus.

Pulmonary Problems

- Often due to oropharyngeal incoordination and reflux.
- Recurrent pneumonia due to aspiration, weak cough; restrictive lung disease due to scoliosis.

- Wheezing/reactive airway disease, especially in setting of aspiration, and history of prematurity.
- Tracheostomy tubes
- Most pediatric tubes are uncuffed.
- Common complications include infection, obstruction, and dislodged tube.
- May temporarily replace with an endotracheal tube (ETT).
- If replacing, have smaller tubes ready in case stoma has started to close or swelling is present.
- Extend neck and lubricate the cannula before replacing.
- Assume obstruction if patient is in respiratory distress. Suction and, if needed, irrigate with sterile saline; it inner cannula, may remove and clean.

Tracheostomy Tube Replacment Size Estimates

Shiley Tracheostomy Tube Size	ETT Size
2	4-4.5
3	4.5-5
4	5-6
5	6-7
6	7-7.5

GI Problems
- Feeding problems (due to hypotonia, weak oropharyngeal muscles, poor swallowing ability)
- Reflux and esophagitis are common.
- Failure to thrive due to feeding problems and increased caloric needs
- May develop rapid dehydration with mild gastroenteritis (therefore, have a low threshold for labs, IV fluids, and admission).

Superior Mesenteric Artery Syndrome
- Recurrent vomiting; may be bilious
- Due to intermittent or functional obstruction of the duodenum
- Management: improve nutrition; prone position after meals; patients may need surgery.

Gastrostomy Tube Problems

- Connect to suction in a patient with vomiting or respiratory distress.
- Obstruction is the most common malfunction.
- Tubes may dislodge; can develop cracks, fractures, and leaks; and may migrate to esophagus or intestines.
- If dislodged, be careful when replacing a new g-tube (it may take 2 weeks to 3 months for a fistula to mature).
- May use a Foley catheter to temporarily replace g-tube, but because catheter can migrate, it should be secured to abdominal wall.
- Jejunostomy tubes should be replaced by an interventional radiologist, surgeon, or gastroenterologist, but a g-tube can be temporarily inserted to keep the stoma patent.
- Excess drooling is mainly a cosmetic problem, but it may impair swallowing.

Constipation

- Often severe
- May require hospitalization for disimpaction.
- Worsened by dehydration and meds for spasticity.
- May cause abdominal pain, rectal tears, decreased appetite, increased reflux.

GU Problems

- Hygiene problems due to lower extremity spasticity.
- Incontinence and UTIs are common.

HEENT Problems

- Chronic otitis media and dental caries common.

Other

- At increased risk of child abuse
- Mental retardation in 50%-60%

Spina Bifida/Neural Tube Defects/ Meningomyelocele

Neurologic Problems

- Disturbances in neural plate formation during development.
- Dysplastic neural elements protrude through unfused vertebral arches; may be open or closed.

Neurologic Problems

- Seizures occur in 14%-29% of NTD patients.
- Chiari malformation (prolongation of the cerebellar vermis and fourth ventricle into the c-spine)
  - ▶ In over 90% patients with open NTD; results in hydrocephalus requiring VP shunt.
  - ▶ Patients may develop "Chiari crisis" (vocal cord paralysis, stridor, apnea, hypoxia).

VP Shunt Malfunction

- Young children may present with irritability, lethargy, bulging fontanelle, or vomiting.
- Older children may present with HA, N/V, change in intellectual capabilities, cardiovascular instability, seizures, apnea, or coma.
- First evaluate for "routine" etiologies of symptoms (i.e., more likely causes of symptoms such as viral syndrome, otitis media, febrile illness), but consider shunt malfunction in the differential.
- Shunt series (plain x-rays of shunt tubing); limited utility, but may show disconnected tubing.
- CT scans are most useful for diagnosing if there is a prior study for comparison.
- Shunt tap is the most definitive test.
- Consult neurosurgery if shunt malfunction is suspected, even if imaging is normal.
- Infections are most common 1-2 months after placement.

Musculoskeletal Problems

- Lower extremity weakness or paralysis
- Bowel or bladder dysfunction

- At risk of hip subluxation
- Increased risk of pathologic fracture, often with increased systemic response to pain (fever, tachycardia, hypertension, or hypotension)
- Foot deformities
- Scoliosis

GU Problems
- Over 90% of NTD patients have significant urologic problems (incontinence, UTI).

GI Problems
- Constipation is common.

Other
- Dental caries
- Skin breakdown
- Intubation may be difficult due to short trachea.
- Latex allergy extremely common

Review Questions

1. **Symptoms of VP shunt malfunction can include which of the following?**

   A. Headache
   B. Vomiting
   C. Altered mental status
   D. A and C
   E. All of the above

2. **Medical problems to which children with spina bifida are predisposed include all of the following EXCEPT?**

   A. UTI
   B. Hip subluxation
   C. Seizures
   D. Bowel obstruction
   E. Latex allergy

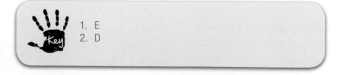

1. E
2. D

Urological Emergencies

Brittany Shutes, MD

Acute Hemiscrotum

The differential to consider in the acute hemiscrotum is broad, but a detailed history and physical will help determine the true etiology and allow for rapid and appropriate treatment to avoid long-term complications in the pediatric patient. Always consider doing a genital exam in patients complaining of abdominal pain, regardless of age.

Differential Diagnosis

- Testicular torsion
- Torsion of the appendix testis and appendix epididymis
- Infection: epididymitis/orchitis
- Hydrocele, varicocele
- Hernia
- Trauma
- Tumor
- Vasculitis (HSP)

Testicular Torsion

Critical Knowledge

- A true urologic emergency.
- Twisting and strangulation of the spermatic cord results in loss of blood supply to the testicle, leading to ischemia and necrosis.
- Remember, "castration by procrastination." If this diagnosis is considered, immediate urology consultation is mandatory from the emergency department.
- The typical history is an acute, severe, unilateral, painful and swollen hemiscrotum associated with nausea and vomiting.
- Intermittent torsion presents as vague abdominal discomfort or intermittent pain lasting from hours to days.

Epidemiology/Anatomy

- Incidence is bimodal with peaks during infancy and between 12-18 years of age.
- An abnormal attachment of the tunica vaginalis results in a predisposition for testicular torsion.
- Physical exam may reveal a high-riding testicle with a transverse lie instead of the normal vertical lie.
- The entire testicle will be exquisitely tender and swollen, making it difficult to distinguish from orchitis and epididymo-orchitis.

Diagnosis

- This is primarily a clinical diagnosis based on history and physical findings suggestive of torsion.
- Normal cremasteric reflex: Lightly stroking the superior medial thigh elicits contraction and elevation of the cremasteric muscle and the ipsilateral scrotum. This is a normal reflex mediated at L1.
- Lack of the ipsilateral cremasteric reflex is sensitive, but not specific, for the diagnosis of torsion. In other words, if the reflex is absent, it may or may not be torsion. If the reflex is present, however, it is *unlikely* to be torsion.
- Systemic symptoms (nausea and vomiting) favor torsion vs. other diagnosis. This is especially useful when there is diagnostic uncertainty.
- A color-flow Doppler should not delay definitive management and is most helpful in unclear cases such as patients with long-standing, intermittent pain.
- Decreased or lack of blood flow to the testicle suggests torsion.

Treatment

- The emergency physician may attempt manual detorsion. Turn testis outward and laterally 180 degrees up to 3 times. Classic teaching is to turn the testicle outward like "opening a book." The end point is pain relief, indicating reestablished perfusion.
- Definitive management will be surgical exploration, detorsion, and fixation of the tunica to avoid recurrence.
- Depending on the source cited, studies indicate that the salvage rate approximates 95%-100% when detorsion is performed within 4-6 hours from the onset of symptoms.

- Administer opiate analgesics and antiemetics as needed.
- The "blue dot sign" in the lateral and superior scrotal wall represents a cyanotic appendix testis and is pathognomonic for torsion of the appendix testis, a mullerian duct remnant. This is *not* an emergency and conservative management with analgesics is typically sufficient.

Epididymitis

Critical Knowledge

- An inflammation of the epididymis.
- Caused by organisms ascending from the prostatic urethra up the ejaculatory duct, through the vas deferens and into the epididymis.
- The typical history is a gradual pain and progressive swelling over several days. Acute onset of pain is less likely and more worrisome for torsion.
- Penile discharge is often present in older and sexually active males.
- Systemic symptoms are uncommon and suggest torsion as the leading diagnosis.

Epidemiology/Anatomy

- Etiology is age-dependent.
  - ▶ In young children, congenital anomalies may result in urinary reflux with a chemical epididymitis or coliform infection.
  - ▶ In adolescents and adults age <35, the causative organisms are usually *N. gonorrhea* and *C. trachomatis*.
  - ▶ Age >35 is usually due to *E. coli, pseudomonas, proteus,* and other coliforms.
- Risk factors include indwelling urinary catheters, recent instrumentation, congenital anomalies of the urinary system, and any activity that increases the risk of acquiring a sexually transmitted disease.
- Pain is initially localized to the posterior and superior poles of the testicle over the area of the epididymis. This inflammatory process may also progress to epididymo-orchitis, resulting in diffuse testicular tenderness, thereby making the distinction with torsion more challenging.

Diagnosis

- This is a clinical diagnosis that may be supported by laboratory evidence.
- Positive Prehn's sign: Elevation of the involved hemiscrotum alleviates pain, suggesting epididymitis. This sign is considered unreliable by itself, and should be used in conjunction with other findings.
- Dysuria, urgency, frequency, and pyuria all favor epididymitis vs. testicular torsion.
- Increased blood flow on color-flow Doppler suggests epididymitis.
- Consider orchitis and inquire about recent infections (post-infectious epididimytis) and immunization status (mumps).

Treatment

- Obtain a urinalysis with culture and a urethral swab for *C. trachomatis*/*N. gonorrhea* cultures.

Table 1. The Treatment of Epididymitis

	Children (Rare)		Adolescents
Symptomatic	Scrotal support with elevation, NSAIDS, and local ice packs		
N. gonorrhea	Ceftriaxone 50 mg/kg IM × 1		Ceftriaxone 250 mg IM × 1
C. trachomatis	<8 yr	Azithromycin 10 mg/kg PO × 1 ***THEN*** 5 mg/kg PO × 4 d	1 g azithromycin once ***OR*** Doxycycline 100 mg PO BID × 10 d
	>8 yr	Doxycycline 5 mg/kg/day PO div BID	
Other considerations	First-line treatment should cover coliforms in infants and prepubertal children (UTI section). Consider urology consult – high incidence of urinary tract congenital anomalies. Screen for sexual abuse.		Treatment as above is FIRST line for sexually active males. Don't forget to treat sexual partners!

Table 2. Acute Non-Traumatic Hemiscrotum Differential

Diagnosis	History	Physical/Exam Findings	Treatment
Testicular Torsion	Acute, severe, unilateral, painful and swollen hemiscrotum associated with nausea & vomiting	High-riding testicle with a transverse lie, lack of the ipsilateral cremasteric reflex, exquisitely tender and swollen testicle	Turn testis outward and laterally 180 degrees up to 3 times ("opening a book"). Surgical exploration, detorsion, and fixation
Torsion of Appendix	Acute, severe, unilateral testicular pain with limited swelling	"Blue dot sign" in the lateral and superior scrotal wall	Conservative management with analgesics
Epididymitis	Initial pain in posterior and superior poles with progressive swelling over several days, +/- penile discharge. Dysuria, urgency, and frequency	Prehn's sign: Elevation of the involved hemiscrotum alleviates pain; Increased blood flow on color-flow Doppler, +pyuria	*See table above*
Orchitis	Possible viral prodrome with swelling and pain of testis	Tender and swollen testis without involvement of epididymitis	Supportive care
Hydrocele	Nonacute, usually painless swelling of testicle	Transillumination of testis, ultrasound rules out other possible causes of fluid and inflammation	None (majority of infantile hydroceles spontaneously resolve within a year)
Varicocele	Nontender enlargement of testis that improves when lying down	Palpable twisted mass (pampiniform plexus) along the spermatic cord – "bag of worms"	Nonemergent surgical repair; be leary of unilateral right sided varicocele and an association with a possible retroperitoneal process
Hernia (incarcerated)	Previously enlarged; testicle more apparent with crying, coughing, or standing; becomes painful acutely and now size is fixed and enlarged; new constipation or vomiting	Nonreducible, painful, tense mass	*Incarcerated hernia:* emergency surgery *Non-incarcerated:* Educate parents about warning signs of incarceration and non-emergent surgical repair.

Penile Emergencies

- Remember to always examine the genitourinary system as part of the detailed pediatric exam of a fussy or crying child, especially when there is no other explanation.

Paraphimosis

Critical Knowledge

- A true urologic emergency.
- Paraphimosis is the inability to retract the prepuce (foreskin) distally over the glans penis.
- Paraphimosis prevents appropriate venous return, leading to engorgement of the glans and compromised arterial blood flow. This can lead to ischemia, necrosis, and gangrene.
- Causes include infection, masturbation, vigorous sexual activity and urethral foreign bodies. Many cases are iatrogenic during physical examination, urethral instrumentation and with urinary catheters.
- Complications: penile necrosis with auto-amputation, acute urinary obstruction with risk of renal failure, infection, severe pain.
- In contrast, phimosis is the inability to retract the foreskin proximally over the glans.
  - ► Normal infant anatomy (<5% of uncircumcised infants will have a retractable prepuce).
  - ► Non-emergency and does not require intervention (90% resolve by age 3).

Epidemiology/Anatomy

- Highest incidence is in infants and adolescents.
- Flaccid proximal penis with a collar of swollen and tender prepuce causing distal strangulation, engorgement, pain, and discoloration.
- Look for evidence of trauma, irritation, foreign bodies, and infection (i.e., cellulitis).

Differential Diagnosis

- Hair or clothing tourniquet
- Localized urticaria

Diagnosis

- This is a clinical diagnosis based on physical exam findings. Parents will often point out the problem.
- The prepuce will not retract to its normal position over and distal to the glans in the uncircumcised or improperly circumcised male.

Treatment

- Pain management and or sedation are crucial to success of reduction. Options include:
  - ► Topical 2% lidocaine gel
  - ► Parenteral morphine or midazolam
  - ► Dorsal penile block
    - Insert a 25-gauge needle directed into the dorsal base of the penis and towards the anterior and inferior pubic symphysis; then inject half bupivacaine and half of 1% lidocaine without epinephrine in either side of the suspensory ligament.
    - Innervation of the penis is by the left and right dorsal nerves (branches of the pudendal nerve).
- Reducing the swelling prior to manipulation with local ice, circumferential manual compression, or plastic wraps facilitates reduction.
- Using both of your thumbs, apply gentle and steady pressure on the glans while the other fingers are fixed proximal to the prepuce. Success rates are generally very high.
- For refractory cases, you may attempt an emergency dorsal slit procedure or even the puncture method, although it is recommended that you do these in consultation with urology.
- Consult urology stat from the ED for any failed manual reductions or complicated cases. An emergency circumcision may be necessary.
- Do not discharge until you verify that patient is able to void spontaneously.
- Provide teaching on proper prepuce care to parents and patients, along with urology follow up prior to discharge.
- Antibiotics are not routinely indicated unless there is evidence of an infection.

Priapism

Critical Knowledge

- This is a prolonged (>4 hours) and pathologic penile erection (tumescence) occurring in the absence of sexual stimulation.
- There are two types:
  - ▶ *Low-flow (ischemic) priapism* is painful and secondary to decreased venous outflow; this is by far the more common of the two types. It represents a true surgical emergency and is most commonly caused by sickle cell events or leukemia.
  - ▶ *High-flow (nonischemic) priapism* is painless or less painful and secondary to excessive arterial inflow. This is generally not a true surgical emergency, although initial expeditious management is still encouraged when there is diagnostic uncertainty. Straddle/groin injuries and spinal cord injuries account for most cases.
- Other causes include compressive tumors, illicit drug use, malaria, and medications – especially immunosuppressive agents.
- Irreversible tissue injury ensues within 24-48 hours of onset. Without timely management, ischemia, necrosis, and gangrene occur.

Epidemiology/Anatomy

- Distribution is bimodal.
  - ▶ 5-10 years of age: usually secondary to sickle cell disease
  - ▶ 20-50 years of age: most often secondary to medications and drugs
- With low-flow priapism, engorgement of the dorsal corpus cavernosum results in a dorsal penile erection, while the ventral surface and glans remain flaccid.
- With high-flow priapism, there is a semi-rigid shaft with an engorged glans.

Diagnosis

- A clinical diagnosis based on a detailed history in conjunction with physical exam findings; parents and patients will often point out the pathologic erection.
- No imaging studies are necessary to establish the diagnosis, although they help in localizing the problem, thereby guiding definitive management. These studies include a color-flow Doppler, MRI, technetium-99m scan, and angiography.

- Consider a complete blood count, reticulocyte count, and drug screen.

Treatment

- Determine the type of priapism and obtain a stat urology consultation.
- *Low-flow (ischemic) priapism:* Identify and target the underlying disease process.
  - ► Administer supplemental oxygen, intravenous fluid hydration and opiate analgesics as needed.
  - ► A dry corpus cavernosum (intracavernous) aspiration may be attempted, followed by aspiration with irrigation.
  - ► Intracavernous injections with dilute sympathomimetics such as phenylephrine will exert a potent alpha-mediated arterial constriction.
  - ► The use of oral systemic therapies such as terbutaline and pseudoophedrine are controversial.
  - ► Various surgical shunts are used for those who fail initial therapeutic measures.
- *High-flow (nonischemic) priapism:* Observation is generally sufficient unless there is diagnostic uncertainty, in which case intracavernous injections and aspiration may be acceptable.
  - ► Certain cases may require arterial embolization.
- The goal in all cases of priapism is to re-establish normal penile perfusion while preserving function.
- Always forewarn parents and patients that complications with or without management include future impotence, although there is a higher incidence with low-flow (ischemic) priapism.

Review Questions

1. Which of the following favors testicular torsion when there is diagnostic uncertainty?
   A. Dysuria
   B. Gradual pain
   C. Fever
   D. Vomiting

2. Which physical finding suggests testicular torsion?
   A. The "blue dot sign"
   B. Lack of the ipsilateral cremasteric reflex
   C. Pain localized to the superior and posterior testis
   D. Pain relieved with elevation of the hemiscrotum

3. A patient presents with an exquisitely tender and acutely swollen hemiscrotum. You should first:
   A. Attempt manual detorsion inward and medially.
   B. Attempt manual detorsion outward and laterally.
   C. Send the patient for a stat color-flow Doppler.
   D. Call urology only if the onset of pain is within 1 hour.

4. Which of the following is most consistent with epididymitis when compared to testicular torsion?
   A. Pyuria
   B. Hematuria
   C. Acute onset of pain
   D. Abdominal pain

5. Young children with recurrent testicular pain attributed to epididymitis should be considered for:
   A. Sexual abuse
   B. Congenital anomalies
   C. Intermittent torsion
   D. All of the above

6. **What is the most common cause of epididymitis in infants and young children:**

    A. *Gonococci*

    B. *Pseudomonas*

    C. *E. Coli*

    D. *Chlamydia*

7. **Which is of the following is TRUE?**

    A. Phimosis is usually a true medical emergency.

    B. Most cases of paraphimosis are successfully reduced without complications.

    C. A patient may be discharged immediately after successful reduction.

    D. Lidocaine with epinephrine can be used to perform a dorsal nerve block.

8. **Treatment of paraphimosis may include:**

    A. The puncture method

    B. Circumferential manual compression of the edematous prepuce while applying steady pressure to the glans

    C. The dorsal slit procedure

    D. All of the above

9. **Which of the following is NOT considered a true urologic emergency?**

    A. Paraphimosis

    B. Low-flow priapism

    C. Testicular torsion

    D. Torsion of the appendix testis

10. **Treatment modalities for ischemic or low-flow priapism include:**

    A. Dry aspiration of corpus spongiosum

    B. Intracavernous phenylephrine

    C. Intracavernous pseudoephedrine

    D. Arterial embolization

11. **Common causes of ischemic priapism include:**

    A. Sickle cell disease

    B. Perineal saddle injuries

    C. Penile trauma

    D. Spinal cord injuries

Key

1. D
2. B
3. B
4. A
5. D

6. C
7. B
8. D
9. D
10. B
11. A

Toxicologic Emergencies

Farshad "Mazda" Shirazi, MD, PhD
Mi Jin Kim-Ley, PharmD
Ryan Young, MD

General Approach

Initial Life Support

- ABCDs: airway patency, protective reflexes (gag reflex), adequate air entry, perfusion, GCS
- IV fluids, electrolytes, ABG, FSBG, oxygen
- Skin decontamination or eye flush for topical caustic agents
- GI decontamination (airway must be protected due to risk of aspiration or esophageal tear; contraindicated in the ingestion of corrosive substances or hydrocarbons, ileus, bowel obstruction or perforation, foreign body, aspiration, hypernatremia, or hypermagnesemia)
  - ▶ Activated charcoal does not alter the clinical course of most toxicities.
  - ▶ Whole bowel irrigation: osmotically balanced polyethylene glycol electrolyte solution 30 mL/hr up to 500 mL/hr until stool is clear

History

If Known Intoxication, 4 Es:

- Estimate amount
- Elapsed time since ingestion
- Early symptoms
- Early interventions by patient of family

If Suspected, but Unknown Intoxication

- Symptoms
- Timing of onset of symptoms
- Medications at home
- Recent illness treatments
- Visitors, travel
- Acute altered mental status

If history is unknown, admit and observe overnight.

Physical Exam

- Vital signs, GCS
- Skin color, bullae, piloerection, diaphoresis
- Eyes/pupils, EOMI, fundi
- Mouth odors
- CV (perfusion)
- Respiratory (air entry, rate)
- GI (motility)

Labs

- CBC, ABG, CMP (BMP w/LFTs), ECG, chest x-ray, KUB, UA, AND complete toxicology screen
- Aspirin and acetaminophen levels for suspected toxicity
- Pregnancy test for females of reproductive age

Hemodialysis may need to be considered for AA STUMBLE.

- Alcohol (Isopropyl)
- Atenolol
- Salicylates
- Theophylline
- Uremia
- Methanol
- Barbiturates
- Lithium/heavy metals
- Ethanol/ethylene glycol

Radio-Opaque Toxins (CHIPES)

- Chloral hydrate
- Heavy metals
- Iron
- Phenothiazines
- Enteric coating
- Salicylates

Seizure-Inducing Toxins

- Glyometra (mushrooms)
- Heavy metals
- Sympathomimetics (cocaine, amphetamines)
- Beta-blockers
- TCA antidepressants
- SSRIs
- Methylhydrosine or isoniazide treated with pyridoxine

Evaluation

6-hour rule: "If nothing has occurred during the first 6 hours after ingestion, nothing will happen" with the exception of acetaminophen, hydrocarbon ingestion, and delayed release pharmaceuticals.

Warning

For a poison emergency in the U.S., call 1-800-222-1222

One Pill Kills: Drugs that may be fatal for a 10-kg child upon ingestion of one commercially available dose unit. (At 1 year of age, an infant can grasp a single pill with a pincer grasp, but only later has the ability to manage a handful of pills.)

Drug	Symptoms	Management
Iron pills	*Phases:* 1: (6 hrs) Mucosal injury-n/v, diarrhea, GI blood loss 2: (6-24 hrs) Recovery-child appears well 3: (>24 hrs) Metabolic acidosis, coma, seizures, shock	ABCs, labs. serum Fe levels >500 ug risk for phase III UGI x-ray, whole bowel irrigation, IV defuroxamine 15 mg/kg/hr
Beta blockers, Ca+ channel blockers	Bradycardia, hypotension, AV block, hypoglycemia with BBs, and hyperglycemia with BBs in CCBs metabolic acidosis in CCBs	ABCs, atropine, fluid bolus, pressors, charcoal, calcium infusion for CCBs
Clonidine	Altered mental status, lethargy, hypothermia, miosis, respiratory depression, coma	ABCs, respiratory support, activated charcoal, naloxone
Hypoglycemics (glucophage)	Hypoglycemia, lethargy, metabolic acidosis	ABCs, charcoal, infusion of hypertonic glucose, octreotide 1-2 µg per kg per dose q6 hrs

| Theophyline | Headache, seizures, PVCs, tachycardia, extra systoles, arrhythmias | ABCs, close monitoring, antiarrhythmics, seizure precautions |
| **Methylsalicylate (Icy Hot, oil of wintergreen – also a nontoxic hydrocarbon)** | Cerebral edema, coma, lethargy, seizures, tinnitus, electrolyte imbalance, pulmonary edema | ABCs, close monitoring, correction of fluid and electrolyte imbalances, if severe hemodialysis or hemoperfusion. |

Common Toxins

Toxins	Clinical Presentation	Management
Opioids Codeine Fentanyl Hydrocodone Hydromorphone Meperidine Methadone Morphine Oxycodone Diamorphine (heroin)	CNS depression Respiratory depression Pupillary miosis Ventricular arrhythmias Mental status changes Agitation Bradypnea Hypotension	**Naloxone** ≤20 kg = 0.1 mg/kg >20 kg = 2 mg/dose (May want to consider giving increments of 1/10th of total dose.)
Acetaminophen *Toxicity generally from >200 mg/kg (150 mg/kg × 2 days or 100 mg/kg × 3 days in children) or can be from chronic use of acetaminophen-containing products* Liver damage can occur 18-24 hrs after ingestion.	Nausea Vomiting Abdominal pain Elevated LFTs Liver failure Coagulopathy Encephalopathy Hyperglycemia Lactic acidosis	BMP LFTs Coagulants Activated charcoal Acetaminophen level – Refer to Rumack-Matthew Nomogram *Treat immediately without levels if >6-8 hrs after ingestion, severe symptoms, staggered overdoses, or extended-release formulations* **N-acetylcysteine oral solution**: 140 mg PO LD, *THEN* 70 mg/kg PO Q 4 hrs × 17 doses **N-acetylcysteine injection**: 150 mg/kg IV over 60 min, *THEN* 50 mg/kg IV over 4 hours, *THEN* 100 mg/kg IV over 16 hours *Call poison center for recommendations.*

Alpha-Adrenergic Agonists Clonidine	CNS depression Lethargy Coma Early transient hypertension Hypotension Early tachycardia Bradycardia Cardiac dysrhythmias (AV block) Respiratory depression Apnea Hypothermia Miosis	Activated charcoal[1] Whole bowel irrigation for patch ingestion Supportive therapy Naloxone for CNS depression Atropine for severe bradycardia (may consider norepinephrine, dopamine)
Amphetamines Atomoxetine Dextroamphetamine Methylphenidate Modafinil Pemoline Phendimetrazine Phentermine	Euphoria Anxiety Restlessness Agitation Psychosis Seizures (status epilepticus) Coma Sweating Tremor Muscle rigidity Tachycardia Hypertension Acute MI Cardiac infarction Ventricular arrhythmias Pulmonary hypertension (with chronic use)	*Acute ingestion of 1 mg/kg of dextroamphetamine (or equivalent) should be considered life-threatening.* Amphetamine level BMP CK ECG (monitor for at least 6 hours) ECHO for pulmonary hypertension Activated charcoal[1] Supportive care: Benzodiazepines, droperidol, or haloperidol (antagonizes CNS dopamine) for agitation *Olanzapine or risperidone also may be used.* Benzodiazepines for seizures Sedation, or phentolamine, nitroprusside for hypertension Labetalol or esmolol for tachyarrhythmias

Anticholinergics	Anticholinergic effects:	ECG
Antihistamines	Mydriasis	CK
Diphenhydramine	Flushing	ABG
Dimenhydrinate	Fever	
Brompheniramine	Dry mouth	Activated charcoal
Chlorpheniramine	Decreased bowel	
Cetirizine	sounds	Benzodiazapines for agitation and delirium
Meclizine	Somnolence	
Promethazine	Tachycardia	***Physostigmine may be used for***
Trimeprazine	Mild hypertension	***diagnosis or for severe symptoms, but***
Astemizole	Nausea/vomiting	***generally not recommended. Close***
Cyproheptadine	Agitation	***monitoring needed; do not give if TCAs***
Desloratadine	Confusion	***also ingested.***
Fexofenadine	Hallucinations	Children = 0.02 mg/kg IV and repeat every
Loratadine	Agitated delirium	5-10 min (max rate = 0.5 mg/min, max
Terfenadine	Psychosis	dose = 2 mg)
		Adults = 2 mg IV, may repeat every 10 to
Antispasmodics	Seizures	30 min, max rate 1mg/min
Dicyclomine	Coma	
Glycopyrrolate	Hypotension	Sodium bicarbonate for myocardial
Oxybutynin	QRS widening	depression and QRS intervals
Tolterodine	Ventricular	
Belladonna alkaloids	dysrhythmias	Lidocaine if sodium bicarbonate
Belladonna		unsuccessful
Atropine		
Tolteridine		
L-Hyoscamine		
Scopolamine		
Salicylates	GI upset	Arterial or venous blood gas
Aspirin	Tinnitis	Salicylate level
Bismuth subsalicylate	Lethargy	LFTs
Oil of wintergreen	Agitation	Coagulants
1 tsp contains 5 gm of	Confusion	
methylsalicylate	Tachycardia	Activated charcoal [1]
(= 7.5 gm ASA)	Tachypnea	
	Respiratory alkalosis	Ingestion:
	Metabolic acidosis	150-300 mg/kg = mild toxicity
	Hyperpnea	300-500 mg/kg = moderate-severe toxicity
	Hyperthermia	>500 mg/kg = severe toxicity
	Hypoglycemia	For ASA level >30 mg/dL –
		Urine alkalinization with D5W + 150
		mEq/L sodium bicarbonate @ 1-1.5 ×
		maintenance (goal UOP >2 mL/kg/hr and
		urine pH >7.5)
		Hemodialysis – if unresponsive acidosis,
		serum level >100 mg/dL, seizures, coma or
		chronic intoxication and levels >60 mg/dL

Barbiturates Phenobarbital Pentobarbital Primidone	CNS depression Respiratory depression Respiratory failure Hypotension Decreased myocardial contraction Hypothermia Confusion Nystagmus Ataxia	Activated charcoal[1] Supportive therapy Cardiac monitoring Urine alkalinization – sodium bicarbonate 1-2 mEq/kg, **THEN** 150 mEq/L in D5W @ 1.5-2 × maintenance (goal urine pH 7.5-8) Hemodialysis
Benzodiazepines Clonazepam Clorazepate Diazepam Flurazepam Lorazepam Midazolam Triazolam	Coma (with normal vital signs) CNS depression Confusion Hallucinations Ataxia Amnesia Dizziness Blurred vision Unresponsiveness Agitation Weakness	Flumazenil Children: 0.01 mg/kg (max dose = 0.2mg), repeat every minute to a max of 2 mg (Continuous infusion 0.005-0.01 mg/kg/hr has been used.) Adults: 0.2 mg, **THEN** 0.3 mg after 30 sec, **THEN** 0.5 mg every 30 sec to a maximum of 3 mg in adults in 1 hr *Use cautiously in chronic uses (can precipitate withdrawal, seizures, cardiac arrhythmias).*

Beta-Blockers
Atenolol
Metoprolol
Nadalol
Propranolol
Sotalol
	Bradycardia
	Hypotension
	Heart block
	Ventricular
	  dysrhythmias (seen
	  with propranolol)
	Congestive heart
	  failure
	CNS depression
	Coma
	Cardiac arrest
	Seizures
	  (with propranolol)
	Wheezing
	Cyanosis
		Activated charcoal[1]
		
		Supportive care (cardiac monitor, fluids for
		hypotension, atropine for bradycardia)
		
		Glucagon (if not responsive to fluids)
		Children 30-150 mcg/kg bolus, **THEN** 70
		mcg/kg/hr infusion
		
		Calcium
		Calcium gluconate 60 mg/kg IV
		OR calcium chloride 20 mg/kg IV
		
		Vasopressors (dopamine, norepinephrine,
		epinephrine) *Use as last line due to worse
		outcomes documented.*
		
		Insulin 1 unit/kg bolus, **THEN** 0.1-1 unit/kg
		with glucose 0.25 gm/kg. Titrate insulin until
		hypotension corrected (max 2 units/kg)
		
		Intravenous lipid therapy[2]

Calcium-Channel Blockers Amlodipine Diltiazem Felodipine Isradipine Nifedipine Nisoldipine Verapamil	Bradycardia Hypotension Heart block AV nodal depression Dysrhythmias Lethargy Syncope Altered mental status Seizures Cerebral ischemia Nausea/vomiting Ileus Bowel ischemia Renal failure Metabolic acidosis Hyperglycemia Coma	Similar to beta-blocker ingestion (refer to above) with the exception of whole bowel irrigation for sustained or extended-release preparations. Norepinephrine is the vasopressor of choice.
Carbamazepine	Nausea/vomiting Nystagmus Ataxia Hyperreflexia CNS depression Dystonia Sinus tachycardia Anticholinergic symptoms Seizures Coma Respiratory depression Rhabdomyolysis Renal failure Cardiac conduction defects	Carbamazepine level every 4 hours ***Can cause false positive for TCAs on urine tox screen.*** ECG BMP, CBC Provide supportive care. Activated charcoal[1] if drug still in GI. Whole bowel irrigation for sustained release formulation. Gastric lavage for large overdoses. Hemodialysis for severe, life-threatening overdose.

Carbon Monoxide	Headache	CO-Hbg level (Conventional pulse oximeter
Binds to hemoglobin with affinity 250x that of O2, producing a left shift of the oxygen dissociation curve	Nausea Dizziness Drowsiness Confusion Angina or MI (in patients with coronary disease)	can be falsely normal.) ECG Electrolytes Blood gas Neurologic exams
Decreased O2 delivery to tissues (especially heart and brain)	Syncope Coma	100% O2 via non-rebreather mask until CO-Hgb <5% *(CO half-life approx 30-90 min vs >200 min on room air.)*
Smoke inhalation Fires Stoves Portable heaters Automobile exhaust Charcoal grills	Convulsions Cardiac arrhythmias Hypotension Metabolic acidosis Cerebral edema	Hyperbaric oxygen in severe cases CO-Hgb >25% Loss of consciousness Severe metabolic acidosis Abnormal neuro exam Cardiovascular dysfunction
	CO-Hgb level >25% significant levels, mild symptoms except in patients with heart disease, >40% shows obvious intoxication	CO exposure >24 hours *(Decreases CO half-life to 15-20 min.)* Call the local poison control center!
Hydrocarbons	Coughing	Respiratory support
Low viscosity, low surface tension = high aspiration risk Halogenated Aromatic Alcohols Ethers Ketones	Gagging Choking Respiratory distress Wheezing Hypoxia Hypercarbia Chemical pneumonitis Drooling	Skin and eye decontamination Blood gases BMP and LFTs ECG monitoring
Aliphatic (lower risk for toxicity unless aspirated) Lighter fluid Kerosene Furniture polish Gasoline	Tachypnea Vomiting Altered mental status Ataxia Lethargy Headache Syncope Coma Respiratory arrest Dysrhythmias	

| Iron
Ferrous gluconate
Ferrous fumarate
Ferrous sulfate
Vitamin (containing iron) | **Phase I** – 0.5-2 hrs
Abdominal pain
Vomiting
Diarrhea
Hematemesis
Lethargy
Metabolic acidosis
Shock
Coagulopathy

Phase II – Apparent recovery

Phase III – 2-12 hrs
Profound shock
Severe acidosis
Cyanosis
Fever | Iron levels
(>300 mcg/dL usually symptomatic)
CMP, CBC
Abdominal x-ray for retained tablets
Whole bowel irrigation

Desferoxamine *(for severe toxicity)*
15 mg/kg/hr for 12-24 hours (max = 6 gm/day; >24-hour infusion can be associated with acute lung injury) |
| Digoxin | Nausea
Vomiting
Abdominal pain
Lethargy
Bradycardia
Heart block
Vomiting
Shock
Hyperkalemia
Cardiac arrest
  (increased with dose
  >4 mg in children
  and >10 mg in
  adults)

Chronic toxicity:
bradycardia, malaise,
nausea, anorexia,
delirium, vision
changes, ventricular
dysrhythmias, heart
block | Digoxin level
BMP (especially potassium every hour)
Cardiac monitoring, ECGs

Digoxin immune fab (for severe toxicity, dysrhythmias, hyperkalemia >5 mEq/L)

For known mg ingestion:
Dose (in # of vials) =
$$\frac{\text{Ingested dose of capsules}}{0.5}$$
OR
$$\frac{\text{Ingested dose of tablets} \times 0.8}{0.5}$$

For known serum digoxin level:
Dose (in # of vials) =
$$\frac{\text{Serum digoxin level (ng/mL)} \times \text{wt (kg)}}{100}$$

Infuse over 30 min w/ 0.22 μ in-line filter

Watch for allergic reactions, precipitation of CHF, and rebound hypokalemia. |

Antidepressants (Tricyclic) Amitriptyline Amoxapine Clomipramine Desipramine Doxepin Imipramine Maprotiline Nortriptyline Protriptyline Trimipramine	CNS depression Respiratory depression Anticholinergic effects (dry mouth, blurred vision, urinary retention, tachycardia) Hallucinations Seizures Coma QRS prolongation with ventricular dysrhythmias Hypotension Decreased GI motility	TCA levels Cardiac monitoring (Cardiac toxicity generally is seen within 6 hours and can last >48 hours.) Activated charcoal[1] if <2 hours Consider lipid therapy [2] early for ventricular dysrhythmias or hypotension for fat-soluble drugs (e.g., clomipramine). Serum alkalinization +/- hypoventilation **For QRS prolongation:** Sodium bicarbonate 1-2 mEq/kg bolus, **THEN** continuous infusion (goal serum pH = 7.45-7.55) Hypertonic saline (if not responsive to alkalinization) Vasopressor support (norepinephrine, vasopressin, epinephrine-dopamine is generally ineffective)
Antidepressants (non-TCA) **SSRI** Citalopram Escitalopram Fluoxetine Fluvoxamine Paroxetine Sertraline Serotonin norepineph- rine reuptake inhibitor Desvenlafaxine Venlafaxine MAOIs **Miscellaneous** Buproprion Duloxetine Mirtazapine Nefazodone Trazodone	Serotonin syndrome *(unlikely with* *single agents-* *hyperreflexia, clonus,* *altered mental* *status, hemodynamic* *instability, seizures)* Sedation Dizziness, nausea Constipation Diarrhea Tachycardia Bradycardia Hypertension Hyperthermia Mydriasis CNS depression	Activated charcoal[1] Lipid therapy[2] if patient develops significant cardiovascular toxicity Benzodiazepines for serotonin syndrome **Cyproheptadine** (for moderate cases) Children – 0.25 mg/kg/day divided q 6 hrs; max dose = 12 mg/day Adults = 12 mg loading dose, then 2 mg every 2 hours until symptoms improve

Antipsychotics	Sedation	Activated charcoal[1]
Typical	Ataxia	Whole bowel irrigation (for sustained-release
Chlorpromazine	Extrapyramidal effects	preparations)
Fluphenazine	Tachycardia	ECG
Haloperidol	Miosis	
Thioridazine	Nystagmus	Supportive therapy (norepinephrine or
Atypical	Seizures	phenylephrine if vasopressor therapy
Risperidone	Delirium	needed)
Ziprasidone	Coma	
Olanzapine	Respiratory depression	Torsades de pointes – magnesium sulfate
Aripiprazole	Hypotension	
Clozapine	Prolonged QTc	QRS prolongation – sodium bicarbonate
Iloperidone	Oculargyric crisis	injection
Paliperidone	Central diabetes	
Loxapine	insipidus	Lipid therapy[2] for lipid soluble drugs
Molidone		
Thiothixine		
Quetiapine		
Paliperidone		
Trifluoroperazine		
Botulism Toxin	Hypotonia	Supportive care
(in infants)	Difficulty feeding	EMG
Honey or corn syrup	Diminished gag,	Serum and stool analysis
Home-canned	sucking, and	
vegetables, fish, meats	swallowing reflex	**Botulism immune globulin**
Fresh garlic in olive oil		**(Baby-BIG)** – for infants <1 year =
Chamomile tea	Constipation	1.5 mL/kg (75 mg/kg)
Newly constructed areas	Tachycardia	**Contact the poison control center!**
	Poor head control	
	Ptosis	
Lead	With large acute	Activated charcoal – efficacy unknown –
	ingestion:	binds poorly to lead
	Levels 25-60 mcg/	Lead level (whole blood)
	dL:	
	Headache	Free erythrocyte protoporphyrin (reflects
	Irritability	chronic exposure)
	Difficulty concentrating	— X-ray to look for lead deposition
	Slowed reaction time	— Whole bowel irrigation if
		radiographic evidence in GI tract
	Levels of 60-80	
	mcg/dL:	IV fluids to maintain adequate urine output
	Abdominal pain	(1-2 mL/kg/hr)
	Hemolytic anemia	
	Toxic hepatitis	Monitor for increased ICP

Lead (continued)	*Levels >80 mcg/dL:*	Increased ICP: ventilation, mannitol, dexamethasone
	Abdominal pain (lead colic)	
	Nephropathy	**Chelation Therapy**
	Parasthesias	(Recommended for levels >45 mcg/dL in children and >50 mcg/dL in adults):
	Levels >100 mcg/dL:	*Note: when using dimercaprol, urine should be alkalinized to prevent lead reabsorption*
	Encephalopathy	
	Neuropathy	
	Seizures	Encephalopathy:
		BAL (dimercaprol)
	With subacute or chronic exposure:	*Watch for peanut allergy.*
	Fatigue	450 mg/m²/day IM (75 mg/m² every 4 hrs) × 5 days
	Malaise	**Calcium EDTA**
	Irritability	*Only with adequate urine output*
	Anorexia	After 2ⁿᵈ dose of BAL – 1500 mg/m2/day
	Insomnia	(50 mg/kg/day) continuous infusion *OR*
	Arthralgias	2-4 divided doses × 5 days
	Myalgias	
	Abdominal cramping	Level >70 mcg/dL w/ symptoms:
	Nausea	**BAL (Dimercaprol)**
	Constipation	450 mg/m³/day IM (75 mg/m² every 4 hrs) × 5 days
	Developmental delay	**Calcium EDTA**
	Cognitive deficits	After 2ⁿᵈ dose of BAL – 1500 mg/m2/day
	Peripheral neuropathy	(50 mg/kg/day) continuous infusion *OR* 2-4 divided doses × 5 days
		Lead level 45-69 mcg/dL w/o symptoms:
		Succimer (DMSA)
		350 mg/m2 (10 mg/kg) PO q 8 hours × 5 days, *THEN* q 12 hours × 2 weeks
		OR
		Calcium EDTA
		1000 mg/m2/day continuous infusion *OR* 2-4 divided IV doses for 5 days
		OR
		D-penicillamine (last line)
		25-35 mg/kg/day in 3-4 divided. Start at 25% of dose and increase by 25% weekly as tolerated (Do not use if patient has a penicillin allergy or renal dysfunction.)

Organophosphates (Cholinesterase inhibitors)	*Central effects* CNS depression Agitation Confusion Delirium Coma Seizures	Symptomatic supportive care for cholinergic excess, airway management
		Plasma +/- RBC Cholinesterase levels
		Electrolytes, lipase, ECG
	CHOLINERGIC side effects *(less predominant in children)* *Muscarinic* **D**iarrhea **U**rination **M**iosis **B**ronchospasm **B**ronchorrhea **B**radycardia **E**mesis **L**acrimation **S**alivation/Sweating Also bronchorrhea, acute lung injury	Decontamination (removal of clothing, scrub skin, irrigate mucous membranes)
		Activated charcoal with large ingestions, gastric lavage in hospital setting only due to risk of aspiration
		Atropine (for muscarinic symptoms) 0.02 mg/kg IV, double dose if inadequate response every 3-5 min until respiratory secretions clear; may need to start continuous infusion at 10%-20% of loading dose for hours to days, depending on severity of symptoms. *Watch for atropine toxicity.
	Nicotinic Tachycardia Hypertension Mydriasis Muscle fasciculations Muscle cramps Weakness Respiratory failure	**Pralidoxime** (neuromuscular blockade reversal, moderate to severe toxicity) *Most effective if given within 48 hrs; continue for 24 hrs after symptoms resolve.* Loading dose 30-50 mg/kg (total of 1-2 gm) IV over 30 min, *THEN* 8-20 mg/kg/hr infusion
		Use inhaled ipratropium or gycopyrrolate in addition to atropine for bronchospasm.

[1]Activated charcoal (only if patient can protect airway)

Infants = 1-2 g/kg every 4-6 hrs

Children = 1-2 g/kg or 15-30 gm every 2-6 hrs

Adolescents and adults = 25-60 gm every 2-6 hrs

[2]Intravenous lipid therapy = 20% Lipids 1-1.5 mL/kg bolus over 2-3 min (may repeat every 3- 5 min × 3 doses) *THEN* 0.25-0.5 mL/kg/min (generally for 30-60 min)

Common Drugs of Abuse

Alcohols Ethanol Methanol Ethylene glycol (antifreeze)	Intoxication Euphoria Ataxia Nystagmus Aggressive behavior Vomiting SVTs Atrial fibrillation Respiratory depression Coma Pulmonary aspiration Hypoglycemia Hypothermia Cardiac arrest **Ethylene glycol** Coma Hypotonia Hyporeflexia Cerebral edema Anion gap metabolic acidosis Renal failure	Ethanol concentration Ethylene glycol concentration Blood gas Serum and urine ketones Supportive care Dextrose for hypoglycemia, altered mental status ***For methanol or ethylene glycol level >20 mg/dL or metabolic acidosis or potentially toxic ingestion:*** **Fomepizole** 15 mg/kg loading dose, ***THEN*** 10 mg/kg IV every 12 hrs × 4 doses until symptoms improve or levels <20 mg/dL. 2nd option **Ethanol** 5%-10%-0.8 g/kg loading dose over 20-60 min, then 80-150ml/ kg/hr. continuous infusion to maintain serum ethanol concentration of 100-150 mg/dL May consider hemodialysis
Amphetamines (hallucinogenic) (phenylethylamines) Methylamphetamine ***("Crank," "Speed," "Ice")*** 3,4-methylene- dioxyphenyl- ethylamine ***MDMA, "ecstasy"*** Paramethoxy- amphetamine ***PMA, "Death"*** Mescaline (Peyote)	Mydriasis Dizziness Hypertension Tachycardia Agitation Delirium Psychosis Bruxism (MDMA) Nausea/vomiting (Peyote) Hypothermia (PMA) Hyperkalemia (PMA) QRS prolongation (PMA) Hypoglycemia Seizures Rhabdomyolysis Coma Ventricular dysrhythmias End-organ damage Serotonin syndrome	ECG CK levels Activated charcoal if substantial ingestion Benzodiazepines for delirium Antipsychotics for agitation

Synthetic Cathinones	Agitation	Supportive care
Bath salts	Aggressiveness	(similar to cocaine and amphetamines)
Plant food	Sweating	
Khat (Natural plant)	Palpitations	Benzodiazepines for sympathomimetic
	Shortness of breath	symptoms
	Chest pain	
	Abdominal pain	
	Nausea/vomiting	
	Tinnitis	
	Headache	
	Muscle twitching	
	Dizziness	
	Vertigo	
	Short-term memory loss	
	Hallucinations	
	Hyponatremia	
Cocaine	Anxiety	**Do NOT give activated charcoal unless symptomatic body stuffer (increased risk of seizures)!**
	Hallucinations	
	Chest pain	
	Hypertension	Troponin if chest pain
	Palpitations	ECG
	Agitation	BMP
	Seizures	CK
	Hyperthermia	
	Rhabdomyolysis	Aggressive cooling for hyperthermia
	Decreased myocardial function	Benzodiazepines for agitation and seizures
	Dysrhythmias	
		Do NOT use beta-blockers.
		Sodium bicarbonate 1-2 mEq IV every 5 min for wide-complex dysrhythmias
		Lidocaine if unresponsive to bicarbonate
		Epinephrine or norepinephrine for refractory hypotension
		Consider lipid therapy with dysrhythmias, hypotension, or severe CNS toxicity.

Gamma Hydroxybutyrate (GHB) *Liquid "Ecstasy"*	Hallucinations Abrupt onset of sleep (15 min after ingestion) Enuresis Myoclonic movements Delirium agitation Bradycardia Coma (30-40 min after ingestion up to 8 hours – alcohol can prolong effects)	Supportive care Activated charcoal and gastric lavage are not helpful due to rapid absorption.
Ketamine	Sedation Respiratory depression Tachycardia Altered mental status Anxiety Palpitations Slurred speech Hallucinations Nystagmus Mydriasis Hypertension Chest pain	Symptomatic care ECG Can produce false positive on urine toxicology for phencyolidine (PCP). Benzodiazepines for agitation and seizures
Marijuana *Inhaled form is 3x more potent than enteral* **Synthetic cannabinoids** *("Spice")* *Have similar effects except for increased agitation and potential for seizures.*	Somnolence Euphoria Time/space distortion Mood alterations Decreased motor coordination Lethargy Muscle jerking Ataxia Pulmonary irritation Mydriasis Hypotonia	Supportive care Albuterol for bronchospasm

Note: *This chapter is designed as a guide for treatment and an aid for acute toxicologic emergencies. It is not the definitive or complete source of information. Your local poison control center should be consulted with any questions and to simply double-check management.*

Review Questions

1. A 5-year-old male is brought to the ED after a suspected overdose. While in a private car on the way over, the patient has "shaking movements" and is seen to have tonic-clonic activity while presenting to triage. Which of the following is LESS likely to be associated with seizures?

   A. Opioids

   B. B-blockers

   C. Anticholinergics

   D. Sympathomimetics

   E. Acute heavy metal ingestion

2. A 4-year-old male with a known seizure disorder presents to the ED with acute mental status change. Father states the patient has been irritable for a couple of weeks. During the morning he was unable to wake from sleep, and was unresponsive to voice and stimulation. Upon arrival, the patient is obtunded; has agonal breathing; and a GCS of 8, moaning only to painful stimulus. After the initial ABCs, the patient is intubated and put on a CV monitor; IV access is obtained and the patient is resuscitated. The patient has a temperature of 36.4°C; a BMP shows a sodium of 118; and the patient has a very brisk urine output. You suspect SIADH. What toxidrome can give you the above symptoms?

   A. Benzodiazepines

   B. ACE inhibitors

   C. Anticholinergics

   D. Tegretol

   E. Phenobarbital

3. A 9-year-old boy is brought to the ED after he was found on his family's farm confused and disoriented. He presents having urinated his pants, is doubled over holding his stomach, and has multiple bouts of emesis. Upon physical exam, he is wheezing with respiratory distress, has moist skin, muscle twitching, and miosis bilaterally. What is the best management for this patient after assessing ABCDs?

   A. ABCs, remove clothing, atropine and pralixocime until symptoms resolve

B. ABCs, activated charcoal, benzos or haldol, IV fluids with alkalinization, and cooling measures

C. ABCs, gastric lavage, UGI x-ray, whole bowel irrigation, IV defuroxamine 15 mg/kg/hr

D. ABCs, serial EKGs, glucagon, and respiratory support

E. ABCs, supportive care, diazepam for seizures, external cooling, sedatives, and airway management for hyperthermia up to 72 hours

4. A 12-month-old girl is hospitalized for ingesting what her mother thinks is approximately 2 tablespoons of vitamin E oil. You observe her for approximately 6 hours and perform a chest x ray, which is normal. At this point, the best course of action is:

A. Perform a gastric lavage with whole bowel irrigation.

B. Send her home with close follow up.

C. Hospitalize and observe overnight with serial chest x-rays.

D. Trial her on room air for another 3 hours; if no symptoms, then send her home.

E. Provide supportive care with PICU admission for possible pneumonitis.

5. A 15-month-old boy arrives in the ED lethargic, with poor respiratory effort, and a slight tremor. The boy's parents are divorced, and the father administered a medication for the first time that evening. He knows that his son was recently hospitalized for an extended period of time and was intubated for acute respiratory failure. What is the next step in management of this child?

A. Intubate, provide supportive care, and admit to the PICU.

B. Administer the appropriate dose of flumazanil.

C. Call poison control to consult.

D. Provide supportive care, diazepam for seizures, external cooling, sedatives, and airway management for hyperthermia up to 72 hours.

E. Gastric lavage, UGI x-ray, whole bowel irrigation, IV defuroxamine 15 mg/kg/hr.

Suspected Non-Accidental Trauma 35

Stephen Charbonneau, MD, JD
Dale Woolridge MD, PhD

Critical Concepts

- Always suspect nonaccidental trauma when evaluating an injured or severely ill pediatric patient.
- Treat emergent injuries first.
- Physicians are mandated to report *all* suspected cases of child abuse and neglect.
- Develop a multidisciplinary team for patient care and child abuse reporting.
- Document and record all pertinent information.
- Establish appropriate follow-up and child safety.
- The risk of pediatric death greatly increases if the initial presentation of child abuse is not recognized.

Epidemiology

- In 2010, U.S. state and local child protective services (CPS) received an estimated 3.3 million reports of children (43.8 per 1,000) being abused or neglected.
  - ► CPS estimated that 695,000 children (9.2 per 1,000) were victims of maltreatment.
  - ► Of the child victims, 78% were victims of neglect; 18% of physical abuse; 9% of sexual abuse; and 8% of emotional abuse.
- In 2010, an estimated 1,560 children died from child maltreatment (rate of 2.1 per 100,000 children).
- More than 740,000 children and youth are treated in hospital emergency departments as a result of violence each year.
- The total lifetime cost of child maltreatment is $124 billion each year.

Differential Diagnosis of Physical Abuse

Injury	Differential Diagnosis
Bruises	Accidental or nonaccidental bruise, cultural practices, dermatologic disorders, genetic disorders (e.g., Ehlers-Danlos syndrome), hematologic disorders, Henoch-Schönlein purpura, salicylate ingestion, Mongolian spots
Burns	Accidental burn, cultural practices such as cupping, phytophotodermatitis, impetigo, inflicted burn, skin infection, Stevens-Johnson syndrome
Fractures	Accidental or intentional fracture, birth trauma, congenital syphilis, leukemia, osteogenesis imperfecta, osteomyelitis, physiologic changes, rickets, scurvy
Head Trauma	Accidental or inflicted trauma, birth trauma, hemorrhagic disease, infection, intracranial vascular anomalies, metabolic disease (e.g., glutaric aciduria type I)

Critical Concepts

- Take a detailed history from those involved and interview the patient separately if time and circumstances allow.

Indicators of Physical Abuse by History
• No history given for the injury
• Conflicting history given by caretakers
• History/injury is inconsistent with the developmental level of the child
• History is inconsistent with the injury
• Delay in seeking medical care
• Seeking health care from multiple providers

- Pay close attention to injuries that cannot be explained by the history; a history that changes; or a delay in seeking medical treatment.
- If the patient presents with obvious signs of nonaccidental trauma, the history may be taken in conjunction with law enforcement and child protective services.
- A child who is lethargic, overly reserved, apneic, or convulsing should raise higher suspicion of abuse.

- The initial assessment of the pediatric patient should include a primary survey including airway, breathing, circulation, and a careful examination of the patient's vital signs adjusted for age.

Closed Head Injury

- Head injury is the leading cause of death in abused children under 2 years of age.

- The clinical manifestations of nonaccidental head trauma can be difficult to recognize, and more than 30% of cases are missed on initial presentation. Suspect this diagnosis with any change in mental status, vomiting, apnea, seizures, bradycardia, irritability, or other unexplained injuries.

- CT of the head without contrast is the preferred imaging study in any infant or child in whom head trauma is suspected.

- Ophthalmology should be consulted to examine the retinas for hemorrhage.

- The physical exam should include assessment of the Pediatric Glasgow Coma Score *(Table 1)*, examination of the pupils, fundoscopic exam, and a complete neurologic exam with reflexes; explore lacerations, assess fontanel, palpate for asymmetry or step-offs, evaluate for hemotympanum, CSF otorrhea or rhinorrhea, Battle's sign, or raccoon eyes.

- Types of intracranial bleed
  - ▶ Subdural hematoma
  - ▶ Epidural hematoma
  - ▶ Subarachnoid hemorrhage
  - ▶ Diffuse axonal injury

- Shaken baby syndrome is a significant source of morbidity and mortality in infants. Approximately 25% of victims die from injuries, and almost 50% have significant morbidity, including neurologic, visual, motor, and cognitive impairment.

Clinical Findings of a Shaken Baby
• Retinal hemorrhages
• Intracranial trauma (particularly subdural hemorrhage)
• Diffuse axonal injury
• Secondary cerebral edema
• Fractures of the posterior and anterolateral ribs

Fractures

- Fractures are present in as many as 55% of physically abused children.
- Fractures are the second-most common injury identified in physical abuse. Soft tissue injuries are the *most* common.
- The estimated annual incidence of fractures attributable to abuse is 36 cases per 100,000 children younger than 12 months, and 5 cases per 100,000 children between 12 and 35 months.
- Palpate all joints and extremities for clinical evaluation of suspected injuries.
- Any pediatric fracture can be the result of physical abuse.
- There are no absolutely pathognomonic fracture patterns; however, certain fractures are more likely to be associated with abuse.

Fracture Types and Their Association with Child Abuse
Likelihood of Nonaccidental Trauma

Low	Moderate	High
Clavicular fracture	Multiple fractures	Metaphyseal, including bucket-handle fracture
Long bone shaft fracture	Epiphyseal separation	Posterior rib fracture
Linear skull fracture	Vertebral body fracture/subluxation	Scapular fracture
	Digital fracture	Spinous process
	Complex skull fracture	Sternal fracture

Bruises

- Infants who do not "cruise" rarely bruise. Bruises anywhere on the body are extremely uncommon in infants younger than 6 months.
- Bruising is rare in healthy children on the hands, buttocks, cheek, nose, neck, forearms, lumbar region, or chest.
- Bruising resembling the shape of an instrument or hand, "pinch mark," or linear on the buttocks are more likely nonaccidental.
- Bilateral black eyes are almost always nonaccidental unless significant trauma is involved with the injury.

- Bruises that resemble human bites should be photographed and measured for evaluation. Adult bite marks can be distinguished from bites inflicted by other children by the maxillary intercanine distance, which is at least 2.5 to 3 cm.

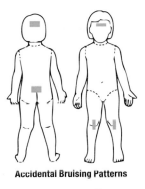

Accidental Bruising Patterns

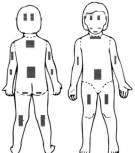

Nonaccidental Bruising Patterns Suggestive of Abuse

Burns

- Approximately 40,000 children younger than 15 years of age are hospitalized each year because of burns.
- More than 2,000 children die from burn injuries each year.

- Approximately 10% to 25% of pediatric burns result from abuse, and most occur in children younger than 3 years.
- Scald burns comprise 85% of all burns.
- Immersion in water at 52°C (126°F) takes 2 minutes to cause full-thickness burns, compared to only 5 seconds of immersion in water at 60°C (140°F).

Use the rule of nines to calculate the percent burn area.

- Each arm is 9%.
- The anterior and posterior portions of each leg are 9% each.
- The anterior upper and lower portions of the thorax are 9% each.
- The posterior upper and lower portions of the thorax are 9% each.
- The area including the neck and head is 9%.
- The perineum comprises the remaining 1%.

The Degrees of Burns

- **First-degree (superficial)** burns affect only the epidermis. The burn site is red, painful, dry, and with no blisters.
- **Second-degree (partial thickness)** burns involve the epidermis and part of the dermis. The burn site appears red, blistered, and may be swollen and painful.
- **Third-degree (full thickness)** burns destroy the epidermis and dermis. Third-degree burns may also damage the underlying bones, muscles, and tendons. The burn site appears white or charred. There is no sensation in the area.

Characteristics of Burns Consistent with Nonaccidental Trauma
Hot water immersion scalds involving lower limbs, and/or perineum/buttocks (seen in immersion injuries)
Glove and stocking burns to hands and feet
Burn has clear upper limits
Consistent burn depth
Symmetrical
Burns neglected or older than history indicates
Numerous lesions of varying ages
Pattern of burn matches instrument

Characteristics of Burns Consistent with Accidental Trauma
Usually asymmetric
Have an irregular edge
Irregular burn depth

Neglect

- Most prevalent form of abuse.
- Accounts for more than 50% of child abuse cases reported to Child Protective Services.
- Neglect is defined as the failure of a caregiver to provide adequate safety, food, clothing, shelter, education, protection, medical/dental care, and supervision for a child.
- The evaluation of neglect is accomplished mainly though a careful history and visual observations of caregiver and patient interactions.
- Psychosocial stressors should be addressed that include poverty, unemployment, substance abuse, domestic violence, and varying discipline styles.
- Most clinical findings of neglect are subtle. Physical findings such as a sunken fontanel and the appearance of poor personal hygiene are subtle nuances that should be evaluated during a pediatric examination.

Some Indications of Neglect
Failure to thrive or developmental delay
Starvation or dehydration
Severe, untreated dental caries
School truancy
Injuries caused by a lack of supervision
Untreated illnesses, including infections or fractures
Lack of connection or caring by the guardian

Treatment

- Initial resuscitation should follow ATLS and PALS guidelines.
- Patients with head injury should receive serial neurological exams, head computed tomography, radiographic evaluation of the cervical spine, and pediatric neurosurgery consultation. The majority of pediatric intracranial bleeding is nonoperative.

- Skeletal survey should be completed to evaluate for acute or chronic fractures. The skeletal survey is mandatory for all children younger than 2 years of age in whom child abuse is suspected.
- Laboratory analysis, if indicated, includes CBC, coagulation studies, CMP, lactate, and ABG if airway is compromised.
- If intra-abdominal injury is suspected, prompt evaluation via ultrasound, radiography, laparoscopy, or laparotomy is needed.
- Ophthalmology consultation to evaluate for retinal hemorrhage.
- Documentation should be done thoroughly, as the medical record may become evidence in a criminal prosecution.
- Medical or legal photography as soon as patient is stabilized.
- The key to treating nonaccidental trauma is *recognition*.

Long-Term Care/Social Care

- Every state has mandated reporting laws with an established multidisciplinary task force consisting of social work, law enforcement, and child abuse specialists, etc.
- Every state has standardized protocols that help ensure that all information is documented and reported correctly.
- Review state laws to determine the information that should be documented with each reported case of child abuse.
- After recognition, report to Child Protective Services or similar agency under the Child Abuse Prevention and Treatment Act.
- The agency will perform the following tasks:
  - ▶ Intake of information
  - ▶ Investigation and assessment, which can include a home visit
  - ▶ Case decision with voluntary or involuntary recommendations
  - ▶ Treatment and case management
- Placement of the child in the home, removal to foster care, or other court-mandated action is based on the estimated risk of danger to the child.
- Case closure occurs when the family has addressed all CPS needs or the child is permanently removed from the home.

Review Questions

1. **What is the most common fracture associated with child abuse?**
   - A. Bucket-handle fracture
   - B. Linear skull fracture
   - C. Long bone shaft fracture
   - D. Posterior rib fracture

2. **Which age-injury relationship is most correct?**
   - A. Infants more likely to present with head trauma, toddlers with abdominal trauma, and abuse-related injuries decrease for school age children.
   - B. Infants more likely to present with head trauma, toddlers with abdominal trauma, and abuse-related injuries increase for school age children.
   - C. Infants more likely to present with abdominal trauma, toddlers with head trauma, and abuse-related injuries decrease for school age children.
   - D. Infants more likely to present with abdominal trauma, toddlers with head trauma, and abuse-related injuries increase for school age children.

3. **Which of the following is true regarding child abuse reporting?**
   - A. All 50 states have mandated reporting laws.
   - B. Failure to report suspected child abuse can result in criminal liability.
   - C. The *Child Abuse Prevention and Treatment Act* protects any individual who reports suspected child abuse in good faith from civil or criminal liability.
   - D. All of the above.

4. **All of the following are common findings in infants who are victims of shaken baby syndrome EXCEPT:**
   - A. Posterior rib fractures
   - B. Retinal hemorrhages
   - C. Intra-abdominal injury
   - D. Subdural hematomas

Sexual Assault

Dale Woolridge MD, PhD
Elizabeth Weinstein, MD

Critical Knowledge

- Generally, any child presenting with alleged assault *within* the preceding 72 hours requires immediate evaluation and complete exam, including genital exam and consideration for forensic evidence collection.

- Any child presenting with alleged assault *outside* of the 72-hour window and without signs or symptoms of acute injury, infection, or pregnancy, or a compelling reason to believe there may be recoverable forensic evidence may have the genital exam deferred to a child advocacy specialist at a later date; but, the patient should have a full medical screening exam. Appropriate authorities should be notified, and the child's safety and safety of other potentially at-risk children must be ensured.

- The interview should be conducted by someone trained in forensic interviewing and, whenever possible, deferred to an advocacy center or similar facility. Physician interview of the patient should include pertinent medical history only, as the physician may otherwise inadvertently contaminate the historical evidence and damage any legal case.

- Virginity CANNOT be determined from an exam, and penetrating injury cannot be excluded by the absence of physical findings.

- Prepubertal children SHOULD NOT undergo a speculum exam. Post-pubertal girls do not necessarily require a speculum exam.

- Children should NOT undergo a forced genital exam, *unless* there is concern for significant injury (i.e., forensic evidence collection alone does not warrant an exam under anesthesia). When there is concern for significant injury, an exam under anesthesia may be appropriate.

- *Most* pediatric victims of sexual assault have NORMAL exams. ("Normal" in this case is defined by the absence of findings.)

- Highly suspicious injuries include transections of the posterior hymen (from 3 to 9 o'clock in the dorsal lithotomy or frog-leg position), bruising, or bleeding of the posterior fourchette, acute laceration or bruising of the hymen, vaginal lacerations, deep perianal lacerations, and bruising of the penis.[1]

- Infection with chlamydia, gonorrhea, or syphilis in a prepubertal child outside of the perinatal period is considered diagnostic of sexual contact, and depending on the age of the child, constitutes sexual abuse.

Definition

Sexual abuse occurs when a child is engaged in sexual activities that he or she cannot comprehend, for which he or she is developmentally unprepared and cannot give consent, and/or which violate the law or social taboos of society. [These] may include all forms of oral-genital, genital, or anal contact by or to the child or abuse that does not involve contact, such as exhibitionism, voyeurism, or using the child in the production of pornography.[2]

Epidemiology

- 12%-25% of girls and 8%-10% of boys in the U.S. have been victims of sexual assault by the age of 18.[2]

- Children less than 18 years comprise two-thirds of all victims of sexual abuse reported to law enforcement in the U.S. One-third are under age 12.[3]

- Adolescents comprise the largest group of victims.[4] Most know their perpetrators.

Anatomy
Figure 1. Normal Hymenal Patterns

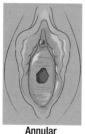

Annular

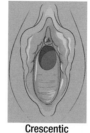

Crescentic

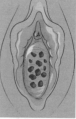

Cribriform

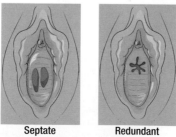

Septate   Redundant

Chief Complaint

- Reasons for referral for exam for suspected abuse:
  - ▶ The child has made a disclosure.
  - ▶ The child has exhibited a change in behavior.
  - ▶ The child has been noted to have an abnormal physical exam.
  - ▶ The child has been exposed to an abuse situation or possible abuse situation.
- Behavioral changes that may prompt referral include:
  - ▶ Sexualized behavior or knowledge inappropriate for age
  - ▶ Masturbation that is beyond normal developmental expectations
  - ▶ New onset enuresis/encopresis
  - ▶ Sleep/appetite disturbances
  - ▶ Other behavioral changes such as declining school performance or aggression

The History

- *Medical history* should be obtained by the physician to include: menstrual history (including tampon use and frequency/length of cycle), surgeries and previous illnesses/chronic illnesses; thorough review of systems including GI, GU (including history of enuresis, encopresis, hematuria, or hematochezia), hematology, and dermatology. Time of last shower/bath, last urination/defecation or brushing of teeth should be obtained if evidence collection is going to be attempted. Any changes in sleeping, eating, or school performance should also be documented.

- *Sexual history* is NOT indicated.

- *Family history* should be obtained.

- History of the allegation/events and thorough *social history* may be obtained from the accompanying adult with the child absent for this portion of the interview. History should include who lives in the home, other adult contacts, history of previous sexual maltreatment, and other previous contacts with Child Protective Services or law enforcement.

- Improper questioning of children can have catastrophic results for legal proceedings. Consequently, history of events/allegations by the child should be obtained by a specialist trained to perform pediatric forensic interviews – often at a child advocacy center or by law enforcement.[5] Any spontaneous disclosures made by the child should be documented verbatim with the use of quotation marks.

The Exam

Timing and Location

- In general, immediate exam is indicated if the alleged event occurred within the preceding 72 hours, or if there is concern for injury. The exam should include forensic evidence collection and a complete medical screening exam.

- Any child with alleged assault outside of the 72-hour window and without signs or symptoms of acute injury, infection, or pregnancy, or compelling reason to believe there may be recoverable forensic evidence, may have the genital exam deferred to a child advocacy specialist at a later date; but the patient should have a full *medical* screening exam. Appropriate authorities should be notified, and the child's safety and safety of other potentially at-risk children must be ensured.

Preparing for the Exam

- Explain the exam to the patient beforehand.

- The child should be allowed to have a trusted adult accompany him or her in the exam room if the child chooses.

- At a minimum, one additional medical staff member should be in the exam room with the examiner. This provides a chaperone and helps facilitate the exam and evidence collection.

Step-by-Step Exam

- Begin with general and nonthreatening exam components that are more familiar to children (listening to the heart and lungs, looking in the ears and mouth, etc.) and progress to the genital exam as the child becomes more comfortable.

- Perform a comprehensive exam for any indications of physical abuse. Evaluate the child's skin and document any bruising. Be specific about size and location. Do NOT estimate age of bruising or other trauma. Evaluate the oropharynx with particular attention to any palatal petechia or tears of the labial or lingular frenula. Evaluate the medial thighs for any injury or bruising. All bruises, bite marks, or other lesions should be photographed with a ruler included in the frame for reference.

- Positioning the child for ano-genital exam: Position of choice is child-dependent. Younger children are generally examined in a supine frog leg position on an exam table or in a caregiver's lap. Adolescents may prefer a stirrup position. Boys can have an adequate exam in the lateral recumbent position, which may be less stressful than knee-chest; however, on occasion, further evaluation of possible injury is best performed in the knee-chest position.

- Visualization of the hymen, vestibule, and vaginal opening is achieved by applying gentle outward labial traction to the labia majora; in pubertal patients, a cotton swab moistened with preservative-free saline can be used to help fully visualize the hymen when hymenal folds are present.

- In prepubertal children, the hymen is very sensitive; touching it can be painful for the patient. In these patients, labial traction can often provide adequate views.

- Photo documentation of the ano-genital exam with colposcopy should be obtained whenever possible.

- Digital rectal exam is not indicated.[5]

- Document Tanner staging (see *Table 2*).

- If swabs are indicated, care should be taken to insert the cotton swab into the vaginal canal without touching the hymenal walls. Cervical swabs are unnecessary in prepubertal children and may not be necessary in the adolescent patient. A genital wash may also be employed. Fill syringe with saline and wash the perineum, catching the run-off on a 2x2.

Forensic Evidence Collection

General Rules

- Follow guidelines of your specific evidence collection kit, as these can vary.

- Urine should be collected AFTER the genital exam so as not to eliminate possible forensic evidence.

- **Maintain chain of evidence.** Seal, label, and initial all samples; mark date and time on everything, including times of transfer of custody; document agency and name of individual accepting forensic evidence for police custody.[6]

- **Avoid transfer of trace evidence**. Separate all collected items; change gloves when changing sites of collection.[6]

- **Protect integrity of samples.** Do not heat-dry samples; air-dry only. Refrigerate any blood and body fluid samples. Use only paper and glass; do not use plastic.[6]

What to Collect

- UPT should be obtained, even in the absence of reported onset of menarche, if the child is Tanner stage-appropriate.
- History, timing, nature of contact, and sex of perpetrator help to determine if a child needs to be swabbed for forensic evidence.[1] In general, children should be swabbed if there has been genital-genital contact, oral-genital contact, and/or anal-genital contact, or if there is a history of ejaculation.
- Black light (Wood's lamp) should be used to evaluate for other areas to swab for secretions.
- Collect the child's clothing or bedding; forensic evidence is frequently collected from these sources.[1]
- Scrape underneath the child's fingernails if there appears to be any material, or if there is any report of the child scratching the alleged perpetrator.
- If there is report of genital contact, comb pubic hair, if present.
- Use floss sticks to collect evidence that may be trapped between teeth in cases of oral-genital contact.

Testing for STDs

- Approximately 5% of abused children acquire an STD. Numbers are higher in the adolescent population, but STDs do occur in prepubertal abuse.[2,7]
- Testing in prepubertal children should be obtained if the child is symptomatic (e.g., discharge, dysuria); the perpetrator is known to have an STD or risk factors for STD; there is history of genital-to-genital contact; or there is genital injury.[8]
- In prepubertal children, infection with chlamydia, gonorrhea, or syphilis outside of the perinatal period is considered diagnostic of abuse. Infection with HIV without other identified risk factors is similarly considered diagnostic. Trichomonas vaginalis infection is considered highly suspicious. Condylomata acuminate and genital herpes are considered suspicious.[8]
- Adolescent victims should be tested for STDs.[9]
- Adolescents who have been raped should have serum samples testing for HIV, syphilis, and HBV (to demonstrate lack or presence of pre-existing infection.) HBV and syphilis testing needs to be repeated at 6 weeks; HIV at 3-6 months.[8,9]
- If STD testing is indicated, vaginal/urethral swabs should be sent for *C. trachomatis* and *N. gonorrhea* culture. (*Note: PCR is inadequate to*

establish legal proof of infection in prepubertal children. In adolescents, PCR may be sufficient as long as there is a confirmatory test of a different part of the genome. Meatal specimen discharge in place of intra-urethral swab is considered adequate in boys.) Vaginal swabs should be sent for culture for *Trichomonas* vaginalis and wet mount. If history indicates oral-genital or anal-genital contact, swabs from the oropharynx and anus should also be obtained.[2]

- Any lesions suspicious for herpes should be cultured for HSV 1 and 2.
- Testing for HIV, hepatitis B and C, and syphilis may vary depending on exposure, age of the child, knowledge of the perpetrator's risk factors, local prevalence, and family wishes.
- Prophylactic/empiric therapy should NOT be instituted unless cultures have been obtained; it is generally not recommended for asymptomatic prepubertal children.[6,0]

Differential Diagnosis: Findings *Confused* with Sexual Abuse

- Traumatic: straddle injuries (there should be NO injury to the hymen as this is a very internal structure, but there may be labial bruising),[6] toilet lid injuries to penis, self-inflicted injuries
- Dermatologic: lichen sclerosis, Henoch-Schönlein purpura
- Non-specific vaginitis: irritant (bubble bath, soaps, fecal contamination, etc.)
- Infectious vaginitis: *Staphylococcus aureus,* group A streptococcus, candida, etc.
- Urinary tract infections
- Anal fissures
- Pre-pubertal vaginal bleeding: arteriovenous malformations, foreign body, hormonal glitches, urethral prolapse.
- Peri-anal group A streptococcal infections

Myth-Busting

- Virginity CANNOT be determined from physical exam.
- The size of the hymenal opening changes with relaxation and position; it does NOT prove penetration.
- In the vast majority of established cases of sexual abuse, even those in which penetration has taken place, the examination is NORMAL.[10,11,12]

Treatment

Chlamydia/GC/Trichomonas

- Prophylaxis for GC/chlamydia and *Trichomonas* should be provided for adolescent assault victims.[8]

- Prophylaxis for asymptomatic pre-pubertal children is not generally recommended, though may be instituted because of familial wishes or other concerns.[6,8]

Table 1. Selected Treatment Options[13]

	Weight <45 kg	Weight >45 kg
Gonorrhea	Ceftriaxone 250 mg IM, single dose	Ceftriaxone 250 mg IM, single dose
Alternative therapy	—	Cefuroxime 1 gm PO, single dose
Chlamydia trachomatis	Azithromycin 20 mg/kg (maximum 1 gm) PO, single dose	Azithromycin 1 gm PO, single dose
Alternative therapy	Erythromycin base 50 mg/kg/day divided QID for 14 days	Doxycycline 100 mg PO BID for 7 days duration (must be at least 8 years old)
Trichomoniasis and bacterial vaginosis	Metronidazole 15 mg/kg/day PO divided TID for 7 days	Metronidazole 2 g PO, single dose

HIV

- HIV infection has been reported in children with sexual abuse as the *only* established risk factor.[8,9]

- Efficacy of post-exposure prophylaxis in the setting of sexual assault is theoretical and based on reduction of transmission of HIV in occupational exposures and in the reduction of vertical transmission from HIV-positive mothers to the fetus.[8,14]

- Prophylaxis may be indicated depending on risk assessment.

- **Risk assessment:** Receptive anal intercourse and receptive vaginal intercourse carry the highest risk for infection. Risk is elevated in the presence of mucosal injury. Risk assessment should include HIV serostatus of the perpetrator if known, or risk factors of the perpetrator (IVDA, incarceration history, etc.) if known. Number of assailants and history of ejaculation should also be considered.[8,14]

- Compliance with medication continuation and follow up is very poor. A frank discussion with the family regarding risk-benefit and drug toxicities should take place before therapy is initiated.[14]

- There are no evidence-based guidelines for initiation of therapy and drug regimen in this population; however, if the child presents within the initial 72 hours following potential exposure baseline HIV testing in the ED, an initiation of a 4-week course of two-drug therapy (generally zidovudine and lamivudine) may be employed.[14,15] In very high-risk situations, a third agent – generally a protease inhibitor – may be added. **Side effects dramatically increase with the addition of a third agent.**

- Two-drug therapy costs approximately $1,000 for a 1-month supply, and may or may not be covered by insurance.[14]

- If treatment is being considered, consultation with a specialist in treating HIV in children is recommended.[8] Baseline complete blood count and blood chemistries, including transaminases, should also be obtained.

- If treatment is initiated, the family should be provided with sufficient medication to last until follow up within 3-7 days. At that time, the child should be reassessed for side effects and tolerance.

- **National Clinician's Post-Exposure Hotline (PEPLine): 888-448-4911.**

Hepatitis B

- HBV vaccination is recommended for those with an incomplete vaccination series and for those who have negative-surface antibodies; however, serologies may not be ordered in cases in which the contact would not warrant concern of transmission (e.g., fondling).[8]

Pregnancy Prevention

- Emergency contraception should be offered in assaults that could potentially result in pregnancy.[9]

Follow Up

- Children reporting sexual assault need to be believed, protected, and supported. Treatment should include follow up with a primary care physician as soon as is reasonable following the event, and referral for counseling/support services.

- For STD concerns in children who do not receive empiric therapy, additional follow up for re-examination should be arranged for 2 weeks and 12 weeks.[8] For adolescents, follow up for STD check should occur in 1-2 weeks.

- Any child with injury should have urgent follow up to ensure that the injury is healing properly. This may be with a child abuse specialist or with the child's primary care physician.

Legal Issues

Mandatory Reporting

- All 50 states have mandatory reporting laws that include medical personnel. These laws protect the reporter from civil litigation in good faith reports. Failure to report, in cases in which there is concern, has resulted in law suits. Any child with complaint of assault or concern for maltreatment or neglect *must* be reported. Reporting requirements for sexual activity between consenting minors varies from state to state. You should be aware of your state's individual reporting requirements.

- HIPAA does *not* trump mandated reporting laws.

- HIPAA *does* allow for the release of information related to child abuse and neglect of ongoing criminal investigations; however, you MUST document to whom you are disclosing information.

Documentation

- Document what questions were asked and what answers were given and by whom. Try to use direct, complete quotes whenever possible and use quotation marks when charting.

- Draw specific diagrams, including location and sizes of all lesions.

- Document chain-of-evidence information as previously detailed.

Working with Child Protective Services

- Once Child Protective Services (CPS) has been involved, clarify what conditions need to be met before the child can be released from the hospital and to whom the child may be released.

- Guidelines may vary by state or jurisdiction. Generally, social workers can help determine the guidelines where you practice.

Table 2. The Tanner Stages

Tanner Stage	Female Breast	Male Penis/Scrotum	Pubic Hair
1	Prepubertal; no glandular tissue	Prepubertal (testicular volume less than 1.5 mL; small penis)	None
2	Breast bud forms with small area of surrounding glandular tissue; areola begins to widen	Penile length unchanged; testicular volume increases (1.6 and 6 mL) skin on scrotum thins, reddens and enlarges	Scant long, downy, slightly pigmented hair at the base of the penis and scrotum or on the labia majora
3	Breast becomes more elevated, and extends beyond the borders of the areola; areola further widens	Penis lengthens; scrotum further enlarges; testicular volume (6-12 mL)	Hair becomes more course and curly and extends laterally
4	Further increased breast size and elevation; areola and papilla form a secondary mound projecting from the contour of the surrounding breast	Penis increases in length and circumference; scrotum enlarges and darkens; testicular volume 12-20 mL	Adult like hair, but spares medial thigh
5	Adult pattern. Areola returns to contour of the surrounding breast.	Adult pattern	Adult pattern

Review Questions

1. Which of the following is appropriate testing in a 9-year-old child complaining of vaginal discharge and sexual assault?

   A. Vaginal swab for GC/chlamydia PCR and trichomonas; serum for hepatitis B and C.

   B. Cervical swab for GC/chlamydia culture and trichomonas; serum for hepatitis B and C.

   C. Cervical swab for GC/chlamydia PCR and trichomonas; serum for hepatitis B and C

   D. Vaginal swab for GC/chlamydia culture and trichomonas; serum for hepatitis B and C

2. A child presents to the emergency department after disclosing to her teacher that she has been touched inappropriately by her mother's boyfriend on several occasions. The last assault was more than 72 hours ago. Which of the following is NOT true?

   A. You should avoid questioning the child about her disclosure and defer this aspect of the history to someone trained in forensic interviewing.

   B. Genital exam can almost always be deferred to a child protection specialist if alleged assault occurred more than 72 hours prior.

   C. If the child refuses a speculum exam, it is appropriate to perform an exam under anesthesia for evidence collection.

   D. Child Protective Services must be notified and the child's safety ensured prior to release.

3. Which of the following statements regarding reporting is TRUE?

   A. A physician is a mandated reporter. Failure to report may be actionable.

   B. HIPAA prevents physicians from sharing information regarding child abuse to law enforcement without guardian consent.

   C. You may be sued by a party for reporting suspected abuse if the party is subsequently found to be innocent of any wrongdoing.

1. D
2. C
3. A

Ultrasound: Common Emergency Presentations

37

Kimberly Leeson, MD
Ben Leeson, MD

Introduction

Bedside ultrasound (US) was introduced to assess patients with traumatic injuries. Over the last several decades, many new US applications have evolved. Ultrasound is an ideal imaging modality for children. Ease of use, portability, lack of radiation exposure, and excellent image resolution because of children's smaller body habitus make ultrasound useful. Many US scanning techniques easily translate from adults to the pediatric population, and emergency ultrasound (EUS) is becoming commonplace in emergency departments.

Special considerations

- Pediatric patients have unique diseases not seen in the adult population (i.e., necrotizing enterocolitis, pyloric stenosis, congenital heart disease).

- More cartilage and growth plates in musculoskeletal system

- Larger heads with open fontanels

- Smaller body parts, sometimes incompatible with adult-sized US probes

- Increased sensitivity to radiation exposure

Common Uses

Trauma

Traumatic injury remains the leading cause of death for children outside of infancy. US is used to evaluate for hemoperitoneum, hemopericardium, and hemothorax during the assessment of trauma patients. A focused assessment with sonography in trauma (FAST) exam consists of obtaining images of these areas:

- Right upper quadrant (Morison's pouch)

- Left upper quadrant (splenorenal junction)

- Subxiphoid cardiac view

- Pelvis

The right and left upper quadrant views should include the diaphragm to evaluate for hemothorax. A FAST exam is considered positive if free fluid is visualized. This is represented by the presence of black (fluid) surrounding grey tissue and organs.

Figure 1. US Image of the Right Upper Quadrant, Demonstrating Positive Free Fluid (Arrow).

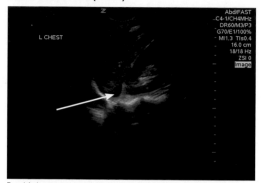

Panel A demonstrates a right upper quadrant view. The arrow indicates free fluid interposed between the right kidney and liver.

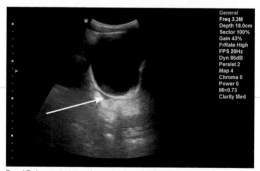

Panel B demonstrates a short axis view of the urinary bladder. The arrow indicates free fluid located posterior to the bladder.

An extended fast or EFAST exam evaluates the thorax for pneumothorax in addition to traditional images.

Benefits to US use in trauma include rapid, repeatable imaging, no need to leave the trauma bay, no exposure to radiation.

Several challenges to the use of FAST in children as a screening tool:

- Children with intra-abdominal injuries are more often managed nonoperatively than adults

- Children have a higher incidence of solid organ injury without free fluid; a negative FAST exam may not exclude the need for a CT or surgery.

- Lower sensitivity, high specificity of FAST exam in children (best used in trauma patients in addition to the history and physical exam).

Abdominal Pathology

A number of abdominal US applications have developed. US has become the initial imaging modality for a number of causes of belly pain. Sonographic features that may be seen with several abdominal conditions include:

- **Acute appendicitis:** an appendiceal diameter greater than 6 mm, echogenic periappendiceal inflammatory fat changes, noncompressible lumen, and appendicolith or periappendiceal free fluid.

- **Pyloric stenosis:** a muscle wall thickness of >3.5-4 mm and a pyloric channel length of 15 mm or longer.

- **Intussusception:** a soft tissue mass in the right mid abdomen with the classic "target" or "donut" sign, "crescent" sign, and "pseudokidney" signs.

- **Urologic applications:** assessing bladder volume prior to urinary catheterization to ensure successful specimen collection, identifying hydronephrosis associated with obstructing renal calculi (dilated black renal pelvis in US).

Cardiac

Indications: chest trauma, unexplained hypotension/shock, dyspnea, tachycardia, cardiovascular collapse and arrest

Key Findings

- Pericardial effusions: appears as black surrounding heart chambers, may lead to tamponade

- Global cardiac function: normal, hyperdynamic, hypokinetic

- Cardiac standstill: absence of organized contractility on EUS

- Volume status: too much or too little blood volume within ventricles
- Right heart strain: increased size of right ventricle and/or right atria compared to left heart

Procedures

- Vascular access: Advantages = decreased time to access, increased success rate, fewer needle redirections, and fewer complications; becoming the standard of care with central-line placement; can be used for peripheral IV placement, arterial line placement, and to confirm intraosseous line placement.
- Soft-tissue procedures: US is useful to distinguish cellulitis (cobblestoning) from abscess (dark or black elliptical fluid collection), ID foreign bodies, and determine the size and ideal site of aspiration for peritonsillar aspiration.

Newer Applications

As the scope of EUS continues to expand, new applications continue to be investigated.

- Lumbar puncture: EUS is a convenient tool to locate the lumbar interspace for spinal needle insertion; it is especially helpful after initial failed efforts.
- Nerve block: Many EPs are becoming skilled in regional anesthesia for pain control. EUS allows direct visualization of needle placement and anesthetic infiltration of nerve bundles. Nerve fascicles appear hypoechoic (darker) embedded within a more hyperechoic (brighter) and homogenous perineurium and endoneurium. When grouped together and viewed in a transverse plane, peripheral nerves demonstrate a classic "honeycomb" appearance. Common sites for nerve blocks include interscalene plexus, wrist (radial, median, and ulnar nerve), ankle and foot (tibial, deep peroneal, saphenous, and sural nerve), and femoral nerves.
- Arthrocentesis: used to identify joint effusions (effusions appear black in EUS) and guide needle insertion for fluid aspiration.
- Skull fracture: US can locate and rule out skull fractures in children who sustain minor head trauma. Highly specific. May be useful in conjunction with head trauma decision tools to decrease need for CT scans in low-risk children who present with head injury.
- Fracture diagnosis and management: EUS is useful to diagnose and assist in fracture care (US findings of fracture include subperiosteal hematomas, bending or plastic deformity, cortical disruption and reverberating echoes).

Has been used to localize clavicle, long bone, and rib fractures. Becomes less sensitive near joints. Also helpful in anesthesia and reduction of fractures. Can ID fracture line to guide hematoma block placement. May be used in real time for assessment for adequate fracture reduction prior to immobilization.

Conclusion

- EUS can be used to diagnose and treat many conditions seen in children who seek emergency care. It is fast, repeatable, convenient, and does not expose patients to ionizing radiation.

- Consider taking an EUS course.

- Put the US probe on your patients, especially those patients who will receive additional diagnostic tests, and compare your results with those "expert" reads.

- Deepen your knowledge with some EUS educational resources:

  ► Textbook: *Ma & Mateer's Emergency Ultrasound*

  ► Podcast: Ultrasound Podcast

  ► Website: ACEP's Ultrasound Guide for Emergency Physicians www.sonoguide.com

  ► Smartphone Apps: One Minute Ultrasound, Emergency Ultrasound, Sonoaccess

Review Questions

1. **Advantages of using bedside ultrasound in the pediatric population include:**

    A. Takes a short time to perform

    B. Avoids exposure to ionizing radiation

    C. Repeatable as patient condition changes

    D. All of the above

2. **Free fluid on bedside ultrasound appears:**

    A. White

    B. Black

    C. Light gray

3. **The sensitivity of the FAST exam in children is the same as in the adult population.**

    True or False?

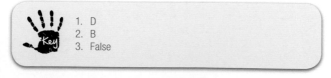

1. D
2. B
3. False

References and Resources

Chapter 1. The Normal Newborn Examination

1. Bland RD. The Newborn Infant. In: Rudolph CD, Rudolph AM, et al. editors. *Rudolph's Pediatrics*, 21st edition, New York: McGraw-Hill; 2003. p.55 222.

2. Hay WW, Levin MJ, Sondheimer JM, et al., editors, *Current Diagnosis and Treatment in Pediatrics*, 18th edition, New York: Lange Medical Books/McGraw-Hill; 2007.

3. Jones KL, *Smith's Recognizable Patterns of Human Malformation* Philadelphia: Saunders; 1997.

4. Fleisher GR, Ludwig S, Henretig FM, editors. *Textbook of Pediatric Emergency Medicine*, 5th edition, Philadelphia: Lippincott Williams and Wilkins; 2006

5. Gunn, VL, Nechyba C, *The Harriet Lane Handbook*, 17th edition, Philadelphia: Mosby; 2005.

6. http://commons.wikimedia.org/wiki/Image:Scalp_hematomas.jpg

Chapter 2. Apparent Life-Threatening Event

1. *Infantile apnea and home monitoring*. National Institutes of Health Consensus Statement, 1986. 6(6): p. 1 10.

2. Brooks, J.G., Apparent life-threatening events and apnea of infancy. *Clin Perinatol*, 1992. 19(4): p. 809-38.

3. Davies, F. and R. Gupta, Apparent life threatening events in infants presenting to an emergency department. *Emerg Med J*, 2002. 19(1): p. 11-6.

4. Kiechl-Kohlendorfer, U., et al., Epidemiology of apparent life threatening events. *Arch Dis Child*, 2005. 90(3): p. 297-300.

5. Parker K, Pitetti R. Mortality and child abuse in children presenting with apparent life-threatening events. *Pediatr Emerg Care*, July 2011. 27(7): p. 591-595.

6. Milioti, S. and C. Einspieler, The long-term outcome of infantile apparent life-threatening event (ALTE): a follow-up study until midpuberty. *Neuropediatrics*, 2005. 36(1): p. 1-5.

7. Oren, J., D. Kelly, and D.C. Shannon, Identification of a high-risk group for sudden infant death syndrome among infants who were resuscitated for sleep apnea. *Pediatrics*, 1986. 77(4): p. 495-9.

8. Gershan, W.M., N.S. Besch, and R.A. Franciosi, A comparison of apparent life-threatening events before and after the back to sleep campaign. *Wmj*, 2002. 101(1): p. 39-45.

9. Doshi A, Bernard-Stover L, Kuelbs C, Castillo E, Stucky E. Apparent life-threatening event admissions and gastroesophageal reflux disease: The value of hospitalization. *Pediatr Emerg Care*, January 2012. 28(1): p. 17-21.

10. Zuckerbraun NS, Zomorrodi A, Pitetti RD. Occurrence of serious bacterial infection in infants aged 60 days or younger with an apparent life-threatening event. *Pediatr Emerg Care*, January 2009. 25(1): p. 19-25.

11. Pitetti RD, Whitman E, Zaylor A. Accidental and nonaccidental poisonings as a cause of apparent life-threatening events in infants. *Pediatrics*, August 2008. 122(2): p. e359-e362.

12. Kahn, A., Recommended clinical evaluation of infants with an apparent life-threatening event. Consensus document of the European Society for the Study and Prevention of Infant Death, 2003. *Eur J Pediatr*, 2004. 163(2): p. 108-15.

13. Gray, C., F. Davies, and E. Molyneux, Apparent life-threatening events presenting to a pediatric emergency department. *Pediatr Emerg Care*, 1999. 15(3): p. 195-9.

14. De Piero, A.D., S.J. Teach, and J.M. Chamberlain, *E*D evaluation of infants after an apparent life-threatening event. *Am J Emerg Med*, 2004. 22(2): p. 83-6.

15. Brand, D.A., et al., Yield of diagnostic testing in infants who have had an apparent life-threatening event. *Pediatrics*, 2005. 115(4): p. 885-93.

16. Claudius I, Keens T. Do all infants with apparent life-threatening events need to be admitted? *Pediatrics*, April 2007. 119(4): p. 679-683.

Chapter 3. The Febrile Child

1. Royal Children's Hospital Clinical Practice Guidelines, www.rch.org.au/clinicalguide.

2. Emergency Management of Pediatric Patients with Fever www.emedicine.medscape.com/article/801598-overview (accessed 11/11/2012)

3. ACEP: Clinical policy for children younger than three years presenting to the emergency department with fever. ACEP Clinical Policies Committee. *Ann Emerg Med* 2003 Oct; 42 (4): 530-545

4. Emergency Medicine, A Comprehensive Study Guide, 5th edition, Tintinalli, Kelen, *Stapczynski* pg 802-805.

5. Evaluation and management of fever in the neonate and young infant (less than three months of age), Smitherman HF, Macias CG, UpToDate.com accessed 9/9/13.

6. Fever without a source in children 3 to 36 months of age, Allen CH, UpToDate.com accessed 9/9/13.

Chapter 4. Acute Otitis Media

1. Lieberthal AS et al. The Diagnosis and Management of Acute Otitis Media. *Pediatrics*, published online February 25, 2013.

2. Subcommittee on Management of Acute Otitis Media—American Academy of Pediatrics and American Academy of Family Physicians. Clinical practice guideline: diagnosis and management of acute otitis media. *Pediatrics* 2004; 113. 1451-1465.

3. Jones WS, Kaleida PH. How helpful is pneumatic otoscopy in improving diagnostic accuracy? *Pediatrics* September 2003;112:510-3.

4. Rosenfeld RM, Vertrees JE, Carr J, ed al. Clinical efficacy of antimicrobial drugs for acute otitis media: metaanalysis of 5400 children from thirty-three randomized trials. *J Pediatr.* 1994;124:355-367.

5. Del Mar C, Glasziou P, Hayem M. Are antibiotics indicated as initial treatment for children with acute otitis media? A meta-analysis. *BMJ* 1997;314:1526-1529.

6. Glasziou PP, Del Mar CB, Hayem, M, Saunders SL. Antibiotics for acute otitis media in children. Cochrane Database Syst Rev. 2000;4:CD000219.

Chapter 5. The Crying Infant

1. Pawel BB, Henretig FM, Crying and Colic in Early Infancy. In: Fleisher GR, Ludwig S, eds. *Textbook of Pediatric Emergency Medicine*, 4th ed. Philadelphia, PA: Lippencott Williams & Wilkins; 2000: 193-195.

2. Poole et al., The Infant with Acute, Unexplained, Excessive Crying. *Pediatrics* 88:450-455, 1991.

3. Freedman et al., The Crying Infant: Diagnostic Testing and Frequency of Serious Underlying Disease, *Pediatrics* 123:841-848, 2009.

Colic

1. Roberts DM, Ostapchuk M, O'Brien JG. *Infantile Colic.* American Family Physician Volume 70, Number 4, August 15, 2004 735-740.

2. Savino F, Cordisco L, Tarasco V, ed al. Lactobacillus reuteri DSM 17938 in infantile colic: a randomized, double-blind, placebo-controlled trial. *Pediatrics* 2010; 125:e526.

3. Weissbluth M. Colic. In: Burg FD, Gellis SS, Kagan BM. *Gellis & Kagan's Current Pediatric Therapy*. 16th ed. Philadelphia: Saunders, 1999:674–8

4. Garrison MM, Christakis DA. A systematic review of treatments for infant colic. *Pediatrics* 2000;106(1 pt 2):184–90

5. Lucassen PL, Assendelft WJ, Gubbels JW, van Eijk JT, van Geldrop WJ, Neven AK. Effectiveness of treatments for infantile colic: systematic review. [published erratum appears in BMJ 1998;317:171.] *BMJ* 1998;316:1563–9.

6. Metcalf TJ, Irons TG, Sher LD, Young PC. Simethicone in the treatment of infant colic: a randomized, placebo-controlled, multicenter trial. *Pediatrics* 1994;94:29–34.

Chapter 6. Head Injury

1. Bazarian JJ, McClung J, Shah MN, et al: Mild traumatic brain injury in the United States, 1998–2000. *Brain Inj* 19(2): 85, 2005.

2. Greenes DS, Schutzman SA: Clinical indicators of intracranial injury in head-injured infants. *Pediatrics* 104: 861, 1999.

3. Haydel MJ, Shembekar AD: Prediction of intracranial injury in children aged five years and older with loss of consciousness after minor head injury due to non-trivial mechanisms. *Ann Emerg Med* 42(4): 507, 2003.

4. Schutzman SA, Greenes DS: Pediatric minor head injury. *Ann Emerg Med* 37: 65, 2001.

5. Gruskin KD, Schutzman SA. Head trauma in children younger than 2 years: are there predictors for complications? *Arch Pediatr Adolsec Med* 153: 15-20, 1999.

6. Quality Standards Subcommittee, American Academy of Neurology. Practice parameter: the management of concussion in sports (summary statement). *Neurology*; 48(3): 581-5, 1997.

7. McCrory P, Johnson K, Meeuwisse W, et al: Summary and agreement statement of the 2nd International Conference on Concussion in Sport, Prague 2004. *Clin J Sport Med* 15(2): 48, 2005.

8. Thompson MD, Irby Jr JW. Recovery from mild head injury in pediatric populations. *Semin Pediatr Neurol* 10(2): 130-9, 2003

9. American Academy of Neurology, Position Statement on Sports Concussion, October 2010.

10. Barlow KM, Minns RA: Annual incidence of shaken impact syndrome in young children. *Lancet* 356: 1571, 2000.

11. American Academy of Neurology, Assessment and Management of Sports Concussion, 2011

12. Bruce DA, Zimmerman RA. Shaken impact syndrome. *Pediatr Ann* 18: 482-94, 1989

13. Berkowitz, C. (2011). Child abuse and neglect. In J. Tintinalli (Ed.), *Tintinalli's Emergency Medicine* (7th ed., pp. 1975-1980). New York: McGraw Hill Medical,

14. Jenny C, Hymel KP, Ritzen A, et al. Analysis of missed cases of abusive head trauma. *JAMA* 282(7): 621-6, 1999

15. Dunning J, Patrick Daly J, Lomas JP, et al: Derivation of the children's head injury algorithm for the prediction of important clinical events decision rule for head injury in children. *Arch Dis Child* 91: 885, 2006,

16. Kupperman N, Holmes JF, Dayan PS, et al: Identification of children at very low risk of clinically-important brain injuries after head trauma: a prospective cohort study. *Lancet* 374(9696): 1160, 2009.

17. Young KD, Okada PJ, Sokolove PE, et al. A randomized double-blinded placebo-controlled trial of phenytoin for the prevention of early posttraumatic seizures in children with moderate to severe blunt head injury. *Ann Emerg Med* 43(4): 435-46, 2004.

18. Hung, G. (2011). Minor head injury in infants and children. In J. Tintinalli (Ed.), *Tintinalli's Emergency Medicine* (7th ed., pp. 888-892). New York: McGraw Hill Medical.

Chapter 7. GI Abdominal Trauma

1. Rose J. Ultrasound in Abdominal Trauma. *Emerg Med Clin N Am* 22 (2004) 581-599.

2. Fox JC, et al. Test Characteristics of focused assessment of sonography for trauma for clinically significant abdominal free fluid in pediatric blunt abdominal trauma. *Acad Emerg Med.* 2011 May;18(5):477-82.

3. Holmes JF et al. Performance of abdominal ultrasonography in pediatric blunt trauma patients: a meta-analysis. *J Pediatr Surg.* 2007 Sep;42(9):1588-94.

4. McGahan JP et al. The Focused Abdominal Sonography for Trauma Scan: Pearls and Pitfalls. *J Ultrasound Med.* 2002 Jul;21(7):789-800.

5. Scalea TM, Rodriguez A, Chiu WC, et al. Focused Assessment with Sonography for Trauma (FAST): results from an international consensus conference. *J Trauma* 1999;46(3): 466-72.

6. Holmes JF, Identifying Children at Very Low Risk of Clinically Important Blunt Abdominal Injuries. *Ann Emerg Med.* 2013 Jan 29. pii: S0196-0644(12)01743-X [EPub ahead of Print].

7. Pediatric Duodenal Perforation Missed on Computed Tomography, Robert Barandica MD and Mitesh Patel MD.

8. Brasel, Karen J. MD, MPH; DeLisle, Christine M. MD; Olson, Christine J. MD; Borgstrom, David C. MD. Splenic Injury: Trends in Evaluation and Management. *Journal of Trauma-Injury Infection & Critical Care*. 44(2):283-286, February 1998.

9. E-Medicine Abdominal Trauma, Blunt Joseph A Salomone III, MD, Jeffrey P Salomone, MD, NREMT-P.

10. D. H. Jamieson, P. S. Babyn and R. Pearl. Imaging gastrointestinal perforation in pediatric blunt abdominal trauma. *Pediatric Radiology*.

11. Porras-Ramírez G, Ramírez-Reyes F, Hernández-Herrera MH, Porras-Hernández JD. Clinical recognition and management of pediatric blunt abdominal trauma without ultrasound or computed tomography scan in community hospitals in Mexico.

12. Diagnostic and therapeutic consequences of kidney injuries in pediatric blunt abdominal trauma.

13. Wessel LM, Jester I, Scholz S, Arnold R, Lorenz C, Wirth H, Waag KL. *Acedemic Emergency Medicine*. FAST Exams in Pediatric Abdominal Trauma Chris S Kennedy and Jeff Kempf.

Chapter 8. Orthopedic Trauma

1. Carson, S, Woolridge, D: Pediatric Upper Extremity Injuries The Pediatric clinics of North America 2006, vol. 53, no 1.

2. Peterson HA: Physeal & apophyseal injuries. In: Rockwood CA, Wilkins KE,

3. Beaty JH, eds. *Fractures in Children*. 4th ed. Lippincott-Raven; 1996.

4. Bright RW: Physeal injuries. In: *Fractures in Children*. 3rd ed. Lippincott-Raven; 1991: 87-186.

5. Wolfram, W: Pediatrics, Nursemaid Elbow Jan 30, 2013 www.emedicine.com.

6. Blasier RD, Aronson J, Tursky EA: External fixation of pediatric femur fractures. J *Pediatr Orthop* 1997 May-Jun; 17(3): 342-6

7. Harrington KD: Orthopaedic management of extremity and pelvic lesions. *Clin Orthop* 1995 Mar; (312): 136-47

8. Kanel JS: Treatment of fractures of the femur in children and adolescents. *West J Med* 1995; 163(6): 570

9. Biffl WL, Smith WR, Moore EE, et al: Evolution of a multidisciplinary clinical pathway for the management of unstable patients with pelvic fractures. *Ann Surg* 2001 Jun; 233(6): 843-50

10. Hart RG, Rittenberry TJ, Uehara DT: *Handbook of Orthopaedic Emergencies.* Lippincott-Raven; 1999: 277-297

11. Blick SS, Brumback RJ, Poka A, et al: Compartment syndrome in open tibial fractures. *J Bone Joint Surg Am* 1986 Dec; 68(9): 1348-53

12. Goller E: Emergency treatment of the trauma patient. In: Dee R, Hurst LC,
13. Gruber MA, Kottmeier SA, eds. *Principles of Orthopedic Practice.* NY: McGraw-Hill; 1997:379-388.

14. McQueen MM, Christie J, Court-Brown CM: Acute compartment syndrome in tibial diaphyseal fractures. *J Bone Joint Surg Br* 1996 Jan; 78(1): 95-8

15. Dabney KW, Lipton G: Evaluation of limp in children. *Curr Opin Pediatr* 1995 Feb; 7(1): 88-94

16. Lee RW, Demos TC: Limp and altered gait. In: Rosen P, Doris PE, Berkin RM, et al, eds. *Diagnostic Radiology in Emergency Medicine.* 1992:509-40

17. Berkowitz CD: Pediatric abuse. New patterns of injury. *Emerg Med Clin North Am* 1995 May; 13(2): 321-41

18. Ludwig S, Kornberg AE, eds: *Child Abuse: A Medical Reference.* 2nd ed. New York. Churchill Livingston; 1992.

19. Sugar NF, Taylor JA, Feldman KW: Bruises in infants and toddlers: those who don't cruise rarely bruise. Puget Sound Pediatric Research Network. *Arch Pediatr Adolesc Med* 1999 Apr; 153(4): 399-403

20. Brown CV, Antevil JL, Sise MJ: Spiral computed tomography for the diagnosis of cervical, thoracic, and lumbar spine fractures: its time has come. *J Trauma* 2005 May; 58(5): 890-5

21. Hadley MN, Walters BC, Grabb PA: Guidelines for the management of acute cervical spine and spinal cord injuries. *Clin Neurosurg* 2002; 49: 407-98

22. Harris MB, Sethi RK: The initial assessment and management of the multiple-trauma patient with an associated spine injury. *Spine* 2006 May 15; 31(11 Suppl): S9-15

23. Stiell IG, Clement CM, McKnight RD: The Canadian C-spine rule versus the NEXUS low-risk criteria in patients with trauma. *N Engl J Med* 2003 Dec 25; 349(26): 2510-8

24. Morris L. Fracture pain relief for kids? Ibuprofen does it better. *J Fam Pract.* 2010 May; 59(5): 273–275

25. Clarke S, Lecky F. Best evidence topic report. Do non-steroidal anti-inflammatory drugs cause a delay in fracture healing? *Emerg Med J.* 2005; 22:652–653

26. Wheeler P, Batt ME. Do non-steroidal anti-inflammatory drugs adversely affect stress fracture healing? A short review. *Br J Sports Med.* 2005; 39:65–69

27. Swanson C. Postoperative Pain Control After Supracondylar Humerus Fracture Fixation. *Journal of Pediatric Orthopaedics.* July/August 2012; 32(5) p. 452-455

28. Macias, CG. A comparison of supination/flexion to hyperpronation in the reduction of radial head subluxations *Pediatrics.* 1998 Jul;102(1):e10.

Chapter 9. Non-Traumatic Orthopedics

Osteomyelitis

1. Lew DP, Waldvogel FA. Osteomyelitis. *Lancet* 2004; 364-79.

2. Gutierrez K. Bone and Joint Infections in Children. *Pediatr Clin N Amer* 2005; 52: 779-94.

3. Blyth MJ, Kincaid R, Craigen MA, Bennet GC. The changing epidemiology of acute and subacute haematogenous osteomyelitis in children. *J Bone and Joint Surg Br* 2001; 83: 99-102.

4. Martinex-Aguilar G, Avalos-Mishaan A, Hulten K, et al. Community-acquired methicillin-resistant and methicillin susceptible *Staphylococcus aureus* musculoskeletal infections in children. *Pediatr Infect Dis J.* 2004; 23:701-706.

5. Yagupsky P. *Kingella kingae*: from medical rarity to an emerging paediatric pathogen. *Lancet Infect Dis.* 2004;4:358-67.

6. Dagan R. Management of acute haematogenous osteomyelitis and septic arthritis in the pediatric patient. *Pediatr Infect Dis J* 1993;12:88-93.

7. Jaramillo D, Treves S, Kasser J, Harper M, Sundel R, Laor T. Osteomyelitis and Septic Arthritis in Children: Appropriate Use of Imaging to Guide Treatment. *AJR* 1995;165:399-403.

Septic Arthritis

1. Gutierrez K. Bone and Joint Infections in Children. *Pediatr Clin N Amer* 2005; 52: 779-94.

2. Blyth MJ, Kindain R, Craigen MA, Bennet GC. The changing epidemiology of acute and subacuate hematogenous osteomyelitis in children. *J Bone Joint Surg Br* 2001; 83:99-102

3. Martinex-Aguilar G, Avalos-Mishaan A, Hulten K, et al. Community-acquired methicillin-resistant and methicillin susceptible *Staphylococcus aureus* musculoskeletal infections in children. *Pediatr Infect Dis J* 2004; 23:701-706.

4. Yagupsky P. *Kingella kingae*: from medical rarity to an emerging paediatric pathogen.*Lancet Infct Dis* 2004;4:358-67.

5. Luhmann J, Luhmann W. Etiology of septic arthritis in children: An update for the 1990s. *Pediatr Fmerg Care* 1999;15:40-42

6. Kocher MS, Zurakowski D, Kasser JR. Differentiating between septic arthritis and transient synovitis of the hip in children: an evidence-based clinical prediction algorithm. *J Bone Joint Surg Am* 1999;81:1662-70.

7. Kocher MS, Mandiga R, Murphy JM, et al. A clinical practice guideline for treatment of septic arthritis in children: efficacy in improving process of care and effect on outcome of septic arthritis of the hip. *J Bone Joint Surg Am* 2003;85:994-9.

8. Volberg F, Sumner T, Abramson J, et al. Unreliability of Radiographic Diagnosis of Septic Hip in Children. *Pediatrics* 1984;74:118-120.

9. Zawin JK, Hoffer F, Rand F, et al. Joint Effusion in Children with an Irritable Hip: US Diagnosis and Aspiration. *Radiology*;187:459-461.

Transient Synovitis

1. Rickerstaff DR, Neal LM, Brennan PO, Vull MJ. An Investigation Into the etiology of irritable hip. *Clin Pediatr* 1991;30:353-6.

2. Hart J. Transient Synovitis of the Hip in Children. *Amer Fam Phys* 1996; 1587-91.

3. Tolat V, Carty H, Klenerman L, Hart CA. Evidence for a viral aetiology of transient synovitis of the hip. *J Bone and Joint Surg Br* 1993;973-4.

4. Haueisen DC, Weiner DS, Weiner SD. The characterization of "transient synovitis of the hip" in children. *J Pedatr Orthop* 1986;6:11-7.

5. Del Beccaro MA, Champoux AN, Bockers T, Mendelman PM. Septic arthritis versus transient synovitis of the hip: the value of screening laboratory tests. *Ann Emerg Med* 1992; 21:1418-22.

6. Kocher MS, Zurakowski D, Kasser JR. Differentiating between septic arthritis and transient synovitis of the hip in children: an evidence-based clinical prediction algorithm. *J Bone Joint Surg Am* 1999;81:1662-70.

7. Zawin JK, Hoffer F, Rand F, et al. Joint Effusion in Children with an Irritable Hip: US Diagnosis and Aspiration. *Radiology*;187:459-461.

Slipped Capital Femoral Epiphysis

1. Perron AD, Miller MD, Brady WJ: Orthopedic Pitfalls in the ED: Slipped Capital Femoral Epiphysis. *J Emerg Med* 2002;20:484-7.

2. Causey AL, Smith ER, Donaldson JJ, et al: Missed slipped capital femoral epiphysis: Illustrative cases and review. *J Emerg Med* 1995;13:175-189.

3. Richards BS: Slipped capital femoral epiphysis. *Pediatr Rev* 1996;17:69-70.

4. Kelsey JL, Acheson RM, Keggi KJ: The body build of patients with slipped capital femoral epiphysis. *Am J Dis Child* 1972;124:276-281.

5. Weiner D: Pathogenesis of slipped capital femoral epiphysis: Current concepts. *J Pediatr Orthop* 1996;5:67-73.

6. Rattey T, Piehl F, Wright JG: Acute slipped capital femoral epiphysis; a review of outcomes and rates of avascular necrosis. *J Bone Joint Surg Am* 1996;78:398-402.

7. Klein A, Joplin RJ, Reidy JA: Roentgenographic features of slipped apical femoral epiphysis. *Am J Radiol* 1951;66:361-365.

8. Carney BT: Natural history of untreated chronic slipped capital femoral epiphysis. *Clin Orthop* 1996;322:43-47.

Osgood-Schlatter Disease

1. Bloom OJ, Mackler L, Barbee J: Clinical inquiries. What is the best treatment of Osgood-Schlatter disease? *J of Fam Pract* 2004;53:153-6.

2. Dunn JF: Osgood-Schlatter disease. *Am Fam Physician* 1990;41:173-6.

3. Krause BL, Williams JP, Catterall A: Natural history of Osgood-Schlatter disease. *J Pediatr Orthop* 1990; 10: 65-8.

4. Smith JB: Knee problems in children. *Pediatr Clin North Am* 1986; 33: 1439-56.

5. Hussain A, Hagroo GA: Osgood-Schlatter disease. *Sports Exer Injury* 1996; 2:202-6.

Legg-Calve-Perthes Disease

1. Roy DR. Current Concepts in Legg-Calve-Perthes disease. *Pediatr Ann* 1999;28: 748-52.

2. Archives of Disease in Childhood: Epidemiology of Perthes' disease. *Arch Dis Child* 2000;82:385.

3. Salter RB, Thompson GH. Legg-Calve-Perthes disease: the prognostic significance of subchondral fracture and a two-group classification of femoral head involvement. *J Bone Joint Surg Am.* 1984;66:479-489.

4. Kaniklides C. Diagnostic radiology in Legg-Calve-Perthes disease. *Acta Radiol Suppl* 1996;406:1-28.

5. Kaniklides C, Lonnerholm T, Moberg, A. Legg-Calve-Perthes disease.

Comparison of conventional radiography, bone scintigraphy and arthrography. *Acta Radiol* 1995;36:434-9.

6. Herring JA. The treatment of Legg-Calve-Perthes disease: a critical review of the literature. *J Bone Joint Surg Am.* 1994;76:448-458.

Other Causes for Limping in Children

1. Adams, Lehman TJ. Update on the pathogenesis and treatment of systemic onset juvenile rheumatoid arthritis. *Curr Opin Rheumatol* 2005;17:612-6.

2. Ilowite NT. Current treatment of juvenile rheumatoid arthritis. *Pediatrics* 2002; 109: 109-15.

3. Birdi N, Hosking M, Clulow MK, et al. Acute rheumatic fever and post streptococcal reactive arthritis: diagnostic and treatment practices of pediatric subspecialists in Canada. *J Rheumatol* 2001;28: 1681-8.

4. Warren RW, Perez MD, Wilking AP, Myones BL. Pediatric rheumatic diseases. *Pediatr Clin North Am* 1994; 41: 783-818.

5. Edworthy SM. Clinical Manifestations of Systemic Lupus Erythematosus. In: Harris ED, et al, Eds. *Kelley's Textbook of Rheumatology*, 7th Ed. Saunders, 2005, 1201-1224.

6. Bartels CM, Hildebrand J, Mueller D. Systemic Lupus Erythematosus. Emedicine 2006.

7. Nadelman RB, Wormser GP. Lyme borreliosis. *Lancet* 1998, 352. 557-65.

8. Steere AC. Lyme disease. *N Engl J Med* 1989, 321: 586-96.

9. Carola AS, Arndt MD and Crist WM. Common Musculoskeletal Tumors of Childhood and Adolescence. *N Engl J of Med* 1999, 341:342-351.

Chapter 10. GI Medical Emergencies

Acute Pancreatitis

1. Bai HX, Lowe ME, Husain SZ. What have we learned about acute pancreatitis in children? *J Pediatr Gastroenterol Nutr.* Mar 2011;52(3):262-70. doi: 10.1097/MPG.0b013e3182061d75.

Gastroesophageal Reflux

1. Chawla S, Seth D, Mahajan P, Kamat D; Gastroesophageal reflux disorder: a review for primary care providers; *Clin Pediatr.* Jan-Feb 2006;45(1):7-13.

2. Churgay CA, Aftab Z. Gastroenteritis in children: Part 1. Diagnosis. *Am Fam Physician.* Jun 2012 1;85(11):1059-62.

Gastroenteritis

1. Practice parameter: the management of acute gastroenteritis in young children. American Academy of Pediatrics, Provisional Committee on Quality Improvement, Subcommittee on Acute Gastroenteritis. Pediatrics 1996 Mar;97(3):424-35

2. Churgay CA, Aftab Z. Gastroenteritis in children: Part I. Diagnosis. *Am Fam Physician*. 2012 Jun 1;85(11):1059-1062.

3. Churgay CA, Aftab Z. Gastroenteritis in children: Part II. Prevention and management. *Am Fam Physician*. 2012 Jun 1;85(11):1066-70.

Chapter 11. GI Surgical Emergencies

Malrotation/Volvulus

1. Chao HC, et al. Sonographic features related to volvulus in neonatal intestinal malrotation. *J Ultrasound Med*. 2000 June; 19(6): 371-6.

2. Hay, et al. Current Diagnosis & Treatment in Pediatrics, 18th ed. McGraw-Hill 2007.

3. Tintinalli, et al. Emergency Medicine: A Comprehensive Study Guide. 6th ed. McGraw-Hill 2004.

4. http://www.emedicine.com/ped/topic1200.htm

5. http://www.emedicine.com/ped/topic2415.htm

Pyloric Stenosis

1. Hay, et al. Current Diagnosis & Treatment in Pediatrics, 18th ed. McGraw-Hill 2007.

2. Tintinalli, et al. Emergency Medicine: A Comprehensive Study Guide. 6th ed. McGraw-Hill 2004. http://www.emedicine.com/emerg/topic397.htm

Intussusception

1. Bhisitkul, et al. Clinical application of ultrasonography in the diagnosis of intussusception. *J Pediatr*. 1992 Aug; 121(2): 182-6.

2. Hay, et al. Current Diagnosis & Treatment in Pediatrics – 18th ed. McGraw-Hill 2007.

3. Mandeville, et al. Intussusception: clinical presentations and imaging characteristics. *Pediatr Emerg Care*. 2012 Sep; 28(9): 842-4

4. Tintinalli, et al. Emergency Medicine: A Comprehensive Study Guide. 6th ed. McGraw-Hill 2004. http://www.emedicine.com/EMERG/topic385.htm

Appendicitis

1. Doria AS, et al. US or CT for diagnosis of appendicitis in children and adults? A meta-analysis. *Radiology.* 2006 Oct; 241(1): 83-94.

2. Hay, et al. Current Diagnosis & Treatment in Pediatrics – 18th ed. McGraw-Hill 2007.

3. Moore et al. MRI for clinically suspected pediatric appendicitis: an implemented program. *Pediatr Radiol.* 2012 Sep; 42(9): 1056-63.

4. Tintinalli et al. Emergency Medicine: A Comprehensive Study Guide. 6th ed. McGraw-Hill 2004. http://www.emedicine.com/EMERG/topic361.htm

Meckel's Diverticulum

1. Tintinalli et al. Emergency Medicine: A Comprehensive Study Guide. 6th edition. McGraw-Hill 2004. http://www.emedicine.com/ped/topic1389.htm

Necrotizing Enterocolitis

1. Tintinalli et al. Emergency Medicine: A Comprehensive Study Guide. 6th ed. McGraw-Hill 2004. http://www.emedicine.com/ped/topic2601.htm

Hirschsprung's Disease

1. http://www.emedicine.com/ped/topic1010.htm

Chapter 12. Foreign Body Aspiration

1. Hitter A, Hullo E, Durand C, Righini C. Diagnostic value of various investigations in children with suspected foreign body aspiration. Review. *Eur Ann Otorhinolaryngol.* 2001 128:248-52.

2. Fleisher G, Ludwig S, Henreting F, eds. *Textbook of Pediatric Emergency Medicine.* Philadelphia, PA: Lippincott Williams & Wilkins, 2006.

3. Sersar S, Hamza UA, AbdelHameed WA, et al. Abstract Inhaled foreign bodies: management according to early or late presentation. *Eur J Cardiothorac Surg.* 2005 Sep;28(3):369-74.

4. Tan HK, Brown K, McGill T, et al. Airway foreign bodies (FB): a 10-year review. *Int J Pediatr Otorhinolaryngol.* 2000 Dec 1;56(2):91-9.

5. Zhijun C, Fugao Z, Niankai Z, Jingjing C. Therapeutic experience from 1428 patients with pediatric tracheobronchial foreign body. 2008 Apr;43(4):718-21.

6. Rouillon I, Charrier JB, Devictor D, et al. Lower respiratory tract foreign bodies: a retrospective review of morbidity, mortality and first aid management. *Int J Pediatr Otorhinolaryngol.* 2006 Nov;70(11):1949-55.

7. Kadmon G, Stern Y, Bron-Harlev E, Nahum E, Battat E, Schonfeld T. Computerized scoring system for the diagnosis of foreign body aspiration in children. *Ann Oto Rhinol Laryngol* 2008 Nov; 117(11):839-43.

8. Mu LC, Sun DQ, He P. Radiological diagnosis of aspirated foreign bodies in children review of 343 cases. *J Laryngol Otol* 1990;104(10):778-82.

9. Kosucu P, Ahmetoglu A, Koramaz I, et al. Low-dose MDCT and virtual bronchoscopy in pediatric patients with foreign body aspiration. *AJR Am J Roentgenol.* 2004 Dec;183(6):1771-7.

10. Righini CA, Morel N, Karkas A, et al. What is the diagnostic value of flexible bronchoscopy in the initial investigation of children with suspected foreign body aspiration? *Int J Pediatr Otorhinolaryngol* 2007;71(9):1383-90.

11. Oliveira CF, Almeida JF, Troster EJ, et al. Complications of tracheobronchial foreign body aspiration in children: report of 5 cases and review of the literature. *Rev Hosp Clin Fac Med Sao Paulo.* 2002 May-Jun;57(3):108-11.

12. Marx, J ed. Rosen's *Emergency Medicine: Concepts and Clinical Practice*, 6th ed. Philadelphia, PA: Mosby, 2006.

13. Girardi G, Contador AM, Castro-Rodriguez JA. Two new radiological findings to improve the diagnosis of bronchial foreign-body aspiration in children. *Pediatr Pulmonol.* 2004 Sep;38(3):261-4.

14. Metrangelo S, Monetti C, Meneghini L, et al. Eight years' experience with foreign-body aspiration in children: what is really important for a timely diagnosis? *J Pediatr Surg.* 1999 Aug;34(8):1229-31.

15. Swanson KL, Prakash UB, Midthun DE, et al. Flexible bronchoscopic management of airway foreign bodies in children. *Chest.* 2002 May;121(5):1695-700.

16. 2005 American Heart Association Guidelines for Cardiopulmonary Resuscitation and Emergency Cardiovascular Care, Part 11: Pediatric Basic Life Support. *Circulation* 2005;112;156-166.

Chapter 13. Foreign Body Ingestion

1. Bronstein AC, Spyker DA, Cantilena LR, Rumack BH, Dart RC. 2011 Annual Report of the American Association of Poison Control Centers' National Poison Data System (NPDS): 29th Annual Report. *Clinical Toxicology* 2012 50:911-1164

2. Conners GP, Chamberlain JM, Weiner PR. Pediatric coin ingestion: a home-based survey. *Am J Emerg Med.* 1995 Nov;13(6):638-40.

3. Kay M, Wyllie MD. Pediatric Foreign Bodies and Their Management. *Curr Gastoenterol Rep* 2005;7:212-8.

4. Centers for Disease Control and Prevention. Gastrointestinal Injuries from Magnet Ingestion in Children—United States, 2003 2006. MMWR. 2006 55(48); 1296-1300.

5. Fleisher G, Ludwig S, Henreting F, eds. *Textbook of Pediatric Emergency Medicine.* Philadelphia, PA: Lippincott Williams & Wilkins, 2000.

6. Bassett KE, Schunk JE, Logan L. Localizing ingested coins with a metal detector. *Am J Emerg Med.* 1999 Jul;17(4):338-41.

7. Wai Pak M, Chung Lee W, Kwok Fung H, et al. A prospective study of foreign-body ingestion in 311 children. *Int J Pediatr Otorhinolaryngol.* 2001 Apr 6;58(1):37-45.

8. Wahbeh G, Wyllie R, Kay M. Foreign Body Ingestion in Infants and Children: Location, Location, Location. *Clin Pediatr* 2002 41:633-40.

9. Soprano JV, Fleisher GR, Mandl KD. The spontaneous passage of esophageal coins in children. *Arch Pediatr Adolesc Med.* 1999 Oct;153(10):1073-6.

10. Waltzman ML, Baskin M, Wypij D. A randomized clinical trial of the management of esophageal coins in children. *Pediatrics.* 2005 Sep;116(3):614-9.

11. Mehta D, Attia M, Quintana E Glucagon use for esophageal coin dislodgment in children: a prospective, double-blind, placebo-controlled trial. *Acad Emerg Med.* 2001 Feb;8(2):200-3.

12. Emslander HC, Bonadio W, Klatzo M. Efficacy of esophageal bougienage by emergency physicians in pediatric coin ingestion. *Ann Emerg Med.* 1996 Jun;27(6):726-9.

13. Eisen GM, Baron TH, Dominitz JA et al. Guideline for the management of ingested foreign bodies. *Gastrointest Endosc.* 2002 Jun;55(7):802-6.

14. Conners GP, Cobaugh DJ, Feinberg, et al. Home observation for asymptomatic coin ingestion: acceptance and outcomes. The New York State Poison Control Center Coin Ingestion Study Group. *Acad Emerg Med.* 1999 Mar;6(3):213-7.

15. Wong KK, Fang CX, Tam PK. Selective upper endoscopy for foreign body ingestion in children: an evaluation of management protocol after 282 cases. *J Pediatr Surg.* 2006 Dec;41(12):2016-8.

Chapter 14. Dermatology

1. *Dermatology Definitions, Diagnostic Algorithm and List of Essential Diseases,* Peter J. Lynch MD, Department of Dermatology, University of California, Davis. Revised, March 2013. Used with permission.

2. Pediatric Dermatology Emergencies. *Current Opinion in Pediatrics.* 2011 Aug; 23(4): 403-6

3. *Differential Diagnosis in Dermatology.* Second Edition. Richard Ashton, Barbara Leppard. Radcliffe Medical Press. 1993, 2-8.

4. Fitzpatrick's Color Atlas & Synopsis of Clinical Dermatology. 5th ed./Klaus Wolff, Richard Allen Johnson, Dick Suurmond. McGraw-Hill. 2005.

5. *Pediatric Dermatology.* 3rd Ed. Schachner, Hansen. Elsevier, 2003.

Chapter 15. Urinary Tract Infections

1. Hoberman A, Chao HP, Keller DM, et al. Prevalence of urinary tract infection in febrile infants. *J Pediatr* 1993; 123, 17.

2. Shaikh N, Morone NE, Lopez J, Chianese J, Sangvai S, D'Amico F, Hoberman A, Wald ER. Does this child have a urinary tract infection? *JAMA.* 2007 Dec 26;298(24):2895-904.

3. Freedman AL; Urologic Diseases in America Project. Urologic diseases in North America Project: trends in resource utilization for urinary tract infections in children. *J Urol.* 2005;173(3):949-954.

4. Weiss R, Tamminen-Mobius T, Koskimies O, et al. Characteristics at entry of children with severe primary vesicoureteral reflux recruited for a multicenter, international therapeutic trial comparing medical and surgical management. The International Reflux Study in Children. *J Urol*; 1992, 148, 1644.

5. Baraff L. Management of fever without a source in infants and children. *Ann Em Med.* 2000: 36: 602-614.

6. Roberts KB; Subcommittee on Urinary Tract Infection, Steering Committee on Quality Improvement and Management. Urinary tract infection: clinical practice guideline for the diagnosis and management of the initial UTI in febrile infants and children 2 to 24 months. *Pediatrics.* 2011;128(3):595-610.

Chapter 16. Bronchiolitis

1. Hanson, IC, Shearer, WT. Bronchiolitis. In: *Oski's Pediatrics. Principles and Practice*, 4th ed, McMillan, JA, Feigin, RD, DeAngelis, C, Jones, MD (Eds), Lippincott, Williams & Wilkins, Philadelphia 2006. p.1391.

2. McConnochie, KM, Roghmann, KJ. Predicting clinically significant lower respiratory tract illness in childhood following mild bronchiolitis. *Am J Dis Child* 1985; 139:625.

3. Diagnosis and management of bronchiolitis. *Pediatrics* 2006 Oct; 118 (4):1774-93.

4. Bordley, WC, Viswanathan, M, King, VJ, et al. Diagnosis and testing in bronchiolitis: a systematic review. *Arch Pediatr Adolesc Med* 2004; 158:119.

5. Ahluwalia, G, Embree, J, McNicol, P, et al. Comparison of nasopharyngeal aspirate and nasopharyngeal swab specimens for respiratory syncytial virus diagnosis by cell culture, indirect immunofluorescence assay, and enzyme-linked immunosorbent assay. *J Clin Microbiol* 1987; 25:763.

6. Welliver, RC. Bronchiolitis and Infectious asthma. In: Textbook of Pediatric Infectious Diseases, 5th ed, Feigin, RD, Cherry, JD, Demmler, GJ, Kaplan, SL (Eds), Saunders, Philadelphia, 2004. p. 273.

7. Coffin, SE. Bronchiolitis; in-patient focus. *Pediatr Clin North Am* 2005; 52:1047.

8. Allander, T, Tammi, MT, Eriksson, M, et al. Cloning of a human parvovirus by molecular screening of respiratory tract samples. *Proc Natl Acad Sci U.S.A.* 2005; 102:12891.

9. Langley, JM, Smith, MB, LeBlanc, JC, et al. Racemic epinephrine compared to salbutamol in hospitalized young children with bronchiolitis; a randomized controlled clinical trial. *BMC Pediatr* 2005; 5:7.

10. Lind I, Gill JH, Calabretta N, Polizzoto M. Clinical inquiries. What are hospital admission criteria for infants with bronchiolitis? *J Fam Pract.* 2006 Jan; 55(1):67-9.

11. Zhang L et al., Nebulized hypertonic saline solution for acute bronchiolitis in infants, October 2009 Editorial Group: Cochrane Acute Respiratory Infections Group, published online: 7 Oct 2010, DOI: 10.1002/14651858. CD006458.pub2.

12. Liet JM, Ducruet, T et al. Heliox inhalation therapy for bronchiolitis in infants. Cochrane Database Syst Rev. 2010 Apr 14; (4):CD006915. Epub 2010 Apr 14.

Chapter 17. Asthma (Reactive Airway Disease)

1. National Asthma Education and Prevention Program: Expert panel report III: Guidelines for the diagnosis and management of asthma. Bethesda, MD: National Heart, Lung, and Blood Institute, 2007. (NIH publication no. 08-4051). Full text available online: www.nhlbi.nih.gov/guidelines/asthma/asthgdln.htm (Accessed September 1, 2007).

2. Bacharier LB, et al. Diagnosis and treatment of asthma in childhood: a PRACTALL consensus report. *Allergy.* 2008; 63[1]: 5-34.

3. Mitka M. New evidence-based guidelines focus on treatment of children with asthma. *JAMA.* 2008 Mar 12; 299(10): 1122-3.

4. Bass, JL, Corwin M, Gozal D, et al. The effect of chronic or intermittent hypoxia on cognition in childhood: a review of the evidence. *Pediatrics* 2004; 114:805.

5. Rodrigo, GJ, Rodriquez Verde, M, Peregalli, V, Rodrigo, C. Effects of short-term 28% and 100% oxygen on PaCO2 and peak expiratory flow rate in acute asthma: a randomized trial. *Chest* 2003; 124:1312.

6. Robertson, J, Shilkofski, N. Harriet Lane: Pulmonology Table 22-3: Predicted Average Peak Expiratory Flow Rates for Normal Children from Voter KZ. *Pediatr Rev* 1996; 17 (2): 53-63.

7. Hsu, P, Lam, L, et al., The pulmonary index score as a clinical assessment tool for acute childhood asthma. *Ann Allergy Asthma Immunol.* 2010:105:425-429.

8. Carroll, C, Sekaran, A, et al. A Modified Pulmonary Index Score with predictive value for pediatric asthma exacerbations. *Ann Allergy Asthma Immunol.* 2005;94:355-359.

Chapter 18. Pneumonia

1. American Academy of Pediatrics. Red Book: 2012 Report of the Committee on Infectious Diseases. *Haemophilus influenza* Infections; pp 345-352. *Pneumococcal* Infections; pp 571-582. Respiratory Syncytial Virus; pp 609-618.

2. Bradley, S., Byington, C., Shah, S., Alverson, B., Carter, E., Harrison, C., Kaplan, S., Mace, S., McCracken, G., Moore, M., St Peter, S., Stockwell, J., Swanson, S.; Executive Summary: The Management of Infants and Children Older Than 3 Months of Age: Clinical Practice Guidelines by the Pediatric Infectious Diseases Society and the Infectious Diseases Society of America. *Clinical Infectious Diseases.* 2011;53(7):617-630.

3. Brown, K., Gilford, W.; Viral and Bacterial Pneumonia in Children. *Emergency Medicine: A Comprehensive Study Guide* 6th Ed. Ch 123; pp 784-789.

4. Browne, L., Gorelick, M.; *Asthma and Pneumonia.* Pediatric Clinics of North America; 2010;57;1347-1356.

5. Campbell, S., Marrie, T., Anstoy, R., Dickinson, G., Ackroyd-Stolarz, S.; The Contribution of Blood Cultures to the Clinical Management of Adult Patients Admitted to the Hospital With Community-Acquired Pneumonia. *Chest.* 2003;123:1142-1150.

6. Durbin, W., Stille, C.; *Pediatrics in Review:* Pneumonia. 2008; 29:147-160.

7. Elward, A., Warren, D., Fraser, V.; Ventilator-Associated Pneumonia in Pediatric Intensive Care Unit Patients: Risk Factors and Outcomes. *Pediatrics.* May 2002; 109: 758-764.

8. Fleisher, G.; *Infectious Disease Emergencies:* Lower Respiratory Infections. *Textbook of Pediatric Emergency Medicine,* 5th Ed. Ch 84; pp 809-14.

9. Gaston, B.; Pediatrics in Review: *Pneumonia.* 2002; 23:132-140.

10. Gilbert, D, Moellering, R, Eliopoulos, G, Sande, M.; *The Sanford Guide to Antimicrobial Therapy* 2013. v 3.02 online application. Pneumonia in Neonates/Infants/Children; Empiric Therapy.

11. Jadavji, T.; An Evidence-Based Review of Pediatric Pneumonia in the ED. *Pediatric Emergency Medicine Practice.* Feb 2011; Vol 8, Number 2.

12. Kimani, K.; *Microbiology and Infectious Disease.* The Harriet Lane Handbook 17th Ed. Ch 16; p 421.

13. Kollef, M., Morrow, L., Niederman, M., Leeper, K., Anzueto, A., Benz-Scott, I., Rodino, F.; Clinical Characteristics and Treatment Patterns Among Patients with Ventilator-Associated Pneumonia Patterns. *Chest*. 2006;129;1210-1218.

14. Michelow, I., Olsen, K., Lozano, J., Rollins, N., Duffy, L., Ziegler, T., Kauppila, J., Leinonen, M., McCracken, G.; Epidemiology and Clinical Characteristics of Community-Acquired Pneumonia in Hospitalized Children. *Pediatrics*. 2004;113(4);701-707.

15. Neuman, M., Monuteaux, M., Scully, K., Bachur, R.; Prediction of Pneumonia in Pediatric Emergency Department. *Pediatrics*, Aug 2011;128:246-253.

16. Reed, W., Byrd, G., Gates, R., Howard, R., Weaver, M.; Sputum Gram's Stain in Community-acquired *Pneumococcal* Pneumonia: a Meta-analysis. *Western Journal of Medicine*. 1996;165(4):197-204.

17. Tsutomu Yamazaki, Kei Murayama, Atsuko Ito, Suzuko Uehara, and Nozomu Sasaki. Epidemiology of Community-Acquired Pneumonia in Children. *Pediatrics*, Feb 2005; 115: 517.

18. Wardlaw, T., Johansson, E., Hodge, M.; Pneumonia the Forgotten Killer of Children. Online report jointly published by World Health Organization and UNICEF. 2006.

19. Wilmott, R., Kaplan, E., Perez, C., Hardie, W, Chini, B., Daines, C.; *Pediatric Secrets*, 3rd Ed. Ch 18; pp 664-668.

20. Viessman, S., Lorin, M.; *Appleton & Lange Review of Pediatrics: Infectious Disease*. Ch 7 p 132, 144.

Chapter 19. Sedation

1. Tschudy M, Arcara K. *The Harriet Lane Handbook: A Manual for Pediatric House Officers*. 19th ed. Philadelphia: Mosby Elsevier; 2012. Formulary.

2. Green SM, Roback MG, Kennedy RM, Krauss B. Clinical practice guideline for emergency department ketamine dissociative sedation: 2011 update. *Ann Emerg Med*. 2011;57(5):449-461.

3. Krauss B, Green SM. Procedural sedation and analgesia in children. *Lancet*. 2006;367(9512):766-780.

4. Baxter AL, Mallory MD, Spandorfer PR, et al. Etomidate versus pentobarbital for computed tomography sedations: Report from the pediatric sedation research consortium. *Pediatr Emerg Care*. 2007;23(10):690-695.

5. Andolfatto G, Willman E. A prospective case series of pediatric procedural sedation and analgesia in the emergency department using single-syringe ketamine-propofol combination (ketofol). *Acad Emerg Med.* 2010;17(2):194-201.

6. McMorrow S, Abrama T. Dexmedetomidine sedation. *Pediatr Emerg Care.* 2012;28(3):292-296.

7. Bahl FE, Oakley E, Seaman C, Barnett P, Sharwood LN. High-concentration nitrous oxide for procedural sedation in children: Adverse events and depth of sedation. *Pediatrics.* 2008;121(3):e528-32.

8. Lane RD, Schunk JE. Atomized intranasal midazolam use for minor procedures in the pediatric emergency department. *Pediatr Emerg Care.* 2008;24(5):300-303.

Chapter 20. Analgesia

1. Cramton RF, Gruchala NE. Managing procedural pain in pediatric patients. *Curr Opin Pediatr.* 2012; 24(4): 530-538.

2. American Academy of Pediatrics Child Life Council and Committee on Hospital Care, Wilson JM, Child life services. *Pediatrics.* 2006; 118(4):1757-1763.

3. Kennedy RM, Luhmann JD. The "ouchless emergency department." Getting closer: Advances in decreasing distress during painful procedures in the emergency department. *Pediatr Clin North Am.* 1999;46(6):1215-47, vii-viii.

4. Ferayorni A, Yniguez R, Bryson M, Bulloch B. Needle-free jet injection of lidocaine for local anesthesia during lumbar puncture: A randomized controlled trial. *Pediatr Emerg Care.* 2012;28(7):687-690.

5. Kusre SR. Towards evidence based emergency medicine: Best BETs from the Manchester royal infirmary. Bet 4: Is intranasal fentanyl better than parenteral morphine for managing acute severe pain in children? *Emerg Med J.* 2011;28(12):1077-1078.

6. Miner JR, Kletti C, Herold M, Hubbard D, Biros MH. Randomized clinical trial of nebulized fentanyl citrate versus IV fentanyl citrate in children presenting to the emergency department with acute pain. *Acad Emerg Med.* 2007;14(10):895-898.

7. Trott, Alexander, and Alexander Trott. *Wounds and lacerations.* 4. Philadelphia: Elsevier, 2012. Print.

8. Tschudy M, Arcara K. *The Harriet Lane handbook: a manual for pediatric house officers.* 19th ed. Philadelphia: Mosby Elsevier; 2012. Formulary.

Chapter 21. Fluid Resuscitation

1. American College of Surgeons' Committee on Trauma, from *Advanced Trauma Life Support for Doctors (ATLS) Student Manual*. 2004, 7th Edition, American College of Surgeons.

2. Carcillo JA and Tasker RC. Fluid Resuscitation of Hypovolemic Shock: Acute Medicine's Great Triumph for Children. *Intensive Care Med* (2006) 32:958-961.

3. Field JM, Hazinski MF, Gilmore D (editors). Pediatric Advanced Life Support. *Handbook of Emergency Cardiovascular Care for Healthcare Providers*. (2006). American Heart Association.

4. Hillyer CD, Silberstein LE, Ness PM, Anderson KC. *Blood Banking and Transfusion Medicine: Basic Principles and Practice*. (2003). Churchill Livingstone, Philadelphia, PA.

5. Kwok, MY. Fever in the toddler. eMedicine. (2006). http://www.emedicine.com/ped/topic3009.htm.

6. Marino PL and Sutin KM. *The ICU Book* (3rd edition). (2006). Lippincott Williams and Wilkins. Philadelphia, PA.

7. Preston, Richard A. Acid-Base, Fluids, and Electrolytes Made Ridiculously Simple. (2002). MedMaster, Inc., Miami FL.

8. Rice, H. Fluid management for the pediatric surgical patient. (2006). http://www.emedicine.com/ped/topic2954.htm

9. Bailey B, Gravel J, Goldman RD, Friedman JN, Parkin PC. External validation of the clinical dehydration scale for children with acute gastroenteritis. *Acad Emerg Med*. 2010 Jun; 17(6):583-8. doi: 10.1111/j.1553-2712.2010.00767.x.

10. Spandorfer PR, Alessandrini EA, Joffe MD, Localio R, Shaw KN. Oral versus intravenous rehydration of moderately dehydrated children: a randomized, controlled trial. *Pediatrics*. 2005 Feb; 115(2):295-301.

11. Santosham M, Fayad I, Abu Zikri M, et. al. A double-blind clinical trial comparing World Health Organization oral rehydration solution with a reduced osmolarity solution containing equal amounts of sodium and glucose. *J Pediatr*. 1996 Jan;128(1):45-51.

12. Choi PT-L, Yip G, Quinonez LG, Cook DJ. Crystalloids vs. colloids in fluid resuscitation: A systematic review. *Critical Care Medicine*. 1999; 27(1):200-210.

13. Perel P, Roberts I, Pearson M. Colloids versus Crystalloids for fluid resuscitation in critically ill patients (Review). *The Cochrane Collaboration*. Published online 8 July 2009.

14. Upadhyah M, Singhi S, Murlidharan J, Kaur N, Majumdar S. Randomized evaluation of fluid resuscitation with crystalloid (saline) and colloid (polymer from degraded gelatin in saline) in pediatric septic shock. *Indian Pediatr.* 2005 Mar; 42(3):223-31.

15. Boluyt N, Bollen CW, Bos AP, Kok JH, Offringa M. Fluid resuscitation in neonatal and pediatric hypovolemic shock: a Dutch Pediatric Society evidence-based clinical practice guideline. *Intensive Care Medicine.* 2006 Jul; 32(7):995-1003.

16. So KW, Fok TF, Ng PC, Wong WW, Cheung KL. Randomized controlled trial of colloid or crystalloid in hypotensive preterm infants. *Arch Dis Fetal Neonatal Ed.* 1997;76:F43-F46. doi:10.1136/fn.76.1.F43.

17. Lacroix J, Hebert PC, Hutchison JS, et. al. Transfusion Strategies for Patients In Pediatric Intensive Care Units. *N Engl J Med.* 2007; 356:1609-1619.

18. Mink RB and Pollack M. Effect of blood transfusion on oxygen consumption in pediatric septic shock. *Crit Care Med.* 1990; 18(10):1087-1091.

19. Oral Rehydration solutions. URL: http://travel.gc.ca/travelling/health-safety/rehydration. Accessed 31 May 2013.

Chapter 22. Cardiopulmonary Arrest

1. Chameides, L., Samson, R., Schexnayder, S., & Hazinski, M. (Eds.). (2011). *2011 American Heart Association Pediatric Advanced Life Support. Provider Manual.* USA. First American Heart Association Printing.

2. Hazinski, M. (Ed.). (2010) *Highlights of the 2010 American Heart Association Guidelines for Cardiopulmonary Resuscitation and Emergency Cardiovascular Care.* USA. First American Heart Association Printing.

3. Field JM, Hazinski MF, Sayre M, et al. Part 1: Executive Summary of 2010 AHA Guidelines for CPR and ECC. *Circulation.* 2010; 122 [Suppl 3]. S640-S656.

4. Donoghue AJ, Nadkarni V, Berg RA, et al. Out-of-hospital pediatric cardiac arrest: an epidemiologic review and assessment of current knowledge. *Ann Emerg Med.* Dec 2005;46(6):512-522.

5. Young KD, Gausche-Hill M, McClung CD, Lewis RJ. A prospective, population-based study of the epidemiology and outcome of out-of-hospital pediatric cardiopulmonary arrest. *Pediatrics.* Jul 2004;114(1):157-164.

6. Lopez-Herce J, Garcia C, Rodriguez-Nunez A, et al. Long-term outcome of paediatric cardiorespiratory arrest in Spain. *Resuscitation.* Jan 2005;64(1):79-85.

7. Gausche M, Lewis RJ, Stratton SJ, et al. Effect of out-of-hospital pediatric endotracheal intubation on survival and neurological outcome: a controlled clinical trial. *JAMA*. Feb 9 2000;283(6):783-790.

8. Perondi MB, Reis AG, Paiva EF, Nadkarni VM, Berg RA. A comparison of high-dose and standard-dose epinephrine in children with cardiac arrest. *N Engl J Med*. Apr 22 2004;350(17):1722-1730.

Chapter 23. Rapid Sequence Induction (RSI)

1. Bano S, Akhtar S, Zia N, et.al. Pediatric Endotracheal Intubation for Airway Management in the Emergency Department. *Pediatric Emergency Care*. 2012;28:1129-1131

2. 2005 AHA Guidelines for Cardiopulmonary Resuscitation and Emergency Cardiovascular Care. Part 12: Pediatric Advanced Life Support. *Circulation* 2005:112/IV-167-VI-187

3. Berry AM, Brimacombe JR, Verghese C. The laryngeal mask airway in emergency medicine, neonatal resuscitation, and intensive care medicine. *Int Anesthesiol Clin*. 1998;36:91–109.

4. Bledsoe GH, Schexnayder SM. Pediatric Rapid Sequence Intubation – A Review. *Pediatric Emergency Care*. 2004;20:339-344.

5. Choi HJ, Je SM, Kim JH, Kim E. The factors associated with successful pediatric endotracheal intubation on the first attempt in emergency departments: A 13-emergency-department registry study. *Resuscitation*. 2012; 83:1363-1368.

6. Gerardi M J, Sacchetti AD, Cantor RM, Santamaria JP, Gausche M, Lucid W, Foltin GL: Rapid-sequence intubation of the pediatric patient. *Ann Emerg Med July* 1996;28:55-74.

7. Kerrey BT, Rinderknecht AS, Gels GL, Nigrovic LE, Mittiga MR. Rapid Sequence Intubation for Pediatric Patients: Higher Frequency of Failed Attempts and Adverse Effects Found by Video Review. *Annals of Emergency Medicine*. 2012; 60:251-263.

8. Lee BS, Gausche-Hill M. Pediatric Airway Management. *Clinical Pediatric Emergency Medicine*. 1996; 2:91-106.

9. Lee C, Doyle E. Developmental Anatomy of the Airway. *Anesthesia and Intensive Care Medicine*. 2012;13:217-219.

10. Moynihan RJ, Brock-Utne JG, Archer JH, Feld LH, Kreitzman TR. The effect of cricoid pressure on preventing gastric insufflation in infants and children. *Anesthesiology*. 1993; 78: 652–656.

11. Nagler J, Bachur RG. Advanced airway management. *Current Opinions in Pediatrics.* 2009; 21:299-305.

12. Newth CJ, Rachman B, Patel N, Hammer J. The use of cuffed versus uncuffed endotracheal tubes in pediatric intensive care. *J Pediatr.* 2004;144 :333 –337

13. Walls, RM, Murphy MF. *Manual of Emergency Airway Management.* 4th Ed. Philadelphia, PA: Lipponcott Williams & Wilkins, 2012.

14. Weiss M, Dullenkopf A, et.al. Prospective randomized controlled multi-center trial of cuffed or uncuffed endotracheal tubes in small children. *British Journal of Anaesthesia.* 2009;103:867-873.

15. Zelicot-Paul A, Smith-Lockridge A, Schnadower D, et. Al. Controversies in rapid sequence intubation in children. *Current Opinion in Pediatrics.* 2005; 17:355-362.

Chapter 24. Electrocardiography

1. Chan TC, Sharieff GQ, Brady WJ. Electrocardiographic manifestations: pediatric. *ECG J Emerg Med.* November 2008;35(4):421-30.

2. Davignon A, Rautaharju P, Boiseclic L, Soumis F, Megelas M, Choguelle A. Normal ECG standards for infants and children. *Pediatr Cardiol* 1979/1980;1:123-131.

3. Garson, A (1999). Electrocardiography. In: Gillette, PC, Garson, A. *Clinical Pediatric Arrhythmias,* 2nd Ed. (pp.735-788). Philadelphia: Saunders.

4. Goodacre S, McLeod K. Clinical review: ABC of clinical electrocardiography, paediatric electrocardiography. *BMJ.* 2002;324:1382-85.

5. O'Connor M, McDaniel N, Brady WJ. The pediatric electrocardiogram. Part 1: Age-related interpretation. *Am J Emerg Med.* February 2008;26(2):221-8.

6. Park, M. K., & Guntheroth W.G. (2006). *How to read pediatric ECGs.* Philadelphia: Mosby Elsevier.

7. Park, M.K. (2008). *Pediatric cardiology for practitioners.* Philadelphia: Mosby Elsevier.

8. Sharieff GQ, Rao SO. *The Pediatric ECG Emergency Medicine Clinics of North America.* February 2006; 24(1):195-208.

9. Woolridge D, Love J. Congenital heart disease in the pediatric emergency department. Pathophysiology and clinical characteristics. *Pediatr Emerg Med Reports* (2002)7:69-80.

Chapter 25. Congenital Heart Defects

1. Abu-Harb. Death in infancy from unrecognized CHD. *Arch Dis Child* 1994

2. Abu Harb. Presentation of obstructive L heart. *Arch Dis Child* 1994 & Ainsworth: *Arch Dis Child*, Jan 1999 & Richmond, Early diagnosis of congenital heart disease, *Semin Neon* 2001

3. Ferencz C. CHD prevalence at livebirth *Am J Epid* 121(1) 1985.31-36 & Grabitz R CHD incidence in the 1st year of life. *Am J Epid* 128(2) 1988. 381-388 & Richmond, Early diagnosis of congenital heart disease, *Semin Neon* 2001 & Ainsworth: *Arch Dis Child*, Jan 1999 & Wren ADC Presentation of CHD in infancy, ADC 99 vol 80 & Kidd S. The incidence of CHD in the 1st year. *J of Pae* 29(5). 1993

4. Link KM, Loehr SP, Martin EM. et al. Congenital heart disease. *Coron Artery Dis.* 1993;4:340-344.

5. Lin AE: Congenital heart defects in malformation syndromes. *Clin Perinatol* 1990;17:641-673.

6. Pelech AN. Evaluation of the pediatric patient with a cardiac murmur. *Pediatr Clin N Am* 1999;46:167-188.

7. Moss AJ, Clues in diagnosing congenital heart disease. *West J Med.* 1992;156:392-398.

8. Horton LA, Mosee S, Brenner J. Use of the electrocardiogram in a pediatric emergency department. *Arch Pediatr Adolesc Med.* 1994;148:184-188.

9. Flynn PA, Engle MA, Ehlers KH, Cardiac issues in the pediatric emergency department. *Pediatr Clin N Am* 1992;39:955-968.

10. Barone, MA. (ed): *The Harriet Lane Handbook*, 14th ed., Mosby, Baltimore, MD, 1996, p. 137-138.

11. Driscoll DJ, Left to right shunt lesions. *Pediatr Clin N Am* 1999;46:355-368.

12. Pelech AN: The cardiac murmur. *Pediatr Clin N Am* 1998;45:107-122.

Chapter 26. Endocrine Emergencies

Diabetic Ketoacidosis

1. Ellis EN. Concepts of fluid therapy in diabetic ketoacidosis and hyperosmolar hyperglycemic nonketotic coma. *Pediatr Clin N Amer* 37:313-321, 1990.

2. Kitabchi AE, Wall BM. Diabetic ketoacidosis. *Med Clin N Amer* 79:9-37, 1995.

3. Keefer, JR. *The Harriet Lane Handbook: Endocrinology.* 15th Ed;207-211. Eds. Siberry and Iannone. Mosby Inc. 2000

4. Porter. Pediatric Dehydration. *Ann Emerg Med* 41:196-205

5. Rosenbloom AL. Intracerebral crises during treatment of diabetic ketoacidosis. *Diab Care* 13:22-33, 1990.

6. Young GM. Pediatrics, Diabetic Ketoacidosis. www.emedicine.com/emerg/topic373.htm. March 27, 2006

Hypoglycemia

1. Agus, MSD. T*extbook of Pediatric Emergency Medicine:* "Endocrine Emergencies- Hypoglycemia." 5th Ed. Ed's Fleisher GR, et al. Lippincott Williams and Wilkins, Philadelphia, 2001.

2. Cranmer, H. Pediatric Hypoglycemia. www.emedicine.com/emerg/topic384.htm. March 15, 2005.

3. Shah, I. "Hypoglycemia" *Pediatric Oncall.* Jan 7, 2006. www.pediatriconcall.com.

Hypocalcemia/Hypocalcemic Crisis

1. Agus, SD. *Textbook of Pediatric Emergency Medicine*: "Endocrine Emergencies- Hypocalcemia." 5th Ed. Ed's Fleisher GR, et al. Lippincott Williams and Wilkins, Philadelphia, 2001.

2. Choukair, MK. *The Harriet Lane Handbook: Fluids and Electrolytes.* 15th Ed;243-246. Eds. Siberry and Iannone. Mosby Inc. 2000.

3. Muir, A. Care of children with Hypocalcemic crisis. http://www.mcg.edu/pediatrics/pedsendo/hypocalcemia.htm. Feb. 27, 2004.

4. Singhal A, Campbell DE. Pediatric Hypocalcemia. http://www.emedicine.com/ped/topic1111.htm. Sept. 14, 2006.

Adrenal Crisis

1. Agus, SD. *Textbook of Pediatric Emergency Medicine*: "Endocrine Emergencies – Acute Adrenal Insufficiency." 5th Ed.:97;1176-1180. Ed's Fleisher GR, et al. Lippincott Williams and Wilkins, Philadelphia, 2001

2. Keeter, JR. *The Harriet Lane Handbook: "Endocrinology."* 15th Ed.:10;209-211. Eds. Siberry and Iannone. Mosby Inc. 2000

3. Macdougall, P. Adrenal Insufficiency: an Approach. Children's & Women's Health centre of British Columbia. http://www.cw.bc.ca/pediatricresidents/aiapprch.asp, 1997.

4. Muir, A. Management of Children with an adrenal crisis. http://www.mcg.edu/pediatrics/pedsendo/adrenal.html. Feb 27, 2004.

Chapter 27. Sport-Specific Injury

Ligamentous Injury and Dislocations

1. *Pediatrics in Review.* 2000;21:433-434.

Fractures

1. Young, Simon et al. *MJA* 2005; 182 (12:644-648).

Heat Stress Injury

1. Hutchinson, Mark. "Common Sports Injuries in Children and Adolescents" 19 July 2000.

Chapter 28. Sports Dysrhythmias and Sudden Cardiac Death in Athletes

1. American Academy of Family Physicians, American Academy of Pediatrics, American College of Sports Medicine. *Preparticipation Physical Evaluation*, 4th ed, Bernhardt D, Roberts W (Eds), American Academy of Pediatrics, Elk Grove Village, IL 2010.

2. Liberthson RR. Sudden death from cardiac causes in children and young adults. *N Engl J Med.* 1996;334(16):1039.

3. Drezner JA, Fudge J, Harmon KG, Berger S, Campbell RM, Vetter VL. Warning symptoms and family history in children and young adults with sudden cardiac arrest. *J Am Board Fam Med.* 2012 Jul;25(4):408-15.

4. Maron BJ, Thompson PD, Ackerman MJ, et al., American Heart Association Council on Nutrition, Physical Activity, and Metabolism. Recommendations and considerations related to preparticipation screening for cardiovascular abnormalities in competitive athletes: 2007 update: a scientific statement from the American Heart Association Council on Nutrition, Physical Activity, and Metabolism: endorsed by the American College of Cardiology Foundation. *Circulation.* 2007;115(12):1643.

5. Corrado D, Pelliccia A, Bjørnstad HH, et al., Study Group of Sport Cardiology of the Working Group of Cardiac Rehabilitation and Exercise Physiology and the Working Group of Myocardial and Pericardial Diseases of the European Society of Cardiology. Cardiovascular pre-participation screening of young competitive athletes for prevention of sudden death: proposal for a common European protocol. Consensus Statement of the Study Group of Sport Cardiology of the Working Group of Cardiac Rehabilitation and Exercise Physiology and the Working Group of Myocardial and Pericardial Diseases of the European Society of Cardiology. *Eur Heart J.* 2005;26(5):516.

6. Corrado D, Basso C, Pavei A, et al. Trends in sudden cardiovascular death in young competitive athletes after implementation of a preparticipation screening program. *JAMA*. 2006;296:1593–1601.

7. Corrado D, Basso C, Schiavon M, Thiene G. Screening for hypertrophic cardiomyopathy in young athletes. *N Engl J Med*. 1998;339:364-369

8. Corrado D, Basso C, Rizzoli G, Schiavon M, Thiene G. Does sports activity enhance the risk of sudden death in adolescents and young adults? *J Am Coll Cardiol*. 2003;42(11):1959.

9. Uberoi A, Stein R, Perez MV, et al. Interpretation of the electrocardiogram of young athletes. *Circulation*. 2011 Aug;124(6):746-57.

10. Drezner JA, Fischbach P, Froelicher V, et al. Normal electrocardiographic findings: recognising physiological adaptations in athletes. *Br J Sports Med*. 2013;47:125-136.

11. Maron BJ. Hypertrophic Cardiomyopathy. A Systematic Review. *JAMA*. 2002;287(10):1308-1320.

12. Maron BJ, Shirani J, Poliac LC, Mathenge R, Roberts WC, Mueller FO. Sudden death in young competitive athletes. Clinical, demographic, and pathological profiles. *JAMA*.1996;276(3):199.

13. Eckart RE, Scoville SL, Campbell CL, Virmani R. et. al. Sudden death in young adults: a 25-year review of autopsies in military recruits. *Ann Intern Med*. 2004;141(11):829.

14. Maron BJ, Ackerman MJ, Nishimura RA, Pyeritz RE, Towbin JA, Udelson JE. Task Force 4: HCM and other cardiomyopathies, mitral valve prolapse, myocarditis, and Marfan syndrome. *J Am Coll Cardiol*. 2005;45(8):1340.

15. Mitchell JH, Haskell W, Snell P, Van Camp SP. Task Force 8: Classification of sports. *J Am Coll Cardiol*. 2005;45(8):1364.

16. Graham TP Jr, Driscoll DJ, Gersony WM, Newburger JW, Rocchini A, Towbin JA. Task Force 2: Congenital heart disease. *J Am Coll Cardiol*. 2005;45(8):1326.

17. Corrado D, Basso C, Thiene G, et al. Spectrum of clinicopathologic manifestations of arrhythmogenic right ventricular cardiomyopathy/dysplasia: a multicenter study. *J Am Coll Cardiol*. 1997;30:1512-1520.

18. Morita H, Wu J, Zipes DP. The QT syndromes: long and short. *Lancet*. 2008;372 (9640): 750–63.

19. Zipes DP, Ackerman MJ, Estes NA 3rd, Grant AO, Myerburg RJ, Van Hare G. Task Force 7: Arrhythmias. *J Am Coll Cardiol*. 2005;45(8):1354.

20. Rosner MH, Brady WJ Jr, Kefer MP, Martin ML. Electrocardiography in the patient with the Wolff–Parkinson–White syndrome: diagnostic and initial therapeutic issues. *American Journal of Emergency Medicine*. 1999; 17 (7): 705–14.

Chapter 29. Hyperbilirubinemia

1. American Academy of Pediatrics Subcommittee on Hyperbilirubinemia. Management of hyperbilirubinemia in the newborn infant 35 or more weeks of gestation. *Pediatrics*. 114(1):297-316, 2004 Jul.

2. Bhutani VK, D. S., Johnson LH (2005). Risk Management of Severe Neonatal Hyperbilirubinemia to Prevent Kernicterus. *Clin Perinatol* 32(1):125-39.

3. Brown, A. (1962). Neonatal Jaundice. *Pediatr Clin of North Am* 9: 589.

4. Claudius I, F. C., Boles R (2005). The Emergency Department Approach to Newborn and Childhood Metabolic Crisis. *Emerg Med Clin N Am* 23:843-883.

5. Dennery PA. Metalloporphyrins for the treatment of neonatal jaundice. *Current Opinion in Pediatrics*. 17(2):167-9, 2005 Apr.

6. Dennery PA, S. D. S., Stevenson DK (2001). Neonatal Hyperbilirubinemia. *N Engl J Med* 344(8): 581 - 590.

7. Huang MJ, K. K., Teng HC, Tang KS, Weng HW, Huang CS (2004). Risk Factors for Severe Hyperbilirubinemia in Neonates. *Pediatr Res* 56(5):682-9.

8. Ip S. Chung M. Kulig J. O'Brien R. Sege R. Glicken S. Maisels MJ. Lau J. (American Academy of Pediatrics Subcommittee on Hyperbilirubinemia). An evidence-based review of important issues concerning neonatal hyperbilirubinemia. *Pediatrics*. 114(1):e130-53, 2004 Jul.

9. Monpoux F, Dageville C, Maillotte AM, et al. High-dose intravenous immunoglobulin therapy and neonatal jaundice due to red blood cell alloimmunization. *Arch Pediatr*. 2009;16:1289-1294.

10. Schwartz HP, Haberman BE, Ruddy RM. Hyperbilirubinemia: current guidelines and emerging therapies. *Pediatr Emerg Care*. 2011 Sep;27(9):884-9

11. Wolff M, Schinasi DA, Lavelle J, Boorstein N, Zorc JJ. Management of Neonates with Hyperbilirubinemia: Improving Timeliness of Care Using a Clinical Pathway. *Pediatrics* 2012;130;e1688

12. Yamamoto LG, Killeen J, French GM. Transcutaneous Bilirubin Measurement Methods in Neonates and Its Utility for Emergency Department Use. *Pediatr Emer Care* 2012;28: 380-387

13. Table 2: Total Bilirubin Levels and Phototherapy Initiation, Adapted from: Fig 3. Guidelines for phototherapy in hospitalized infants of 35 or more weeks' gestation. *Pediatrics* Vol. 114 No. 1 July 2004, pp. 297-316.

14. Table 3: Level to Initiate Exchange Transfusion, Adapted from Fig 4. Guidelines for exchange transfusion in infants 35 or more weeks' gestation. *Pediatrics* Vol. 114 No. 1 July 2004, pp. 297-316

Chapter 30. Neurologic Emergencies

1. American Academy of Pediatrics. Subcommittee on Febrile Seizures. Febrile Seizures: Guideline for the Neurodiagnostic Evaluation of the Child With a Simple Febrile Seizure. *Pediatrics* 2011; 127; 389

2. Fuchs, Susan M. "Neurologic Disorders." *Pediatric Emergency Medicine*. Ed. Roger M Barkin. Mosby-Year Book. 1997. 972-1024

3. Pitetti, R. Emergency Department Evaluation of Ventricular Shunt Malfunction Is the shunt series really necessary? *Pediatr Emerg Care*. 2007 Mar; 23(3): 137-41

4. Kim TY, Stewart G, Voth M, Moynihan JA, Brown L. Signs and symptoms of cerebrospinal fluid shunt malfunction in the pediatric emergency department. *Pediatr Emerg Care*. 2006 Jan; 22(1): 28-34

5. Lewis DW. Pediatric migraine. *Pediatr Rev*. 2007 Feb; 28(2): 43-53.

6. De Negri M, Baglietto MG. Treatment of status epilepticus in children. *Paediatr Drugs*. 2001; 3(6): 411-20.

7. Ngo, Bryan G, Holmes, James F. Performance of lumbar puncture in young children with febrile seizures. *Acad Emerg Med* 2004 11(5) 597

8. Meyer PG, Ducrocq S, Carli P. Pediatric neurologic emergencies. *Curr Opin Crit Care*. 2001 Apr; 7(2): 81-7.

9. Sogawa Y, Maytal J. Emergency department admission of children with unprovoked seizure: recurrence within 24 hours. *Pediatr Neurol*. 2006 Aug; 35(2): 98-101.

10. Fleisher G, Ludwig S. *Textbook of Pediatric Emergency Medicine*. 6th ed. Philadelphia, PA: Wolters Kluwer; 2010: 564-570.

11. McMillan J, Feigin R, DeAngelis C, Jones MD. *Oski's Pediatrics*. 4th ed. Philadelphia, PA: Lippincott, Williams & Wilikins; 2006: 2280-2299.

12. Kimia, A. Yield of Lumbar Puncture Among Children Who Present With Their First Complex Febrile Seizure. *The Journal of Pediatrics*. 2010; 126:62-69

Chapter 31. Hematologic Emergencies

1. Adams WG, Geva J, Coffman J, Palfrey S, Bauchner H. Anemia and Elevated Lead Levels in Under-immunized Inner-city Children. *Pediatrics*. 1998 Mar; 101(3):E6

2. Alexander SR. Pediatric Uses of Recombinant Human Erythropoietin: the Outlook in 1991. *Am J Kidney Dis*. 1991 Oct; 18(4):42-53

3. Boutry M, Needlman R. Use of Dietary History in the Screening of Iron Deficiency. *Pediatrics*. 1996 Dec; 6(1):1138-42

4. Fleisher G, Ludwig S. *Textbook of Pediatric Emergency Medicine*. 6th ed. Philadelphia, PA: Wolters Kluwer; 2010: 483-489.

5. DeBenoist, B, McLean, E, Egli, I, et al. Worldwide prevalence of anemia 1993-2005: WHO global database on anemia. Report, World Health Organization; Centers for Disease Control, Geneva, 2008.

6. Goldman SC, Holcenberg JS, Finklestein JZ, Hutchinson R, Kreissman S, Johnson FL, Tou C, Harvey E, Morris E, Cairo MS. A Randomized Comparison Between Rasburicase and Allopurinol in Children With Lymphoma or Leukemia at High Risk for Tumor Lysis. *Blood*. 2001 May; 97(10):2998-3003

7. Ries LA, Kosary CL, Hankey BF, et al. *SEER Cancer Statistics Review*, 1973-1996. Bethesda, Md: National Cancer Institute (http://seer.cancer.gov/csr/1973_1996/)

8. Pui CH, Relling MV, Downing JR. Acute Lymphoblastic Leukemia. *N Engl J Med*. 2004; 350 (15):1535-48.

9. Fleisher G, Ludwig S. *Textbook of Pediatric Emergency Medicine*. 6th ed. Philadelphia, PA: Wolters Kluwer; 2010: 1033-1038.

10. Giampietro PF, Davis JG, Adler-Brecher B, Verlander PC, Auerbach AD, Pavlakis SG. The Need for More Accurate and Timely Diagnosis in Fanconi Anemia: A Report From the International Fanconi Anemia Registry. *Pediatrics*. 1993 June; 91(6):1116-1120

11. Guinan EC. *Aplastic Anemia: The Management of Pediatric Patients*. Hematology: Am Soc Hematol Educ Program Book. 2005:104-109

12. Killick SB, Marsh JC, Gordon-Smith EC, Sorlin L, Gibson FM. Long-term Outcome of Acquired Aplastic Anemia in Children: Comparison Between Immunosuppressive Therapy and Bone Marrow Transplantation. *Br J Haematol*. 2000; 111:321–328.

13. Killick SB, Win N, Marsh JC, et al. Pilot study of HLA Alloimmunization After Transfusion with Pre-storage Leucodepleted Blood products in Aplastic Anaemia. *Br J Haematol*. 1997; 97:677–684.

14. Marsh J, Schrezenmeier H, Marin P, et al. Prospective Randomized Multicenter Study Comparing Cyclosporin Alone Versus the Combination of Antithymocyte Globulin and Cyclosporin for Treatment of Patients with Nonsevere Aplastic Anemia: A Report from the European Blood and Marrow Transplant (EBMT) Severe Aplastic Anaemia Working Party. *Blood.* 1999; 93:2191–2195

15. Constantinescu AR, Bitzan M, Weiss LS, Christen E, Kaplan BS, Cnaan A, Trachtman H. Non-enteropathic Hemolytic Uremic Syndrome: Causes and Short-term Course. *Am J Kidney Dis.* 2004 Jun; 43(6):976-982

16. Safdar N, Said A, Gangnon RE, Maki DG. Risk of Hemolytic Uremic Syndrome after Antibiotic Treatment of *Escherichia coli* O157:H7 Enteritis: A Meta-analysis. *JAMA.* 2002 Aug; 288(8):996-1001.

17. Wong CS, Jelacic S, Habeeb RL, Watkins SL, Tarr PI. The Risk of the Hemolytic-Uremic Syndrome after Antibiotic Treatment of Escherichia coli O157:H7 Infections. *N Engl J Med.* 2000 Jun; 342(26):1930-1936.

18. Fleichor G, Ludwig S. *Textbook of Pediatric Emergency Medicine.* 6th ed. Philadelphia, PA: Wolters Kluwer; 2010: 1118-1119.

19. Bergstein J, Leiser J, Andreoli SP. Response of Crescentic Henoch-Schoenlein Purpura Nephritis to Corticosteroid and Azathioprine Therapy. *Clin Nephrol.* 1998 Jan; 49(1):9-14

20. Trapani S, Micheli A, Grisolia F, Resti M, Chiappini E, Falcini F, De Martino M. Henoch Schonlein Purpura in Childhood: Epidemiological and Clinical Analysis of 150 Cases Over a 5-year Period and Review of Literature. *Semin Arthritis Rheum.* 2005 Dec; 35(3):143-53.

21. Fleisher G, Ludwig S. *Textbook of Pediatric Emergency Medicine.* 6th ed. Philadelphia, PA: Wolters Kluwer; 2010: 1117-1118.

22. Ancona KG, Parker RI, Atlas MP, Prakash D. Randomized Trial of High-Dose Methylprednisolone Versus Intravenous Immunoglobulin for the Treatment of Acute Idiopathic Thrombocytopenic Purpura in Children. *J Pediatr Hematol Oncol.* 2002 Oct; 24(7):540-4

23. Beck CE, Nathan PC, Parkin PC, Blanchette VS, Macarthur C. Corticosteroids Versus Intravenous Immune Globulin for the Treatment of Acute Immune Thrombocytopenic Purpura in Children: A Systematic Review and Meta-analysis of Randomized Controlled Trials. *J Pediatr.* 2005 Oct; 147(4):521-7.

24. Chu Y-W, Korb J, Sakamoto KM. Idiopathic Thrombocytopenic Purpura. *Pediatrics in Review.* 2000; 21:95-104.

25. Fleisher G, Ludwig S. *Textbook of Pediatric Emergency Medicine.* 6th ed. Philadelphia, PA: Wolters Kluwer; 2010: 875-876.

1. Kelly KM, Butler RB, Farace L, Cohen AR, Manno CS. Superior in vivo Response of Recombinant Factor VIII Concentrate in Children with Hemophilia A. *J Pediatr.* 1997 Apr; 130(4):537-40

2. Ljung RC. Prophylactic Infusion Regimens in the Management of Hemophilia. *Thromb Haemost.* 1999 Aug; 82(2):525-30

3. Ludlam CA. The Evidence Behind Inhibitor Treatment with Recombinant Factor VIIa. *Pathophysiol Haemost Thromb.* 2002; 32 Suppl 1:13-8

1. Fleisher G, Ludwig S. *Textbook of Pediatric Emergency Medicine.* 6th ed. Philadelphia, PA: Wolters Kluwer; 2010: 879-883.

Chapter 32. Special Health Care Needs

1. Rogers, EA, Kimia, A, Madsen, JR, et al. Predictors of ventricular shunt infection among children presenting to a pediatric emergency department. *Pediatric Emergency Care* 28(5):405-9, 2012.

2. Geskey, JM, Erdman, HJ, Bramley, HP, et al. Superior mesenteric artery syndrome in intellectually disabled children. *Pediatric Emergency Care* 28(4):351-3, 2012.

3. Lehnert, BE, Rahbar, H, Relyea-Chew, A, et al. Detection of ventricular shunt malfunction in the ED: relative utility of radiography, CT, and nuclear imaging. *Emergency Radiology* 18(4):299-305, 2011.

4. Blumstein H, and Schardt, S. Utility of radiography in suspected ventricular shunt malfunction. *Journal of Emergency Medicine* 36(1): 50-4, 2009.

5. Shirley, KW, Kothare, S, Piatt JH Jr, et al. Intrathecal baclofen overdose and withdrawal. *Pediatric Emergency Care* 22(4): 258-61, 2006.

6. Caterino, JM, Scheatzie, MD, and D'Antonio, JA. Descriptive analysis of 258 emergency department visits by spina bifida patients. *J Emerg Med* 31(1): 17-22, 2006.

7. Heniff, M. Emergency department management of children with cerebral palsy. *Ped Emerg Med Reports* 3(4), 1998.

Chapter 33. Urological Emergencies

1. Cherian J, Rao AR, Thwaini A, et al. Medical and surgical management of priapism. *Postgraduate Medical Journal*. February 2006; 82: 89-94.

2. National Guideline Clearinghouse. *Epididymitis. Sexually transmitted diseases guidelines 2006.* Center for Disease Control and Prevention, August 4, 2006.

3. Marx J, Hockberger R, Walls R. Rosen's Emergency Medicine: Concepts and Clinical Practice. *The Pediatric Patient: Renal and Genitourinary Tract Disorders;* 6th Ed. Philadelphia, PA: Mosby Elsevier; 2006: 2635-2656.

4. Brenner JS, Ojo A. Evaluation of scrotal pain or swelling in children and adolescents. UpToDate.com. 2006.

5. Rosenstein D, McAninch JW. Urologic emergencies. *Medical Clinics of North America.* March 2004; 88: 495-518.

6. Wan J, Bloom DA. Genitourinary problems in adolescent males. *Adolescent Medicine.* October 2003; 13: 717-31.

7. Hatzichristou D, Salpiggidis G, Hatzimouratidis K, et al. Management strategy for arterial priapism: therapeutic dilemmas. *The Journal of Urology.* November 2002; 168: 2074-2077.

8. Luzzi GA, O'Brien TS: Acute epididymitis. *BJU International.* May 2001; 87: 747-55.

9. Blaivas M, Sierzenski P, Lambert M. Emergency evaluation of patients presenting with acute scrotum using bedside ultrasonography. *Academic Emergency Medicine.* January 2001; 8: 90-3.

10. Merlini E, Rotundi F, Seymandi PL, Canning DA. Acute epididymitis and urinary tract anomalies in children. *Scandinavian Journal of Urology and Nephrology.* July 1998; 32: 273-5.

11. Peterson NE. Common urologic emergencies: a logical and practical approach to rapid diagnosis and treatment. *Emergency Medicine Reports.* 1994; 15: 16.

12. Lambert, Sarah. Pediatric Urological Emergencies. *Pediatric Clinics of North America.* Volume 59, Issue 4 , Pages 965-976, August 2012

13. McGrath N, Howell J, Davis J. Pediatric Genitourinary Emergencies. *Emergency Medicine Clinics of North America.* Volume 29, Issue 3, Pages 655-666, August 2011

Chapter 34. Toxicologic Emergencies

1. American Academy of Pediatrics Committee on Drugs: Acetaminophen toxicity in children. *Pediatrics* 2001;108(4): 1020-1024.

2. Ford MD, Delaney KA, Ling LL, Erickson T (eds): *Clinical Toxicology*, 1st ed. Philadelphia, WB Sounders, 2001

3. Jones AL: *J Toxicology* 1998;36:277-285. Tylenol nomogram.

4. Miller K, Chang A: Acute inhalation injury. *Emerg Med Clin North Am* 2003;21(2):533-557.

5. Ousterhoudt KC, Shannon M, Henretig FM: Toxicologic emergencies. In Fleisher GR, Ludwig S (eds): *Textbook of Pediatric Emergency Medicine*, 4th ed. Philadelphia, Lippincott Williams & Wilkins, 2006.

6. Riordan M, Rylance G, Berry K. Poisoning in children 1: General Management. *Arch Dis Child* 2002;87:392-396.

7. Riordan M, Rylance G, Berry K. Poisoning in children 4: Household products, plants, and mushrooms. *Arch Dis Child* 2002;87:403-406.

8. Riordan M, Rylance G, Berry K. Poisoning in children 5 rare and dangerous poisons. *Arch Dis Child* 2002;87:407-410.

9. Tenenbein, M. Poisoning pearls regarding the very young. *Clin Ped Emerg Med* 2000;1:176-179.

10. Temple AR: Acute and chronic effects of aspirin toxicity and their treatment. *Arch Intern Med* 1981;141:366.

Chapter 35. Suspected Non-Accidental Trauma

1. American Academy of Pediatrics: *Visual Diagnosis of Child Abuse,* 2nd Edition. 2003.

2. Christopher NC, Anderson D, Gaertner L, et al. Childhood injuries and the importance of documentation in the emergency department. *Pediatr Emerg Care* 1995 Feb; 11(1): 52-7

3. Council on Scientific Affairs: AMA diagnostic and treatment guidelines concerning child abuse and neglect. *JAMA* 1985 Aug 9; 254(6): 796-800

4. Crume, T, DiGuiseppi, C, Byers, T., Sirotnak, A, & Garrett, C, Under-ascertainment of child maltreatment fatalities by death certificates, 1990-1998. *Pediatrics*, 2002; 110 (2).

5. Duhaime AC, Christian CW, Rorke LB, Zimmerman RA. Nonaccidental head injury in infants – the "shaken-baby syndrome." *New Engl J Med.* 1998;338: 1822-1829

6. Herman-Giddens ME, Brown G, Verbiest S, et al: Underascertainment of child abuse mortality in the United States. *JAMA* 1999 Aug 4; 282(5): 463-7

7. Hornor, G. Physical Abuse: Recognition and Reporting. *Journal of Pediatric Health Care.* 19;1. 2005.

8. Hyden PW, Gallagher TA: Child abuse intervention in the emergency room. *Pediatr Clin North Am* 1992 Oct; 39(5): 1053-81

9. Kleinman PK. Skeletal trauma: general considerations. In: Kleinman PK, ed. *Diagnostic imaging of child abuse.* Baltimore: Williams & Wilkins, 1987;8-25

10. Kocher, MS. Kasser, JR. Orthopaedic aspects of child abuse. *J Am Acad Orthopedic Surgery* 2000, 8.10.

11. Leventhal JM, Martin KD, Asnes AG. Incidence of fractures attributable to abuse in young hospitalized children: results from analysis of a United States database. *Pediatrics* 2008; 122:599.

12. Maguire, S. Which injuries may indicate child abuse. *Arch Dis Child Educ Pract Ed.* 2010 Dec;95(6):170-7

13. McDonald, K. Child Abuse: Approach and Management. *Am Fam Physician.* 2007 Jan 15;75(2):221-228

14. Pressel, D. Evaluation of physical abuse in children. *American Family Physician.* May 2000 15;61 (10).

15. U.S. Department of Health and Human Services, Administration for Children and Families, Administration on Children, Youth and Families, Children's Bureau. *Child Maltreatment* 2010. Washington, DC: Department of Health and Human Services; 2011. Available from www.acf.hhs.gov/programs/cb/pubs/cm10/index.htm.

Chapter 36. Sexual Assault

1. Palusci, VJ, et al., Urgent medical assessment after child sexual abuse. *Child Abuse & Neglect*, 2006. 30(4): p. 367-80.

2. Kellogg, N and N. American Academy of Pediatrics Committee on Child Abuse and, The evaluation of sexual abuse in children. *Pediatrics*, 2005. 116(2): p. 506-12.

3. Howard N. Snyder, P.D., *Sexual Assault of Young Children as Reported to Law Enforcement: Victim, Incident, and Offender Characteristics.* 2000, U.S Department of Justice, Bureau of Justice Statistics. p. ii-14.

4. Young, KL, et al., Forensic laboratory evidence in sexually abused children and adolescents. *Archives of Pediatrics & Adolescent Medicine*, 2006. 160(6): p. 585-8.

5. Bernard, D., P. Melissa, and K. Makoroff, The Evaluation of Suspected Pediatric Sexual Abuse. *Clinical Pediatric Emergency Medicine*, 2006. 7(3): p. 9.

6. Physicians, A.C.o.E., Evaluation and Management of the Sexually Assaulted or Sexually Abused Patient. 1999, Dallas: American College of Emergency Physicians.

7. Siegel RM, S.C.e.a., The prevalence of sexually transmitted diseases in children and adolescents evaluated for sexual abuse in Cincinnati: rationale for limited STD testing in prepubertal girls. *Pediatrics*, 1995. 96(6): p. 5.

8. CDC. Sexually Transmitted Diseases Treatment Guidelines 2006: Sexual Assault and STDs. 2006 [cited; Available from: http://www.cdc.gov/std/treatment/2006/sexual-assault.htm.

9. Kaplan, D.W., et al., Care of the adolescent sexual assault victim. *Pediatrics*, 2001. 107(6): p. 1476-9.

10. Heger, A., et al., Children referred for possible sexual abuse: medical findings in 2384 children. *Child Abuse & Neglect*, 2002. 26(6-7): p. 645-59.

11. Adams, J.A., et al., Examination findings in legally confirmed child sexual abuse: it's normal to be normal. *Pediatrics*, 1994. 94(3): p. 310-7.

12. Kellogg, N., S.W. Menard, and A. Santos, Genital Anatomy in Pregnant Adolescents: "Normal" Does Not Mean "Nothing Happened." *Pediatrics*, 2004. 113(1): p. 3.

13. Pickering LK, B.C., Long SS, McMillan JA, eds., *Red Book: 2006 Report of the Committee on Infectious Diseases* 27th ed. 2006, Elk Grove Village: American Academy of Pediatrics. 992.

14. Schremmer, R.D., D. Swanson, and K. Kraly, Human immunodeficiency virus postexposure prophylaxis in child and adolescent victims of sexual assault. *Pediatric Emergency Care*, 2005. 21(8): p. 502-6.

15. Babl, F.E., et al., Prophylaxis against possible human immunodeficiency virus exposure after nonoccupational needlestick injuries or sexual assaults in children and adolescents. *Archives of Pediatrics & Adolescent Medicine*, 2001. 155(6): p. 680-2.

Resources

National Children's Alliance

www.nca-online.org

Regional Children's Advocacy Centers

Midwest Regional Children's Advocacy Center

www.mrcac.org

(888) 422-2955

(651) 220-6750

Southern Regional Children's Advocacy Center

www.nationalcac.org/professionals/srcac

(800) 747-8122

(704) 285-9588

Northeast Regional Children's Advocacy Center

www.nrcac.org

(800) 662-4124

Western Regional Children's Advocacy Center

(800) 582-2203

Chapter 37. Ultrasound: Common Emergency Presentations

1. Levy and Noble, Bedside Ultrasound in Pediatric Emergency Medicine
   http://www.acep.org/content.aspx?id=33402 Focus On: Ultrasound
   Guided Lumbar Puncture

2. http://www.sonoguide.com/nerve_block.html Ultrasound guided nerve
   blocks.

English–Spanish Glossary of Common Words

Melissa Zukowski, MD, MPH

abdomen abdomen (ab-doh-mehn)
abnormal abnormal (ab-nohr-mahl)
abrasion abrasion (ah-brah-see-ohn)
abscess absceso (ahb-sehs-soh)
accident accidente (ag-see-dent-teh)
acetaminophen paracetamol (pah-rah-seh-tay-mohl)
activated charcoal carbón activado (cahn-bohn ahk-tee-vah-doh)
acute agudo (ah-guh-doh)
adolescent adolescente (ah-doh-leh-sehn-teh)
adrenal gland glándula suprarrenales (glahn-duh-lah-suh-prah-reh-nah-lehs)
adult adulto (ah duhl toh)
adverse effects efectos adversos (eh-fehk-tohs ahd-vehr-sohs)
age edad (eh-dahd)
airborne en la aire (ehn-lah-aye-reh)
airway vías respiratorias (vee-yahs rehs-pee-rah-toh-ree-ahs)
alcohol alcohol (ahl-coh-hohl)
allergy alergia (ah-lehr-hee-ah)
anaphylactic anafiláctico (ah-nah-fee-lahc-tee-coh)
anemia anemia (ah-neh-mee-yah)
anesthesia anesthesia (ah-nehs-teh-see-yah)
aneurysm aneurisma (ahn-yehr-eehs-mah)
angina angina de pecho (ahn-hee-nah-deh-peh-cho)
antibiotic antibiótico (ahn-tee-bee-oh-tee-coh)
anti-inflammatory antiinflamatorio (ahn-tee-ehn-flah-mah-tohr-ee-oh)
anxiety ansiedad (ahn-see-eh-dad)
appendicitis appendicitis (ah-pehn-dee-see-tees)
arm brazo (brah-soh)
aspiration aspiración (ah-spee-rah-see-ohn)
asthma asma (ahs-mah)
attending physician médico adscrito (meh-dee-coh-ahd-scree-toh)

autoimmune autoinmune (ah-toh-een-muhn)

baby bebé (beh-beh)

back espalda (ehs-pahl-dah)

better mejor (meh-hohr)

biopsy biopsia (bee-ohp-see-yah)

birth nacimiento (nah-see-mee-ehn-toh)

bladder vejiga (veh-hee-gah)

blockage bloqueo (bloh-keh-yoh)

blood sangre (sahn-greh)

blood pressure presión arterial (preh-see-ohn-ahr-teh-ree-ahl)

blood type tipo de sangre (tee-poh-deh-sahn-greh)

body cuerpo (kwehr-poh)

bone hueso (weh-soh)

bowel intestine (een-tehs-teen)

brain cerebro (seh-reh-broh)

breast pecho (peh-choh)

breath, to respirar (rehs-pee-rahr)

bronchitis bronquitis (brohn-kee-tees)

bruise moretón (moh-reh-tohn)

burn quemadura (keh-mah-duhr-rah)

cancer carcinoma (kahr-see-noh-mah)

cardiac cardíaco (kahr-dee-ah-koh)

cellulitis celulitis (sehl-yoo-lee-tees)

cervix cuello uterino (kweh-yoh-ooh-teh-ree-noh)

change cambio (kahm-bee-yoh)

chest pecho (peh-cho)

chicken pox varicela (vah-ree-sehl-lah)

child niño (neen-yoh)

choke asfixia (ahs-feek-see-yah)

cholecystitis colecistitis (cohl-lee-seehs-tee-seehs)

chronic persistente (pehr-seehs-tehn-teh)

clear claro (clah-roh)

clinic consultorio (kohn-sool-tohr-ree-yoh)

cold frío (free-yoh)

coma coma (coh-mah)

concussion conmoción (cohn-moh-see-ohn)

conjunctivitis conjunctivitis (cohn-johnk-tee-vee-teehs)

constipation estreñimiento (ehs-treh-nyee-mee-ehn-toh)
contagious contagioso (kohn-tah-gee-oh-soh)
cough tos (tohs)
CT scan tomografía computada (toh-moh-grah-fee-yah-cohm-puh-tah-dah)
cut incision (een-seh-see-ohn)
death muerte (mwer-teh)
dehydration deshidratación (dehs-hee-drah-tah-see-yohn)
depression depression (deh-preh-see-ohn)
diabetes diabetes (dee-yeh-bee-tees)
diaphragm diafragma (dee-yah-frahg-mah)
diarrhea diarrhea (dee-yah-reh-yah)
differential diferencial (dee-feh-rehn-see-yahl)
digestive tract tracto intestinal (trhak-toh een-tehs-tee-nahl)
discharge flujo (fluh-yoh)
disease enfermedad (ehn-fehr-mee-dahd)
dizzy marcado (mah-ree-ah-doh)
dose dosis (doh-sees)
draw blood, to sacar sangre (sah-kahr sahn-greh)
drug droga (droh-gah)
dry seca (seh-cah)
dysuria distrofia (dees-troh-fee-yah)
ear oído (oh-eeh-doh)
earache dolor de oído (doh-lohr-de-oh-eeh-doh)
EKG electrocardiograma (ee-lchk troh-kahr-dee-yoh-grah-mah)
elbow codo (coh-doh)
emergency emergencia (ee-mehr-hen-see-yah)
epilepsy epilepsia (eh-pee-lehp-see-yah)
erythema eritema (eh-ree-teh-mah)
eye ojo (oh-hoh)
face cara (cah-rah)
faint desmayo (dehs-mah-yoh)
family familia (fah-meeh-leeh-yah)
feces las heces (lahs-eh-sehs)
female mujer (muh-hehr)
fever fiebre (fee-eh-breh)
finger dedo (deh-doh)
fluid liquido (lee-kweeh-doh)

follow-up recordatorio (reh-kohr-dah-toh-ree-yoh)

food alimento (ah-lee-men-toh)

foot pie (pee-yeh)

fracture fractura (frahc-tuh-rah)

fungal fúngico (foon-gee-koh)

fussy mimado (mee-mah-dah)

gall bladder vesícular biliar (veh-see-kuh-lahr-bee-lee-yar)

gallstone cálculo biliar (kahl-kuh-loh-bee-lee-yahr)

gas flatulencia (flah-tuh-lehn-see-yah)

good bueno (bweh-noh)

green verde (vehr-deh)

hair pelo (peh-loh)

hand mano (mah-noh)

hard duro (duh-roh)

head cabeza (cah-beh-sah)

headache dolor de cabeza (doh-lohr-de-cah-beh-sah)

head injury daño de la cabeza dahn-yoh-de-lah-cah-beh-sah)

heal, to curar (kuh-rahr)

health salud (sah-lood)

healthy sano (sahn-noh)

heart corazón (koh-rah-sohn)

heart attack infarto de miocardio (een-fahr-toh-de-mee-yoh-kar-dee-yoh)

heart rate frecuencia cardíaca (free-kwen-see-yah-kahr-dee-yah-cah)

hello hola (oh-lah)

hematuria hematuria (he-mah-tuh-ree-yah)

hereditary hereditario (heh-reh-dee-tah-ree-yoh)

hernia hernia (hehr-nee-yah)

hip pelvis (pel-vees)

home casa (cah-sah)

hospital hospital (hohs-see-tahl)

hospital admission ingreso en un hospital (een-greh-soh-en-uhn-hohs-pee-tahl)

hot caliente (kah-lee-yen-teh)

hydration hidratación (hee-drah-tah-see-yohn)

hypersensitivity hipersensibilidad (hee-pehr-sehn-see-bee-lee-dahd)

hypertension hypertension (hee-pehr-tehn-see-yohn)

ice hielo (yeh-loh)

ibuprofen *ibuprofeno* (ee-buh-proh-fee-noh)

illness enfermedad (en-fehr-mee-dahd)

immunization vacunación (vah-cuh-nah-see yohn)

incision incision (ehn-seh-see-yohn)

infant lactante (lahc-tahn-teh)

infection infección (een-fehk-see-yohn)

inflammation inflamacion (een-flah-mah-see-yohn)

influenza gripe (gree-peh)

injury lesion (leh-see-yohn)

intensive care cuidados intensivos (kwee-dah-dohs-een-tehn-see-vohs)

internal interno (een-tehr-noh)

intestine intestine (een-tes-tee-noh)

intubation intubacion (een-tuh-bah-see-yohn)

irregular aberrante (ah-beh-rahn-teh)

ischemia isquemia (ees-keh-mee-yah)

itch prurito (pruh-reeh-toh)

IV intravenoso (een-trah-veh-non-soh)

jaw mandibula (mahn-dee-buh-lah)

joint articulación (ahr-teek-yoo-lah-see-yohn)

kidney riñón (reen-yohn)

knee rodilla (roh-dee-yah)

lab tests exámenes medicos (ex-ah-mee-nehs-med-dee-cohs)

laceration laceración (lah-seh-rah-see-yohn)

left izquierda (eez-kee-yehr-dah)

leg plerna (pee-yehr-nah)

lesion lesion (leh-see-yohn)

liver hígado (ee-gah-doh)

local anesthesia anesthesia local (ah-nehs-teh-see-yah-loh-cahl)

lung pulmón (puhl-mohn)

lymphadenopathy linfadenopatía (len-fah-deh-noh-pah-tee-yah)

malignant maligno (mah-leeg-noh)

mass masa (mah-sah)

medical medico (med-dee-coh)

medication medicación (meh-dee-kah-see-yohn)

meningitis meningitis (mee-neen-gee-tees)

mild ligero (lee-geh-roh)

moderate moderado (moh-deh-rah-doh)

mouth boca (boh-cah)

muscle músculo (moos-koo-loh)

nausea náuseas (nah-seh-ahs)

neck cuello (kweh-yoh)

needle aguja (ah-guh-hah)

negative negativo (neh-gah-tee-voh)

nerve nervio (nehr-vee-oh)

normal normal (nohr-mahl)

nose nariz (nah-rees)

nurse enfermera (en-fehr-mehr-rah)

ointment pomada (poh-mah-dah)

organ órgano (orh-gah-noh)

outpatient clinic centro ambulatorio (sen-troh-ahm-buh-lah-tah-ree-yoh)

pain dolor (doh-lohr)

pain medication analgésico (ah-nahl-geh-seeh-coh)

patient paciente (pah-see-ehn-teh)

pediatric pediátrico (peh-dee-ah-tree-coh)

pelvic exam tacto vaginal (tahc-toh-vah-hee-nahl)

pharyngitis faringitis (fah-reen-geeh-teehs)

physical exam examen medico (ex-ah-mehn-meh-dee-coh)

physician medico (meh-dee-coh)

pill pastilla (pahs-tee-yah)

pneumonia neumonía (new-moh-nee-ah)

poisoning intoxicación (ihn-tohx-see-cah-see-yohn)

positive positive (poh-see-tee-voh)

pregnancy embarazo (ehm-bah-rah-zoh)

prescription prescripción (preh-screep-see-ohn)

problem problema (proh-bleh-mah)

procedure procedimiento (proh-seh-dee-meeh-ehn-toh)

psychiatry psiquiatría (see-kee-ah-tree-ah)

pulse pulso (puhl-soh)

rash exantema (ex-ahn-tee-mah)

red rojo (roh-hoh)

relax, to relajarse (reh-lah-heh-seh)

renal renal (reh-nahl)

respiration respiración (reh-spee-rah-see-yohn)

retina retina (reh-tee-nah)

right derecha (deh-reh-chah)

septic séptico (sehp-tee-coh)
serious injury accidente serio (ahk-see-dehn-teh-seh-ree-yoh)
severe intenso (een-tehn-soh)
shoulder hombro (ohm-broh)
sick, to be estar enfermo (ehs-tahr-ehn-fehr-moh)
skin piel (pee-ehl)
skull cráneo (krah-neh-oh)
spleen bazo (bah-zoh)
sprain torcer (tohr-sehr)
stitches puntadas (poon-tah-dahs)
stomach estómago (ehs-toh-mah-goh)
stool excrementos (egs-kreh-mehn-tohs)
surgery operación (oh-peh-rah-see-yohn)
swollen hinchado (een-chah-doh)
temperature temperatura (tehm-pehr-ah-tuh-rah)
throat garganta (gahr-gahn-tah)
toe dedo de pie (deh-doh-deh-pee-yeh)
tongue lengua (lehn-gwah)
tooth diente (deeh-ehn-teh)
trauma traumatismo (trah-mah-tees-moh)
travel viaje (vee-ah-heh)
ultrasound ultrasonida (ool-trah-sohn-nee-dah)
urine orina (orh-ree-nah)
UTI infección urinaria (een-fehk-see-yohn-oohr-eeh-nah-reeh-yah)
vaccine vacuna (vah-cuhn-nah)
viral disease virosis (veeh-roh-sis)
vitamin vitamina (veeh-tah-meeh-nah)
vomiting vomitos (voh-meh-tohs)
wheeze, to resollar (reh-soh-yahr)
where donde (dohn-deh)
white blanca (blahn-kah)
worse peor (peh-ohr)
wound lesion (leh-see-yohn)
wrist muñeca (moo-nyeh-kah)
x-ray radiografía (rah-dee-yoh-grah-fee-yah)
yellow amarillo (ah-mah-ree-yoh)